Podiatric Medicine

Podiatric Medicine

IRVING YALE, D.P.M., EdD. (Hon.)

Past President, American Podiatry Association
Past President and Fellow, American College of Foot Roentgenologists

Formerly, Chairman, Council on Podiatry Education
Formerly, Chief of Podiatry Service, Orthopaedic Section, Department of Surgery, Yale-New Haven Medical Center
Formerly, Chief of Podiatry Service, Metabolic Clinic, Grace-New Haven Hospital

Member, Editorial Advisory Board, *Journal of the American Podiatry Association*

Fellow, American Public Health Association

Associate Fellow, American College of Foot Surgeons

THE WILLIAMS & WILKINS COMPANY
Baltimore

Made in the United States of America
Reprinted 1974

Library of Congress Catalog Card Number 72-87513
SBN 683-09315-0

Composed and printed at the
Waverly Press, Inc.
Mt. Royal and Guilford Aves.
Baltimore, Md. 21202, U.S.A.

Dedication

To the American Podiatry Association, its Board of Trustees, Past Presidents, Council on Podiatry Education, Association of Colleges of Podiatric Medicine, dedicated Staff, and to the members of the Podiatry Profession who have made it possible for unprecedented growth and firm progress in providing foot health to the Community they serve.

IRVING YALE, D.P.M., ED.D. (HON.)

Foreword

A few more years ago than I care to count I came to know Dr. Yale when he and I were classmates. It is unfortunate for podiatry and the podiatrists who have since entered the field that he chose to enter practice instead of becoming a teacher at a podiatry college. If he had begun his practice nearby one of the colleges, I am confident he would have been recruited for the faculty, for Dr. Yale is at heart a teacher and has devoted much time and effort teaching all podiatrists as much as his practice permitted. Very early in his professional career he became an acknowledged leader in the teaching of clinical and radiographic interpretation through appearances on programs of professional meetings, guest lecture series at all of the colleges, publication of papers, and a textbook on the subject. He later collaborated on the book "Clinical Foot Roentgenology."

Calling on his vast background of clinical experience in private practice and at the University Hospitals of Yale University, he now presents us the present text on the conditions commonly encountered in a podiatry practice. It is the first such American textbook in a quarter of a century or more. It is sorely needed.

The podiatrist in practice will find it a source book—where to begin his search for more information about a particular aspect of a common condition that needs more elucidation. The podiatry student will find it invaluable as a basic text in podiatric medicine—a storehouse of knowledge in one reference that will fire his desire to acquire more. The general physician practicing where there are few if any podiatrists will refer to it again and again—to help his patients who suffer those nagging foot aches and pains that strike such large numbers of our population.

I wish I had written it first.

Abe Rubin, D.P.M., Ed.D. (Hon.), Litt.D.
President
Ohio College of Podiatric Medicine

Acknowledgments

The specialists acknowledged in the references and bibliography are to be commended for their contributions to the literature.

I am particularly appreciative of the encouragement given to me for many years by my dear friend Victor Szanton, M.D., recently deceased. His words of wisdom and humanistic approach to the problems of American medicine and the delivery of health care have found their place in the philosophy of this text.

Billy K. S. Tam, Ph.D., Senior Reference Librarian, Yale Medical Library, and his wife Miriam, a University of Connecticut medical librarian, have provided assistance in editing and authenticating much of the bibliography. Jo-Ellen Yale, Ph.D., my daughter, has given me considerable inspiration and editorial assistance.

My admiration goes to Thomas Parasiliti, D.P.M., R.Ph., for his invaluable aid in compiling some of the background on drugs.

Frank Zeoli, B.S., Director of the Zeoli Medical Laboratory, provided expertise in reviewing the laboratory section. Any controversial views presented are strictly my own.

Phyllis Kaletsky, medical secretary, is responsible for the excellent and careful typing of the final manuscript. Some of the early typing was performed by Jeanne Devenport Szoldra, podiatric assistant, and Meredith Yale Press, podiatric aid.

Many people share the responsibility for preparing the figures. I am grateful for the contributions of Jack Stock and Jeremy Szanton for the completion of my photographic efforts at short notice.

Dwight Miller, M.D., Chief Pathologist, Griffin Hospital, has been most gracious and liberal with his time and knowledge.

Most of the pathologic photomicrographs are from the collection of my son and partner, Jeffrey F. Yale, D.P.M. His interest and assistance in selecting illustrations from our joint extensive collection of slides eased my burden in the last days of writing.

Many of the techniques described are the product of evolution. They are not original. My appreciation extends to all who have contributed. I have endeavored to give credit to individuals who courageously expounded on subjects that show promise of becoming acceptable techniques.

To the many thousands of unnamed scholars who played a part in recording information on foot disorders, I salute you!

The cooperation of my wife, Bernice, was essential and heartwarming, since she had been through this experience on two previous occasions!—Thanks.

I appreciate the concern and able assistance of Sara A. Finnegan and the editorial staff of Williams & Wilkins. A special thanks to Eden Allen Delcher for her dedication in the final editing of my manuscript.

IRVING YALE

Preface

Podiatric educators have recognized the need for a textbook which provides insight into the general day-to-day practice of podiatry. The emphasis on graduate training for special areas of practice has all but dwarfed the 90% of the fine work that podiatrists perform in the everyday practice of their profession. *Podiatric Medicine* is written for the student and for the doctor who will find it a useful reference for reviewing, diagnosing and treating podiatric problems. Other medical disciplines and governmental and insurance agencies as well as the community at large will find this text a factual and inclusive approach to the general practice of podiatry and will recognize the tremendous importance of the podiatry profession as a major provider of health services to the community. The text is based on the author's extensive personal experience as a teacher, consultant, and practicing podiatrist with a critical review of podiatric and medical literature.

The reader will note that there are two different type faces used in the text corresponding as nearly as possible to the divisions of the text itself: diagnosis and treatment. The standard type is used for discussions and descriptive material. The "plain" or "*sans serif*" type is used for discussions of treatments for the various conditions described.

The chapters on podiatric equipment illustrate the need for specialized training for doctors of podiatry. Likewise, the instruments used in podiatry can best be manipulated by the specialized and skilled hand of the Doctor of Podiatric Medicine. The development of many new therapeutic modalities attest to the close liaison between foot doctors and industry in providing specialized instruments of high quality for the patient's good.

One has only to view the many and varied materials being used in the treatment of foot disorders to appreciate the degree of diversified knowledge that the podiatrist needs to practice his profession. Supplies range from pharmaceutical chemicals, dressings, adherents, rubber compounds, plaster, leather, a variety of plastics and countless other materials limited only by the resourcefulness of the operator and his staff.

The practical value of this text to the profession will depend on its everyday use by the doctor in general practice. Here the podiatrist will find a review of podiatric equipment, materials and instruments so necessary to his successful practice. Practical information is included on the clinical considerations, diagnosis, pathology and treatment of the great majority of common foot disorders.

Despite the author's reputation as a diagnostician and foot radiologist, this book treats the radiograph as another tool in the overall armamentarium of the podiatrist. The reader is referred to the specialized texts in foot radiology. Surgery, foot orthopedics, podopediatrics and podogeriatrics are discussed only as they relate to the everyday practice of podiatry by the progressive podiatrist in his well-equipped operatory. This text places the common foot disorders in proper perspective as they relate to systemic disturbances.

It has been a joy to add this text to the other fine books written by podiatrists. It is my fond hope that others will be stimulated to contribute to the literature of Podiatric Medicine in the not too distant future.

IRVING YALE, D.P.M., ED.D (HON.)

Contents

1

The Podiatric Operatory

Podiatry Equipment

The most essential equipment in a podiatrist's practice is the podiatry chair, operating light and the podiatrist's stool. A patient must be seated comfortably with his extremities at a height convenient to the doctor. He should be at rest mentally and physically in order to derive maximum relief from the treatment by his foot doctor.

The Podiatry Chair

The podiatry chair must have marked maneuverability. It should go up and down to allow for easy seating and egress by children, the elderly and the disabled. The movement of the chair should be simple, and an electrically powered chair is desirable. A toe's touch or simple touch by a finger to a switch should carry the chair into a position suitable for proper examination and treatment. Illustrations of modern podiatry chairs are presented in these pages.

Operating Lights

Podiatry operating lights may vary for specific purposes. The first and most necessary requirement for general practice is that the lighting be adequate and cool. Lights must have proper reflection from divergent angles to cover the operative field. A surgical light may be a mobile floor model, or it may be suspended from the ceiling or attached to a wall. Shadows should be kept at a minimum and the infrared rays filtered out. Regular operating lights may be incandescent or fluorescent. Some lights consist of both a 60-watt incandescent and a 22-watt fluorescent bulb. Most of these lights move with the slightest touch and are attached to wall brackets. Other lights are totally fluorescent using two standard T815-watt fluorescent bulbs.

The Podiatrist's Stool

The podiatrist's stool may or may not be used by all podiatrists. Some practitioners prefer to stand while working. The majority of practitioners sit while treating feet. A quality operator's stool is important if the foot doctor expects to have many productive years free of postural problems. The chair should be on sturdy rollers. The seat should be flexible for adjustment to leg length. The backrest must be adjustable to height and flexible enough to yield to back pressure. Seat padding should be comfortable and thick enough to protect the coccyx from repeated trauma. Upholstery may match the rest of the office equipment.

Podiatric Drills

A high speed podiatry cord drill for treatment of a multitude of foot and nail problems is a necessary piece of equipment. It may be mobile or attached to the wall or a cabinet. Its arm must be flexible enough to move about the affected part with ease. One-tenth horsepower is typical for a podiatry cord drill. The handpiece is precision constructed and the drill is moved by a foot rheostat. High speed air or nitrogen powered drills are free of vibration and most efficient for bone work and nail problems. Most offices have two or more cord drills. Hand drills are available for use on house or hospital calls. The minimum specifications for cord drills used by podiatrists is 14,000 r.p.m. idle speed. Higher speed drills are available for specialized needs at 100,000 or more r.p.m. for bone work. The Hall Surgairtome, an ultrahigh speed air drill, and the Stryker equipment operated by nitrogen gas pressure are especially applicable to podiatry. The high speed under control is less traumatizing and minimizes postoperative pain and edema. Môhrle (1966), Berman and Gartland (1971). Jenkinson (1970) used ultrasonics for painless debridement of the nail bed and nail groove. The unit used is similar to current dental equipment with interchangeable inserts. When the machine is turned on, the tip of the insert moves back and forth 25,000 times a second in a 1/1000-in. stroke.

X-ray and Dark Room Equipment

X-ray equipment must be manufactured in accordance with radiation protection specifications of the Radiation Protection Section of the Bureau of Radiological Health. The x-ray machine head should be counterbalanced and maneuverable to within inches of the floor. It should be 100% protected and have a small, fine focal spot and builtin filter to minimize the soft rays. Exacting collimation is essential for good results and proper protection from secondary radiation. Current investigations hopefully will result in the development of x-ray equipment best suited for podiatric use. Present equipment is of a general caliber and not designed specifically for podiatric weight bearing techniques.

Dark room equipment for the podiatrist may be standard medical equipment. A 2½-gallon developing tank is desirable for the busy office. A variety of film sizes, screens, cassettes and film holders are necessary equipment for all offices. The 10- x 12-in. nonscreen film has proven to be the most useful size for full foot radiographs. Intensifying screens will decrease exposure time and may be necessary to cut down radiation exposure without sacrifice of quality.

Other Diagnostic and Therapeutic Equipment

For a modern, well-equipped office, the podiatrist should have available FCC, U/L approved ultrasound units, short wave generators which can be used for surgery such as electrodesiccation, fulgeration, coagulation and section; Hyfrecator, Electrocator and Bove units to destroy pathologic tissue; and low volt multiple wave generators for muscle stimulation, testing and rehabilitation. Low voltage generators also provide currents for iontophoresis, and destruction of pathologic tissue by electrolysis. Many doctors find extensive use for hydrotherapy, ultraviolet irradiation and paraffin baths.

The Horwitron—Variometer is an electrodiagnostic and treatment device used for neuromuscular dysfunction. Evaluations made with this instrument determine the reflex tone of the neuromuscular mechanism. Treatment is based on accurate diagnosis and treatment using a ballistic impulse. Because of the reduced current (1/100 of the usual current) and the rapid ballistic-type impulse, the sensory nerve endings can be bypassed to influence only the motor end-plates.

Precision measuring equipment such as forefoot devices, the Martins Goniometer, the tractograph and a protractor are essential for evaluating the degree of functional and structural alterations and establishing the necessary amount of correction. Clinical diagnostic equipment at every chair should have a lesion measuring device, a tuning fork with brush and needle, a small flashlight for eye reactions to light and a tape measure. A skin thermometer, sphygmomanometer and oscillometer are helpful and essential for proper evaluation of peripheral vascular disease.

The Podiatric Laboratory

A well-equipped podiatry office will have two types of laboratories. One should be equipped to provide for physiologic testing of blood samples and urine. The other should be equipped to construct foot appliances and devices for patients requiring additional support, correction, balancing or protection. The laboratories should have such equipment as a microscope, test tubes, culture media, pipettes, counting chambers, a hemoglobinometer, reagents and the necessary sophisticated electronic devices. The appliance laboratory requires stocks of leather, rubber and plastics capable of being skived by special knives, and a basic grind-wheel for shaping and correcting orthotics to fit the feet.

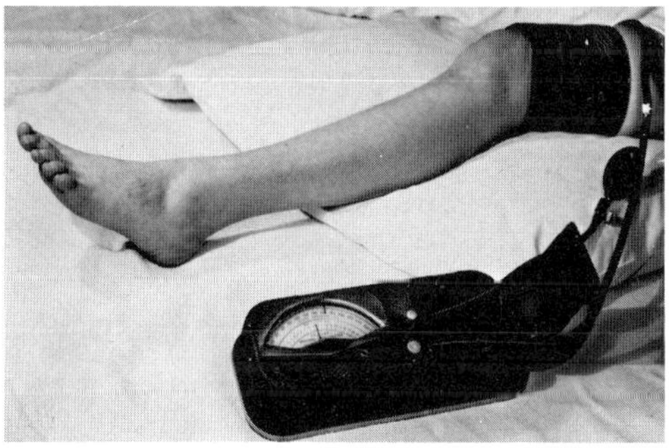

Fig. 1.1. Collens sphygmo-oscillometer. Courtesy of U.M.A. Inc.

No office is complete without a grinder for its orthopedic laboratory. The most popular equipment is the Sani-Grinder, which provides a quiet, efficient vacuum action for dust collection, replacement abrasive sleeves, a grinding drum, stone chuck and taper chuck for buffs, emery cloths and polishing.

Maintenance of Sterile Supplies and Office Aids

Sterilizers are an essential part of podiatric equipment. Despite the disposable materials and syringes available today, no office can function without an autoclave. Surgical packs, instruments, suture removal kits, linens and a host of other specialized supplies are autoclaved. The inside dimensions of the autoclave should be large enough to handle essential supplies and instruments. Steam under pressure units should be of finest quality to insure many years of use.

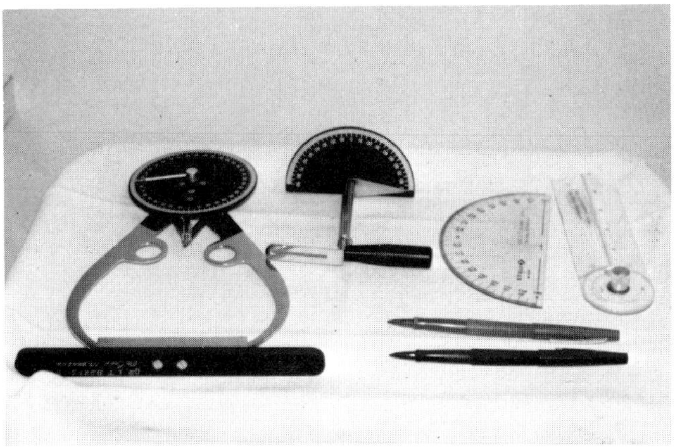

Fig. 1.2. The basic instruments are laid out for the reader's inspection. On the left is the goniometer, next the forefoot varus measuring device, third, the large protractor, next the tractograph and last, but not least, the black and red marking pens for ease in distinguishing the inversion and eversion lines from each other. Courtesy of Burns Podiatric Laboratory.

Cabinets used to house supplies and instruments may be built-in and designed to match the decor of the office. Special wall cabinets are desirable to allow for easy maintenance of floors.

The Locke Sani-Tray is an indespensable heavy gauge stainless steel and aluminum tray that fits under the foot rest of most podiatry chairs. This tray has provided a simple, clean method for capturing debris and excrescences removed from the foot during routine podiatric treatment. It eliminates the old-fashioned stigmatized floor pan, protects the operator's clothing and generally enhances the professional environment of the modern podiatric office.

The well-equipped podiatry office is surgically oriented. As in every specialized field, the operator is a responsible practitioner of the healing arts and recognizes his limitations and scope of practice. One of the foot specialist's responsibilities is to maintain sterile packs and available autoclaved surgical instruments for emergency and daily use in the practice of his profession. Only those operative procedures which may be carried out in the office will be discussed in this text. For further information, the reader is referred to the several texts on foot surgery. We will briefly discuss the surgical instruments, their basic features and use.

Instruments Used in the Practice of Podiatry

The highly specialized practice of podiatry requires special instruments for the successful treatment of podiatric problems. Many instruments are the exclusive product of the imagination and creativity of the podiatrist. Other instruments were originally developed by other specialists for their specific needs. Podiatrists have adopted specialized instruments and adapted them for treatment of unusual foot disorders.

Since most instruments are of the cutting variety, the student in his early days develops the touch and ability to handle instruments skillfully and proficiently. With quality stainless steel surgical hand instruments, the podiatrist becomes a great respecter of the tissues he treats. The student and doctor alike are cautioned about the purchase of inferior instruments. They must use only the finest instruments in an effort to provide the quality service so intimately associated with the practice of podiatry. The skilled operator can actually feel the tissue through his instrument.

Operative instruments for the treatment of skin excrescences, such as heloma, tyloma and nails, may be classified as chisels, knives, special feature instruments and tissue forceps.

Chisels

Chisels may be small, medium or large depending on the width of the blade. The edge of the blade may be slightly curved or straight. The straight blade is generally angulated to varying degrees for the purpose of easier handling of tissues by the podiatrist. The handles of both chisels and knives are either octagonal, rounded or flat in shape. The instrument handle may taper; its surface may be irregular or smooth. Many instrument handles are constructed of stainless steel, aluminum or other metallic alloys. Many foot specialists prefer finest quality stainless steel and replaceable chisel blades. Chisel blade size may be 1/16, 1/4, 3/8, 1/2 or 5/8 in.; a variety of other sizes are available on a special order basis. Good quality instruments constructed by expert manufacturers allow for high quality podiatric treatment.

Replaceable curved or oblique chisel blades are convenient to use. Blade instruments must be sharpened often if sharp and safe instruments are to be available for regular daily use.

Knives

Knives are either straight or curved back. Blades may be small, medium,

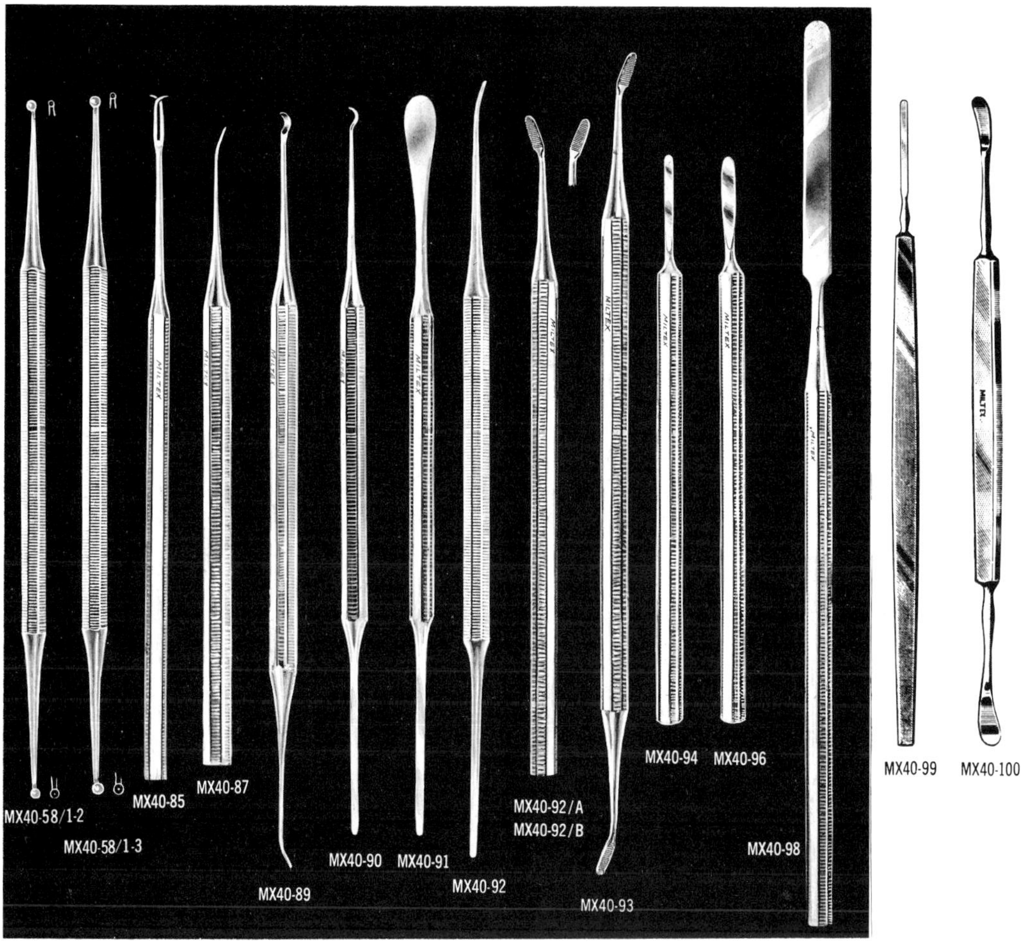

Fig. 1.3. Podiatry hand instruments. MX40-58/1-2: double end curette excavator w/hole 1.5 and 2 mm.; MX40-58/1-3: double end curette excavator w/hole 1.5 and 2.5 mm.; MX40-85: fixator for lifting and holding tissue; MX40-87: probe stainless steel; MX40-89: probe and excavator, double ended; MX40-90: excavator and packer, double ended; MX40-91: spatula and packer, double ended; MX40-92: probe and packer, double ended; MX40-92/A: nail or bone rasp, angular, file inside; MX40-92/B: nail or bone rasp, angular, file outside; MX40-93: double ended nail or bone rasp, angular, file inside and outside; MX40-94: Locke elevator, narrow blade; MX40-96: Locke elevator, wide blade; MX40-98: flexible spatula, 2 x ¼ in.; MX40-99: Dix spud, half round; MX40-100: Green spatula, double ended. Courtesy of Miltex Instrument Corp.

large and extra heavy. These may also be supplied as replaceable blades with suitable handles with the usual advantages of having a sharp blade available. The typical knife is a surgical scalpel. They are available in different sizes.

It is essential to note that one popular instrument called a golf stick embodies the multiple features of being angulated like a chisel, rounded like a regular scalpel knife blade and variable in size to serve a variety of purposes in treatment. As one would suspect, its blade shape is similar to that of a golf club head. The golf stick is commonly used to reduce calluses.

The podiatrist regularly uses the instruments discussed above and he must learn to master them by repeated use under controlled conditions in training clinics. Often the operator feels more comfortable with one type of instrument

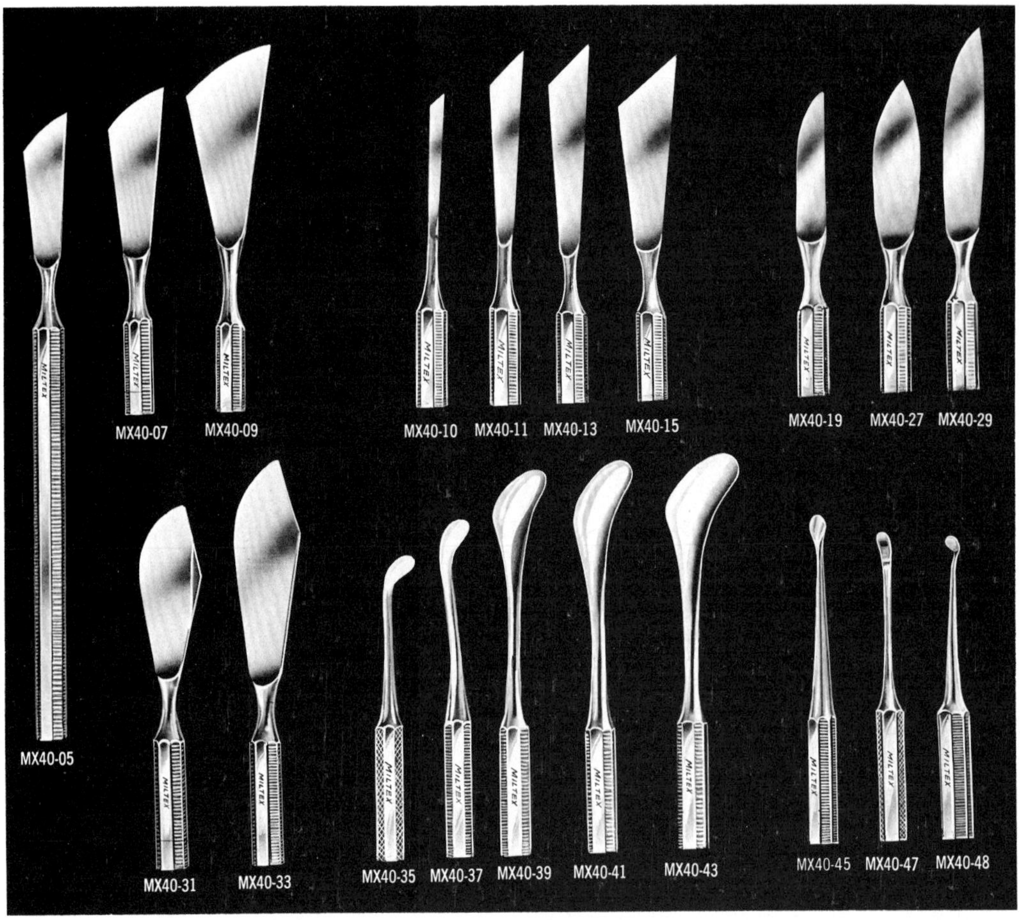

Fig. 1.4. Podiatry hand instruments. MX40-05, MX40-07, MX40-09, MX40-10, MX40-11, MX40-13, MX40-15: chisels used for reduction of hyperkeratosis; MX40-19, MX40-27, MX40-29, MX40-31, MX40-33: scalpels used for surgical incisions and removal of excrescences; MX40-35, MX40-37, MX40-39, MX40-41, MX40-43: golf-stick shaped cutting instruments; MX40-45, MX40-47, MX40-48: curettes. Courtesy of Miltex Instrument Corp.

than with others and can adapt it for use in a variety of conditions. We will discuss the use of instruments for specific operative problems, however, the practical application of the theory of clinical practice will depend on the experience acquired in an academic clinical environment.

Special Feature Instruments

Special feature instruments can be defined as those instruments scientifically designed to be used for specific types of pathology. Instruments for specific purposes may be developed. A useful instrument is a soft corn spoon knife that is either round, oval, slightly curved or angular. A special feature corn chisel may have an oblique edge with a sharp point for special applications. Nucleus knives have a special construction for removal of small hyperkeratotic lesions. They come in a variety of sizes and shapes and require special handling techniques for successful use in practice.

Tissue Forceps

Flat jaw and angle jawed forceps have a variety of uses in the treatment of tylomas, helomas and nail pathology.

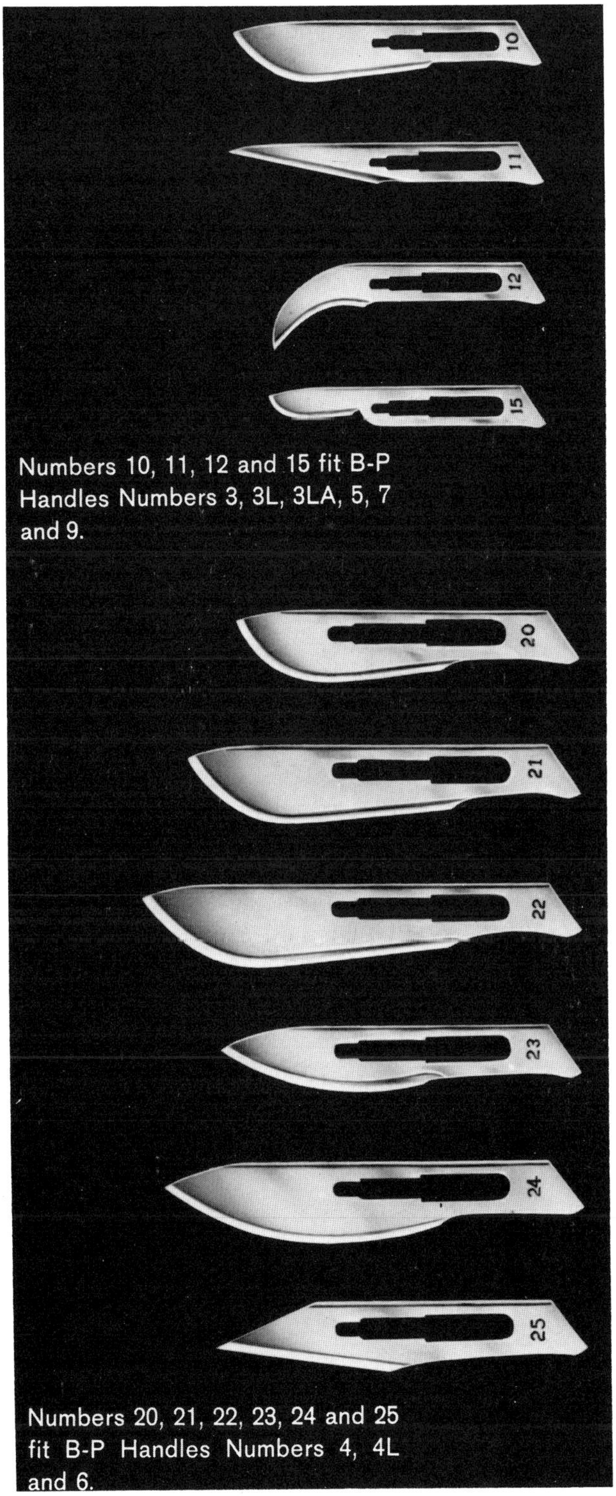

Fig. 1.5. Scalpel blades. Note the variety of scalpel blade shapes. No. 25 suitable for straight incisions of even depth; Nos. 10, 15, 20, 21, 22, 23 and 24 ideal for plantar tylomas. May also be used for surgical incisions and subcutaneous dissections. No. 12 is desirable for snap tenotomy and No. 11 for deep incisions of abscess to facilitate drainage. Courtesy of Bard-Parker.

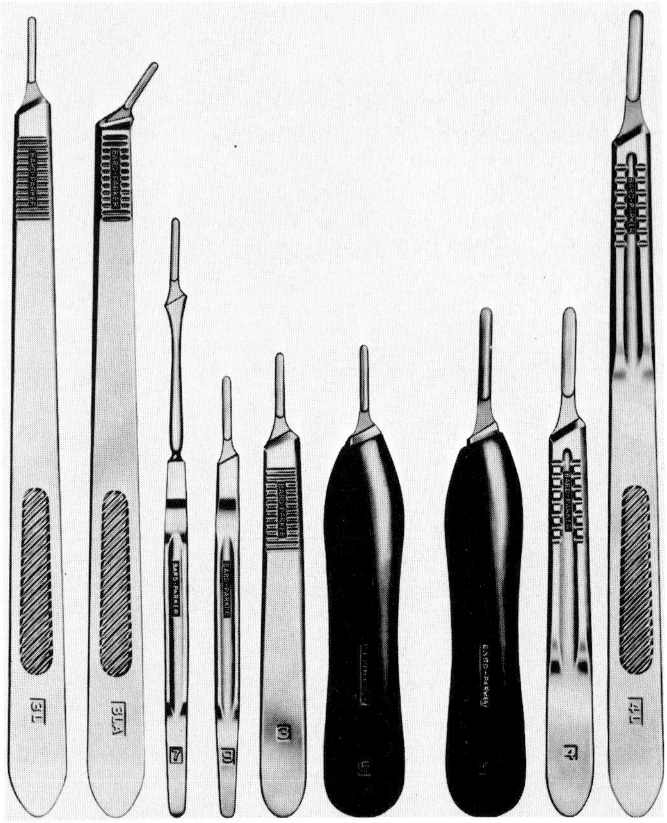

Fig. 1.6. Scalpel handles. Design suitable for handling and deft instrumentation in surgical treatment of most foot disorders. Courtesy of Bard-Parker.

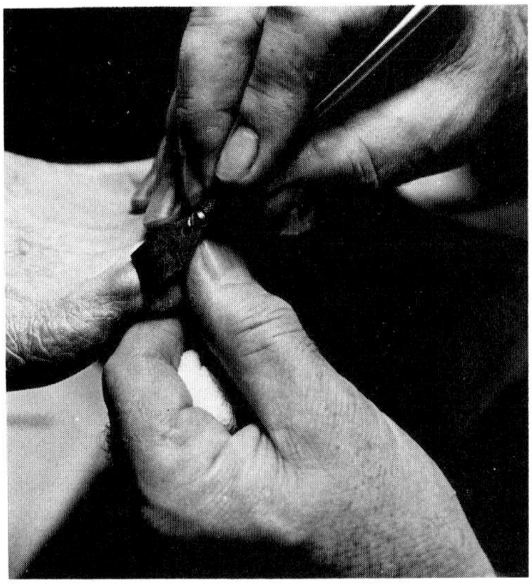

Fig. 1.7. Use of heloma chisel. Observe position of fingers of the left hand grasping the toe and holding skin taut. Note position of instrument and fingers of right hand holding the instrument and resting on the dorsum of the foot for leverage.

The handles on these forceps are different enough to enable the operator to select an instrument that feels comfortable.

Instrument Use

The clinical use of instruments will be illustrated. Holding an instrument is a technique in itself. The movement of the fingers and wrists varies with the instrument being used, the location of the lesion and the assist from the opposite hand. Manual dexterity is developed with frequent use of a variety of instruments.

Chisels

A chisel may be used for the reduction of corns and calluses. The size of the instrument blade should be no wider than the excrescence itself. As a rule, smaller sized chisels are used on helomas and larger ones on plantar tylomas. In the treatment of a corn on a toe, the proper chisel is selected and held between the thumb and forefinger and rests on the third finger as in holding a pencil. The finger motion used to reduce a corn consists of multiple forward and angulated thrusts from the distal end of the heloma backward toward the toe base. The fourth and fifth fingers provide some stability by resting on the unaffected part of the foot. The fingers of the opposite hand maintain a taut skin on the affected toe. They form a steady base of support for the instrument wielding hand. If the heloma is complicated by deep centers of horny tissue, these are removed by dissection with a nucleus knife. The nucleus knife is held in the same hand position as the chisel. The blade is placed at the periphery of the nucleus and with a downward and lateral force a circumscribed incision is made about the lesion. By a forward and lateral push and slight twirl between the fingers, a line of demarcation is made about the lesion and it is gently separated from the surrounding tissue. Often the operator uses a tissue forceps in his left hand to grasp the pathologic tissue while he cuts it away with an instrument in his right hand.

The same type chisel may be used to reduce tylomas. The choice of size and angle of the blade is left to the doctor's experience. It is usually a wider chisel than that used for helomas. The instrument is held in the same fashion as a pencil for calluses overlying the hallux joint or fifth metatarsophalangeal joint. However, plantar calluses may be reduced by chisel as illustrated here. The chisel is held between the thumb and second and third fingers at its neck with the handle resting between the fourth and fifth fingers. The motion used is a semicircular one and is effective in reduction of the excrescence. The third, fourth and fifth fingers may act as a fulcrum either separately or together.

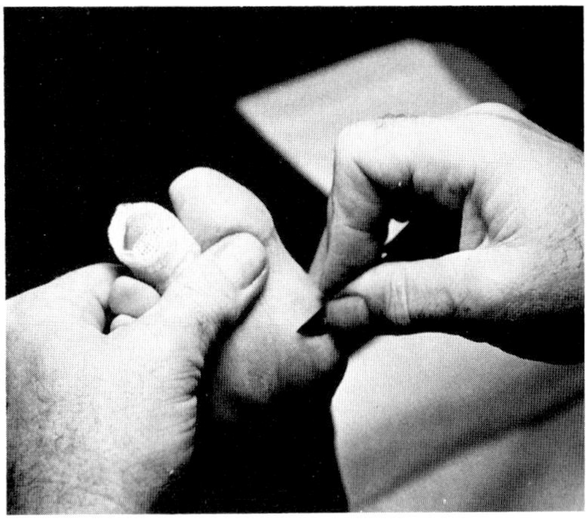

Fig. 1.8. Use of tyloma scalpel. Position of left thumb holds skin taut while the right hand holding the scalpel rests its third, fourth and fifth fingers on the foot proper for leverage.

Knives

The knives, for the most part, are scalpels. They are held and used in the same fashion as the chisel on a callus. In the hands of the skilled podiatrist, the scalpel-type blade is most effective when used in reduction of calluses. The point of the scalpel can be used to enucleate deep lesions.

The soft corn spoon looks somewhat like a miniature spoon with sharp edges. It is used as a spoon with excavation-like motions. The stroke on the soft corn is a pushing and semicircular cutting action on the heloma molle.

Tissue Forceps

Standard instruments used in treating certain skin lesions and nails are essential armamentaria for all podiatrists. Tissue forceps or nippers resemble small surgical nail clippers. They can be used for excising skin lesions and nails. Tissue forceps may have convex or straight edges. In the hands of the skilled operator they can be used to excise corns and calluses. The convex blade is generally useful for this purpose. However, the straight edge blade which is easier to control can be used for excising superficial and deep hyperkeratoses as well as incurvated nail borders.

Curettes

Curettes are used extensively for removal of verrucae, poromas and callused nail grooves. Curettes are sharp and measure from 1 mm. to 2.5 mm. in diameter. The most popular use is in curettage of nail margins and nail grooves. In curettage of nail grooves, the rounded section of the curette is carefully placed on the viable skin while the scooping motion of the sharp margins is directed into the free nail margins or callus in the nail groove. The motion is from the proximal end of the nail forward to distal. Verrucae and poromas are removed by sharp curettage under local anesthesia.

Nail Splitters

Nail splitters have straight and angulated blades. They must be kept sharp to be effective. The skillful use of the nail splitter requires a fine instrument, a feel for the type of tissue being cut, and broad experience in treating nail diseases. The action from the distal to the proximal end of the nail plate is a pushing motion. Some nail splitters are in forceps form.

Excavators, nail probes and soft tissue probes of many sizes, together with a miscellaneous group of specially designed instruments, are necessary for the scientific practice of podiatry.

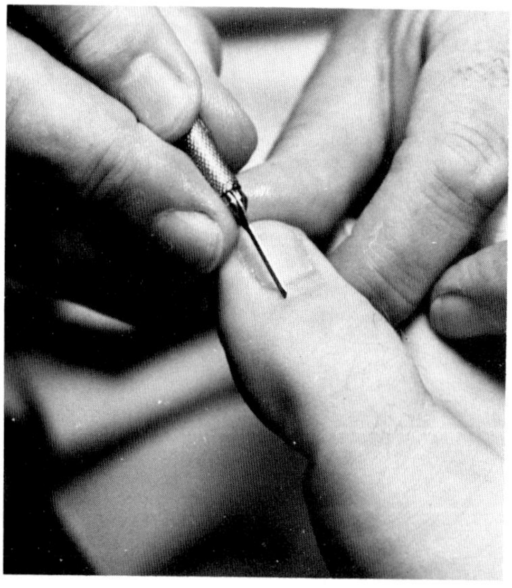

Fig. 1.9. Nail being split in preparation for corrective surgery.

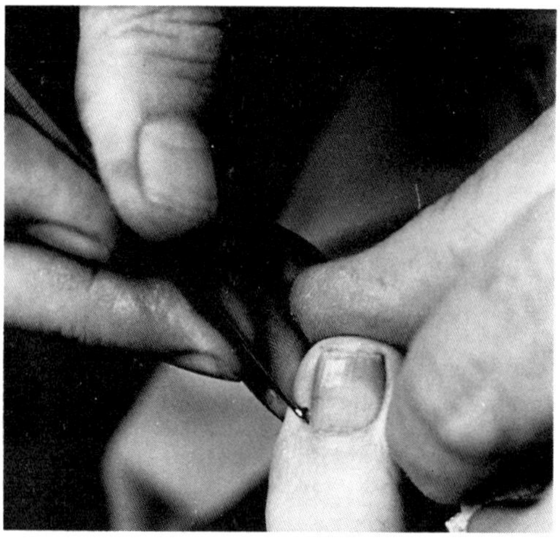

Fig. 1.10. Curettage hallux nail. Note position of fingers holding hallux steady. Observe the position of the curette with the sharp concave surface cutting the margin of the nail and the smooth convexity of the curette moving along the skin margin in the nail groove.

Scissors, Dressing Forceps and Related Instruments

Surgical scissors have a variety of uses. The blades may be curved or straight, short or long, heavy or thin, straight edged or serrated. Some scissors are used for cutting bandages, materials, skin, eponychial tissue and nails; others are designed for removal of sutures. Different types of scissors are used for sharp and blunt dissection. Some have serrated edges for cutting felt materials.

The cutting of adhesive tape is an art that all podiatrists must master. In order to have a firm grip on the instrument and thus assure maneuverability, place the thumb in one opening of the handle and the fourth finger in the other. The second and third fingers assist the fourth finger and are flexed over the handle for additional leverage.

Splinter forceps have a variety of points for grasping foreign bodies.

The Hosch Derm-A-Brade is a surgical

instrument used for the office debridement of corns, calluses and other hyperkeratoses. It consists of two separate cutting blades especially designed for skin and nails, respectively. The Derm-A-Brade attaches to a cord drill or air drill and is used on the dry skin. Its action is much like a scalpel blade and its use is easily mastered by the skilled podiatrist.

Dressing forceps and a variety of thumb forceps for grasping tissue are interesting in design. Ends may be serrated, pointed, mouse tooth and sharp. Forceps are used for skin grasping and also for surgical grasping of subcutaneous tissue for mobilization, dissection and retraction.

Suturing Equipment

Mosquito forceps and Kelly forceps may be straight or curved. They are used for clamping bleeding vessels for hemostasis. Forceps help the operator in sterile instrument suturing. Tissues can be grasped and gently moved with the deft use of hemostats.

There are several types of needle holders and their use in suturing depends on the discrimination of the operator. The Olsen-Hegar holder is a combination needle holder and scissor blade. Other popular models are the Mayo-Hegar and the Mathieu.

Clamps and Retractors

Backhaus and Jones towel clamps are necessary for an orderly and neat draping of the operative field. Working in a small field, the podiatric surgeon may use the 3½-in. clamp to advantage.

Retractors come in a variety of types and sizes. Senn retractors have three sharp prongs and three blunt prongs. Some retractors have two prongs and others have rigid or flexible necks. These instruments can only be used with an extra pair of hands. This, of course, requires an assistant who has scrubbed. Since an assistant may not be available for most office surgery, the operator will find useful the self-retaining retractors that can be applied by the surgeon himself. Proper exposure of the field when operating alone can be achieved by use of the Weitlander, Alm and Miltex retractors. These retractors are self-retaining and meet the rigid specifications for good exposure. They are available in different sizes.

Locke (1963) developed a versatile bone clamp for foot surgery designed to grasp firmly a phalanx, metatarsal or sesamoid. A wide variety of uses have been found for this clamp which causes minimal tissue damage.

Bone Cutting Forceps, Rasps and Related Instruments

Bone cutting forceps and rongeurs are straight or angled to suit the require-

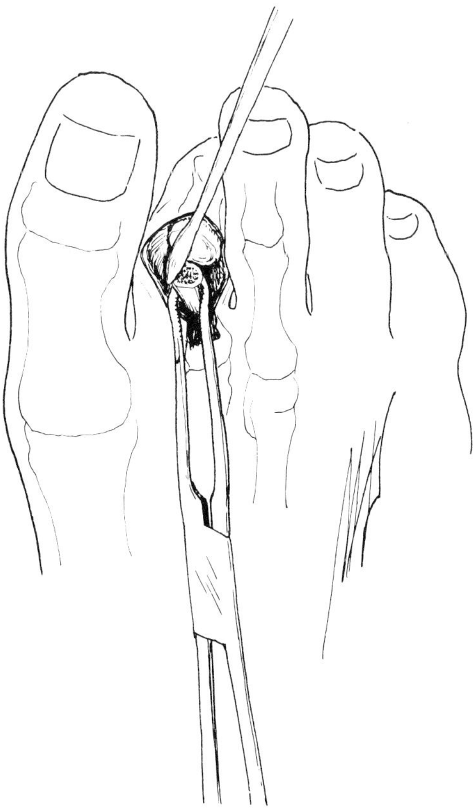

Fig. 1.11. Locke clamp.

ments of the operative procedure. The purchase of these instruments should be based on the necessary size and the practicality of the jaw shape for podiatric procedures. Bizarre designs are unnecessary. Special feature instruments adapted for specific bone lesions are highly desirable and necessary to extensive bone surgery.

Greed (1966) designed a much needed instrument for clamping sesamoids during hallux valgus procedures.

Bone files or rasps have reached greater acceptance and are being used in techniques for removal of exostosis and osteophytic alterations on toe joints. Bone files may be fine or coarse, small, medium or large in size. Bone chisels, saws, osteotomes, elevators and mallets are necessary instruments in the operatory of the podiatric surgeon. Their use will be described in various operative procedures. Electronically controlled rasps are being used with greater frequency in minor foot surgery.

Kaplan and Cornfield (1969) described a micropneumatic surgical instrument operated by a small, powerful pneumatic motor at speeds up to 35,000 r.p.m. They conclude that the use of such an instrument saves time, minimizes trauma, diminishes postoperative pain and

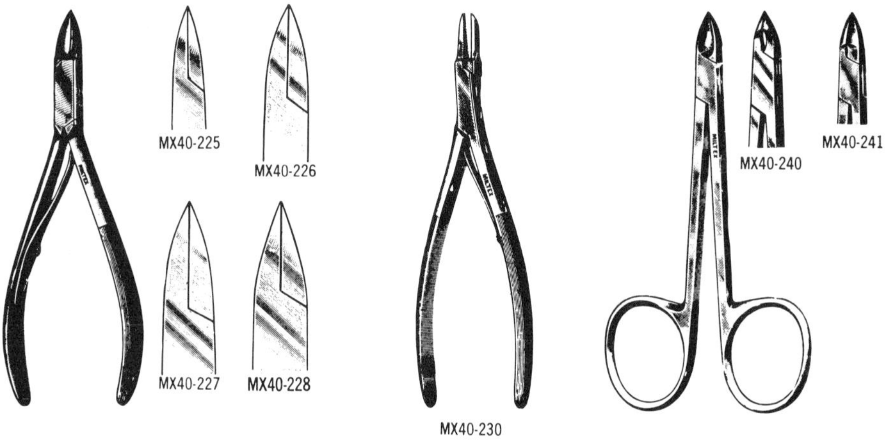

Fig. 1.12. Tissue forceps and nail splitters. Courtesy of Miltex Instrument Corp.

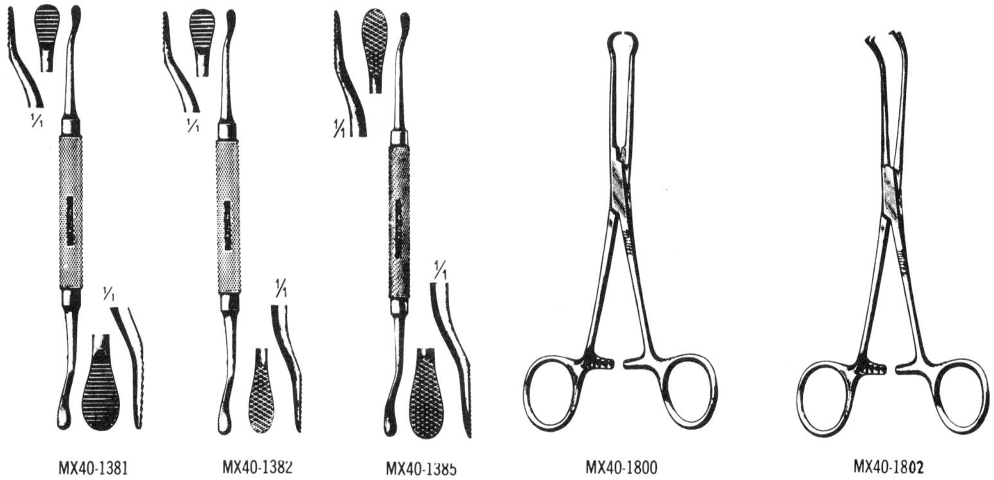

Fig. 1.13. Bone instruments. Courtesy of Miltex Instrument Corp.

provides excellent results in bone surgery. The Roto-Osteotome may use over 30 burrs and drills. A microreciprocating or oscillating saw are also available.

Forceps are podiatrically designed to grasp and clamp sesamoids and phalanges. Other forceps for grasping sponges are necessary instruments in all operatories.

Kurgweil (1961) developed a unique instrument which retracts the extensor tendon and dorsal soft tissue and elevates the head of the proximal phalanx, and is used in hammertoe surgery.

Cast spreaders and cutters may be used in the everyday practice of podiatry. Stryker electric cast cutters are a necessary adjunct to a busy general podiatry practice.

Podiatric Drills and Attachments

Electric drills are an absolute necessity for the proper practice of podiatry. Hand drills are used on house calls by many podiatrists and have their limitations. However, each operatory in the podiatrist's suite must have a high speed electric cord drill for the treatment of hyperkeratosis and hypertrophied nails of whatever etiology. The drill should perform at about 14,000 r.p.m.

The cord drill appears to be the best type for reduction of vibrations. The revolutions are governed by a foot rheostat capable of increasing or reducing speed. A new concept in drills is a handpiece driven by air at low speed and high torque. It can be used instead of conventional chisels, bone rasps or rongeurs. This lightweight handpiece relieves fatigue and improves tactile sensation. It weighs 4½ oz. and operates at speeds of 0 to 8000 r.p.m. forward and reverse at 50/60 lb. of pressure. The attachments can be autoclaved. The need for many shapes and styles of burrs constructed of a variety of materials are needed for podiatric practice. Burrs are made of stainless steel, diamond dust and sand finishes. They may be coarse or fine and are shaped for a variety of purposes. They can be pointed, sharp, broad and narrow.

Syringes and Related Equipment

A variety of syringes and needle sizes are essential to the proper practice of

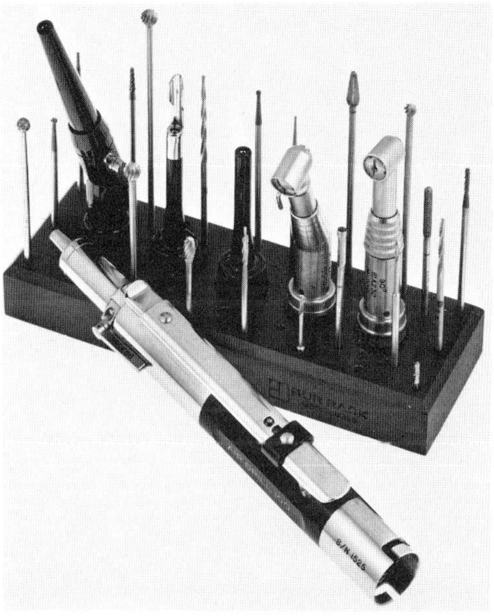

Fig. 1.14. Air drill 100 with attachments and burrs. Courtesy of Hall International Inc.

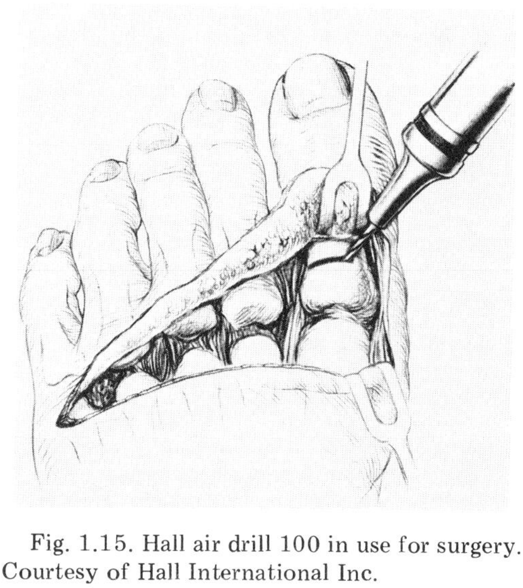

Fig. 1.15. Hall air drill 100 in use for surgery. Courtesy of Hall International Inc.

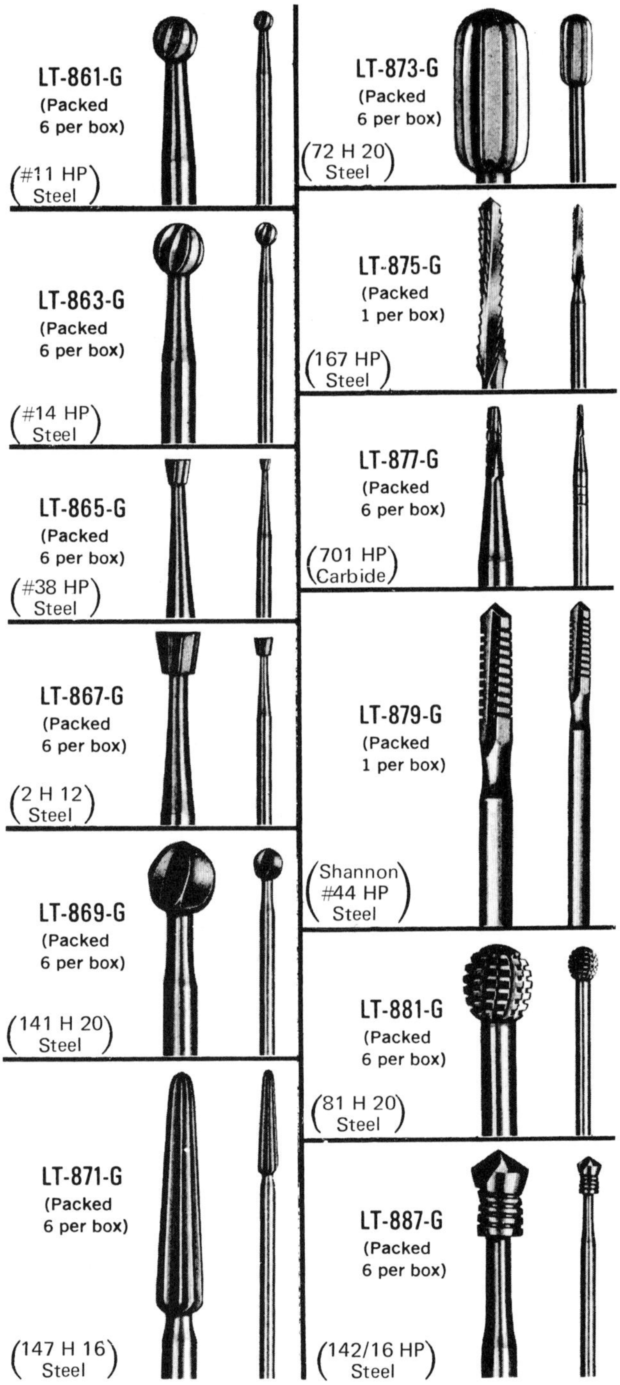

Fig. 1.16. Burrs used in podiatry. Uses are as follows. LT-861-G: Distal extoses, tyloma medial of great toe, brushing or erasure technique; LT-863-G: distal exostoses, tyloma medial of great toe, bunionectomy—ambulatory procedure, brushing or erasure technique; LT-865-G: nail surgery, Perrone matrix erasure; LT-867-G: nail surgery, Perrone matrix erasure; LT-869-G: tyloma medial of great toe, bunionectomy—ambulatory procedure, heel spur, brushing or erasure technique; LT-871-G: capsular elevation or smoothing large bones; LT-873-G: reducing large bones, smoothing large bones; LT-875-G: hallux valgus, sectioning technique, gross removal technique, tailor's bunion; LT-877-G: sectioning—small bones; LT-879-G: heloma durum and molle, tailor's bunion, tibial sesamoid reduction, hallux valgus—brushing technique, hallux valgus—erasure technique, hallux valgus—sectioning, hallux valgus—gross removal; LT-881-G: reducing large bones, smoothing large bones, heloma durum and molle; LT-887-G: heel spur. Pictures courtesy of Weber Co. Burs available from Miltex Instrument Company, Miltex stock numbers in parentheses.

podiatry. Syringes used for aspiration, injection of medication at varying levels of tissue and equipment for local anesthesia must be readily available. Presterilized needles, syringes and combinations of needle length and gauge are a necessary adjunct to other modalities. Kaplan and Weinstock (1967) described

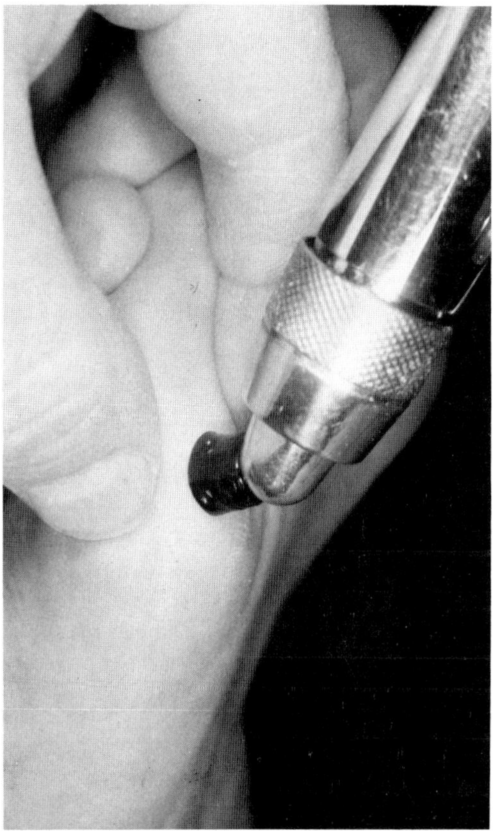

Fig. 1.17. Intralesional jet spray of sclerosing agent into verruca. Penetration 4 to 6 mm. in depth to deposit 0.1 ml. of medication. Courtesy of R. K. Locke, D.P.M.

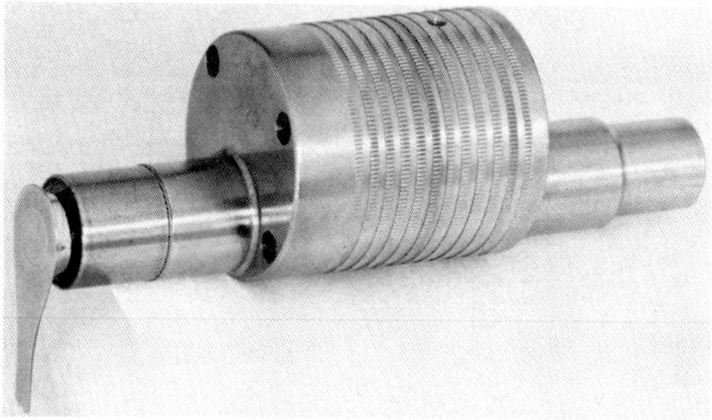

Fig. 1.18. Oscillating saw. Nitrogen driven handpiece. Saw is useful for rapid, smooth excision of exostosis, lipping, osteophytes and arthroplasty. Courtesy of Stryker Co.

the use of the hypospray injector as a precise instrument for administering medication and local anesthesia to a variety of sites on the foot. Their report

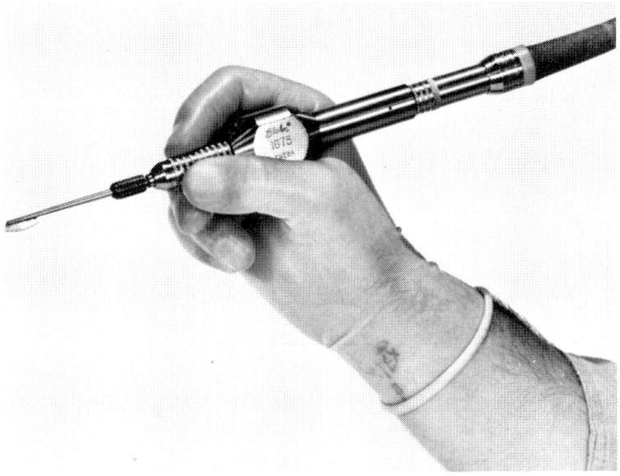

Fig. 1.19. Reciprocal saw. Nitrogen driven saw reduces vibration. Courtesy of Stryker Co.

was based on a study of 100 surgical patients and they conclude that this method of delivering local anesthesia has some distinct advantages over using a needle in selected cases.

In a later paper, Kaplan and Weinstock demonstrated the diffusion of injectable material by the high powered spray, hypospray, using a solution of Hypaque mixed equally with lidocaine. They concluded from this study that pain was less than by use of an ordinary injection with exception of the metatarsal area and toes. Bleeding was minimal. If not properly presented, the noise of injection was objectionable to some patients. There were no serious side effects.

Materials and Their Usage in Podiatric Medicine

A representative group of materials used in podiatric practice may be listed as:

1. Drugs—including anesthetics and other injectables
2. Dressings
   a. Gauze, cotton bandages
   b. Adhesive
   c. Plaster
   d. Rubber
   e. Special
3. Felt and similar materials
   a. Moleskin—thin, medium or heavy

   b. Cotton and wool felt—variety of densities and thicknesses
4. Rubber, foam, polyurethane, cork, styrene and combinations with rubber
5. Celastic—colloid cellulose acetate in a fabric base
6. Leather—various gauges for appliance construction
7. Plastic, thermoplastics, acrylics, polyethylene
8. Latex—natural and synthetic
9. Chemicals
   a. Solvents
   b. Rubber cement
   c. Pharmaceuticals
   d. Skin adherants
10. Plaster of Paris
11. Suture material
12. Antiseptic, germicidal solutions for cold sterilization.

Podiatric Pads and Shields

There are many professional pads and shields that are prefabricated for use by discriminating foot specialists. They prove useful when stocked by the podiatrist in a variety of sizes, shapes and densities. These may be hammertoe correctors, shields and protectors. Precut or fabricated adhesive backed moleskin, foam, sponge or felt pads in a variety of sizes and shapes for heloma dura, heloma molle, tyloma and hallux joint pathology are used extensively as time-savers. Sling pads made of foam or felt in many sizes and densities are available for use over pressure areas. Combinations of foam covered by a closely knit material and other specially shaped removable pads are available for specific problems.

Dallek (1971), in an illustrated catalogue, describes pads for a variety of uses, e.g., toe separators, toe sling pads, half-moon pads, duck pads for corns between the fourth and fifth toes, oval pads, sling bunion pads, tailor's bunion pads, diamond-shaped, kidney-shaped, criss-cross, T-sling, bell sling, combination anterior and longitudinal pads, c-shaped, U-shaped and dancer pads. These pads are available commercially and can be of value in selected cases.

Overlapping and hammertoes may be treated and maintained in correct position by the prefabricated and adjustable Budin toe splints. These splints are especially useful where there is no joint disease or ankylosis and only soft tissues are involved.

A wide variety of appliance accessories are prefabricated for the busy podiatrist who desires to construct his own prosthetic devices. Molded rubber heel wedges, longitudinal, metatarsal raises and special feature pads are useful in shoe therapy.

Molded cork inlays are often used as a base for construction of definitive appliances. Several leather shells with low, medium and high flanges, dual flanges and extensions may be purchased for use as a base for corrective or accommodative removable prostheses. Sponge rubber, acrylics, leather, cork, Celastic, aluminum, steel or steel spring longitudinal raises are available as prefabricated prosthetic materials.

Appliances constructed from these materials may be a flexible, semi-rigid to rigid device or range from a low, medium to high raise. The laboratory assistant follows the doctor's orders for the type of raise and material to be used to construct an appliance for a particular case. This requires considerable forethought and study for best results.

A complete and thorough discussion of materials would result in an extensive volume on physical and chemical properties and their uses.

Should the patient require surgical intervention or orthopedic correction by the foot doctor, it is obvious that more sophisticated techniques, materials and equipment will be necessary. Internal medication may be necessary to relieve pain, prevent infection and relax tissues.

There is no attempt to describe such techniques and materials in this chapter. The reader should refer to the specific disorders discussed in this book for a more sophisticated discussion of their treatment. The creative use of materials will depend on the clinical experience, laboratory skill and personal aptitude of the foot doctor and his staff.

I have attempted in this chapter to give the student and the doctor an appreciation of the dependence of a profession on high quality materials. No profession can improve without the cooperation of the allied sciences and the contributions of material engineers. The materials necessary for the practice of podiatry are the result of painstaking research for their intelligent application.

Suture Materials

The general practitioner in podiatry must have a well-equipped operatory for emergency needs. It is essential to include in surgical pacs a variety of suturing materials and needles.

The basic sutures necessary are as follows:

1. 000 plain catgut, for retention of deep tissues
2. 000 chromic catgut, for deep closure, capsules and tendons
3. 00000 stainless steel, for subcuticular continuous suturing
4. 000 black silk for continuous lock and interrupted suturing
5. 000 and 0000 monofilament nyon for tendon suturing.
6. 000 and 0000 Dexon, for subcuticular suturing.

Office Emergencies

It is also essential that the podiatrist's staff be trained in the handling of medical emergencies. Cerebral hypoxia (fainting) occurs with peripheral vasodilatation due to single or multiple stimuli. Occasional lowering of the blood pressure may stimulate dizziness, cold sweat and pallor with resultant loss of consciousness. It is essential to have smelling salts and oxygen available for immediate use. Application of cold compresses to the head is helpful. With a weak, slow pulse, the doctor must evaluate the need for vasopressor medication. Often a slap or loud noise will stimulate a more rapid pulse and arouse the patient from loss of consciousness. Legs should be elevated and the patient lying down. The staff is alerted to the possibility of vomiting and proper containers should be made available.

Sensitivity to drugs with its alarming symptoms is an ever-present problem which may be avoided by taking a good history that often discloses previous symptoms of reactions to drugs. The patient generally flushes from vasodilatation. Itching, edema, dyspnea and anaphylactic shock are not uncommon. A tourniquet proximal to the injection site slows down absorption. Antihistamines, vasopressors and respiratory dilators are necessary supplies in the well-equipped office. A 1-ml. epinephrine 1/1000 injected into the injection site will slow down absorption of offending medication. Oxygen should be administered, and care should be taken to provide for adequate egress of vomitus. Five-tenths milliliter of 1/1000 epinephrine injected subcutaneously is helpful. Cardiac massage and artificial respiration is essential in the presence of cardiac arrest. Injections of 50 mg. of Benadryl intramuscularly will assist in slowing the release of histamine.

In the presence of occlusion of the blood supply to the brain by thrombosis, embolism or cerebral hemorrhage, there may be a sudden loss of consciousness. Pulse, blood pressure and respiration is noted along with neurologic deficits. With intracranial pressure the pupil is dilated on the affected side. Supporting respiration with clearing of the airways and use of oxygen is helpful. The use of good judgment is most important at this time, and the patient should be removed to a hospital for more definitive treatment if necessary.

2

Guidelines for the Case History

The podiatrist achieves a desired result in treating a specific condition by accurate diagnosis of the problem. The treatment of symptoms alone may provide temporary emergency care but should only be a vehicle for establishing patient rapport until a diagnosis is made.

An inadequate diagnosis may result from a too hurried examination or failure to take a complete history of the case. Insufficient diagnostic equipment or the examiner's lack of knowledge and experience in interpreting the subjective and objective findings are other obstacles to establishing an accurate diagnosis.

It is necessary to understand the practical basis for taking a case history because of its importance in making an accurate diagnosis.

A reliable history depends upon the intelligent cooperation of the patient. If the patient cannot understand why the foot doctor must take a thorough history when he is treating the patient's feet, he must be shown the relationship between general health and foot health. Unfortunately, the average patient has been indoctrinated with the philosophy of "remove your clothes but keep your hose on."

The patient requires sympathetic kindness and understanding in history taking as well as in therapy. Every move and facial expression indicates to the patient your attitude toward his case. There is nothing more potent in successful treatment than having the patient's confidence. The patient receives this feeling in his early contact with the doctor.

The patient knows more than the examiner does about his symptoms. Let him relate his troubles to you. Talking about his problems may help relieve the patient's anxiety. The examiner should keep his eyes, ears and mind open for vital points of the patient's medical history. If the examiner asks too many questions, the patient's responses may confuse interpretation of the main complaint.

Many doctors attempt to use a history form in directing questions at a patient, but a patient who is worried about his particular symptoms may be unable to give the necessary information in a logical and organized way. Skillfully guiding the patient's discussion of himself and his symptoms will bring the best results. The examiner must keep the loquacious patient on the subject, encourage the reticent person to say more and put the nervous individual at ease.

When the diagnosis is obvious, it should be supported by objective findings and then treated accordingly. If a patient complains of pain in certain joints of the feet, especially on arising in the morning, and he has similar pain in the hands, knee or back, etc., an investigation is in order to rule out other complicating factors; but simple complaints of pain of a fifth toe that presents a heloma do not necessarily require elaborate blood studies and sophisticated laboratory examinations.

Taking and Interpreting the General History

Adequate records require that the name, address, and telephone number of all patients be kept. It is also desirable to maintain a record of who referred a patient to you. Whether the patient came to your office through personal, social, business or political affiliations, or whether he was sent by a former patient or another doctor may make a difference in your new relationship with him and with the community you serve. Confidence is so important in patient-podiatrist relationships that this point cannot be overlooked in asking questions for your history. A patient referred by another patient, a colleague or physician immediately has the necessary confidence.

A patient's address may suggest environmental influences as a factor in diagnosis, and racial origins and hereditary factors are often revealed by his family name. Knowing whether he lives near the river or close to a swamp where it is damp, or if he lives near a rat infested dump, in a tenement or in a more desirable locale will often assist in interpreting the patient's symptoms.

Age. Ailments affecting the human body are in many instances related to the age of the individual. Remember that children have wonderful imaginations and enjoy mimicry. Women about menopause age are exceptionally nervous and irritable and they too must be handled with care and understanding. Circulatory involvement would be unlikely in a child, yet injuries to epiphyses are common in children and not seen in adults. Rickets, of course, is a childhood disease and can be suspected in young children. Venereal disease is commonly acquired in the second and third decades of life.

One must refrain from making a snap diagnosis with age as the only basis, however, since many conditions affecting adults with certain characteristic symptoms may be something entirely different in childhood. Dietary deficiencies in children may cause certain skin and bone involvements. Eczematous lesions may be characteristic of the individual's age.

Kravitz and Boehm (1971) note that normal children began to flex their extremities rhythmically within the first 6 months of life. In an older child such symptoms may suggest a neuromuscular disorder.

Gesell notes that children between the ages of 6 and 7 years remove their shoes when coming into the house after school or periods of play. This behavior pattern must not be confused with a sign of discomfort or foot pathology. Yet in the adult one may suspect a neurosis, ill-fitting shoes or definite foot pathology when he has difficulty in wearing shoes.

Tuberculosis is more common in childhood although it may manifest at any age. Infectious diseases, congenital malformations, and many injuries passed unnoticed are seen in children. The cardiovascular diseases of children are commonly rheumatic or congenital; that of middle age diabetic, syphilitic or hypertensive; in old age, arteriosclerotic. Thromboangitis obliterans usually occurs between the ages of 20 and 40.

Subacute combined sclerosis of the spinal cord with numbness, tingling of the hands and feet and with gradual paralysis is seen in individuals between 45 and 55. Multiple sclerosis is often discovered in the age group 15 to 25. Arteriosclerosis is generally thought to be a natural degenerative occurrence in the aged. Predisposing causes are excessive muscular activity, syphilis, alcoholism, lead poisoning, hypertension and renal disease. Arteriosclerosis is described as being a degenerative fibrositis with secondary sclerotic changes in the arteries.

Yale (1954), in a radiographic study of calcification of the medial calcaneal branch of the posterior tibial artery, cited a high incidence of calcification in the age group 20 to 40.

Monckeberg's sclerosis occurs in the aged and in the diabetic. The media is degenerated with the formation of plaques of calcium encircling the vessel. This sclerosis is believed to start at birth.

Other forms of arteriosclerosis are the senile, or atherosclerosis and nodular sclerosis. Calcium deposition within the vessel lumen may occlude circulation with ultimate gangrene and loss of limb.

Progressive muscular atrophy may be seen during childhood and adolescence. It is hereditary and manifests itself early in the feet. The foot is in varus deformity with shortening of the tendo achillis producing an unsteady gait which requires great muscular effort for function. The hands and feet become clawed, the arches abnormally high and the toes hyperflexed.

Friedreich's ataxia usually occurs in adolescence up to the 15th year of age and may affect more than one child in a family. The gait is uncertain, limb movements involuntary, and a widespread leg posture to maintain balance is in evidence. Disturbances in speech, early loss of deep reflexes with abnormal position sense of an extremity are pathognomonic. Equinovarus of both feet occurs later in the disease.

Patients in menopause have varied complaints, some organic and others of psychosomatic origin. Tenderness of the anterior lower third of the tibia in women in the climacteric who have rheumatic pains is a common finding. This has not been found in regularly menstruating women and it does not disappear or change in intensity. It has not been observed in amenorrhea not due to menopause.

A patient in the throes of menopause may develop vague aches and pains in the hands and feet. Stiffness of the small joints of the feet is common. Dry skin with fissures about the heels have been noted. Marked flexion of the toes, night cramps and alternate hot and cold lightning pains in the extremities are common. Treatment may include referral to a gynecologist if the history indicates menopausal etiology. Local symptoms of pain and stiffness may be treated symptomatically; dry, fissured and scaling skin may respond to treatment with moisturizing agents.

Sex. Sex is an important factor in diagnosis since certain conditions are more prevalent in one sex than in the other. For example, diseases of the thyroid, breasts and biliary system are more common in women. Spurs of the heels, apophysitis of the os calcis and many other foot ailments characteristically occur in males, but may occur in females.

Arteriosclerosis obliterans and Buerger's disease are believed to be more common in males. Rheumatoid arthritis, hyperthyroidism and Raynaud's disease are predominant in the young or middle-aged female. Although gout is supposed to be more common in the male, I feel that many cases of gout in the female are being overlooked in diagnosis. Shoes worn by women aggravate foot involvements. Pregnancies, menstrual and menopausal difficulties cause varied foot disturbances. The union of epiphyses takes place about 2 years earlier in the females than in males. A prostatitis must be considered in men as a possible source of infection and pain in the extremities.

A nonsuppurative acute inflammatory cutaneous and subcutaneous nodule formation occurring in females about the second to fourth decade may be erythema nodosum. It is a self-limited disorder of firm somewhat tender nodules, pink to purple in color, usually on the anterior of the legs. Temperature, sore throat and joint pains may accompany this bilateral, symmetrical lesion.

National, Ethnic and Racial Background. The patient's race, nationality and family heredity are important in making a diagnosis. Patients of Mediterranean origin may have a short, stubby and hypermobile type of foot with many minor phalangeal deformities, whereas low-arched feet are common in Semitic peoples. Negroes have a characteristic flat foot, while Caucasians of Nordic ancestry have abnormally high-arched, bony feet. The broad, flexible type of foot with low arch and hallux valgus deformity is typical of the Slavic peoples.

The Negro race shows a high incidence of syphilitic infections and their complicating lesions. Ainhum, also known as dactylolysis spontanea due to its progressive gross pathology, most commonly found in Negroes. A firm constrictive band of fibrous connective tissue covered by a callus creates a cleft in the toe resulting in a swollen, bulbous end. Progressive constriction cuts off circulation causing considerable pain, ulceration and often gangrene followed by spontaneous amputation. Pain can be relieved by early diagnosis and amputation of the toe proximal to the constricting band. The etiology is unknown. Ross (1958) describes a case of ainhum and its treatment. I have seen several cases. A smooth, shiny and elevated massive scar or keloid is also common to the Negro. Occasionally helomas develop in these keloids rendering them painful. Although bone changes rarely affect the extremities, sickle cell anemia is another condition which may be found in Negroes.

People of the Mongoloid race have tiny feet for their size. In Chinese women, especially, this results from the practice of binding the feet for many years. Kaposi's sarcoma commonly affects people originating from the region of the Mediterranean.

Weight. Weight is an important etiologic factor in mechanical foot imbalance. Muscular and ligamentous weakness are affected by being overweight. Improper footgear, poor posture and overwork are aggravating to the feet of individuals who are overweight. Increased weight in pregnancy, carrying of heavy loads and the stress of lifting in certain occupations may produce mechanical foot defects. A rapid increase or decrease in weight may be due to systemic illness or metabolic or endocrine disturbances that may weaken the feet to a point of interfering with normal foot physiology.

Height. Extreme alteration in height may be of anterior pituitary origin. Height has an effect on the individual in proportion to weight and general stature. Frequently an extremely tall individual will develop poor body posture affecting his feet. Short individuals may have metabolic or developmental disturbances with faulty rate of growth in bone.

Occupation. A sedentary occupation may result in atrophy of certain muscular structures as a result of disuse. The use of a foot pedal in certain industries results in strain or inflammation of a part because of repeated trauma to a single area. Lifting of heavy weights and changes from sedentary to active occupations will produce injury to the active part. Dentists, motormen, taxi drivers, bus drivers and persons in like occupations are subject to injury to a single extremity as a result of overuse. Men and women walking long hours on hard surfaces in factories, such as on concrete or metal floors, suffer fatigue readily from lack of a resilient weight bearing surface. Salesladies and countermen, having to stand at one counter for several hours during the day, commonly develop low back pains, poor posture and aching sensations of the feet and legs from overuse or abuse of a single group of muscles.

Psychosomatic difficulties may arise in subconscious fears or dislikes concerned with one's occupation. Allergic reactions and dermatitis venenata may be actively associated with occupational disorders involving feet. Certain eczemas may be directly or indirectly associated with hazardous or irritating occupations.

Working habits, vacations, use of leisure time, diet and use of drugs may influence development of a pathology. Very often secretaries curl their feet about the rungs of a chair while working and this results in pressure over the extensor tendons on the dorsum of the foot. A tenosynovitis is common. If the chair presses forward at the popliteal space or if the legs are pushed back under the chair while working, one may develop a pressure neuralgia or a congestive edema of the foot and ankle.

Family History and Personal Habit. The family history should contain information on the medical background of parents, siblings and other close relatives. If either of the parents is dead, the age of death and the cause should be recorded. The number of siblings and their medical backgrounds should be similarly recorded.

Does the patient smoke, drink or use

narcotics? How much is used? Are these habits moderate or excessive? Smoking may affect the circulatory status of an extremity, alcohol may upset normal mental reactions and morphine or its derivatives may prove to be an excitant.

Environment. An individual accustomed to a cold or warm climate is readily affected by alterations in temperature. Symptoms of Raynaud's disease are more prevalent in the winter.

Arthritics are affected by alterations in atmospheric conditions and they suffer much discomfort in a cold, humid environment. Atmospheric changes cause pain in low-grade inflammatory lesions such as helomas, tylomas and arthritis. Hyperidrosis, bromidrosis, anhidrosis, and sensitivities to nylon, rubber, leather, glue, sock linings, tanning chemicals and dyes are not uncommon causes of foot trouble.

Fungi thrive in a dark, moist, warm and dirty environment. Skin, clothing and bed clothes may become infected by the mite, its eggs and wastes resulting in scabies or the itch.

Typhus fever may cause thrombosis of the blood vessels of the skin. Skin necrosis or gangrene can occur. A scratch or puncture wound on the foot makes a fine avenue of entrance of the virus from fecal deposits.

History of the Chief Complaint

This portion of the history is in the patient's own words. It includes all subjective symptoms and possible etiology.

What the patient reports is of utmost importance. If the condition began suddenly it is acute. If it developed gradually it is chronic in nature. The subacute symptoms lie somewhere between the acute and chronic. How long the condition had been present has much to do with the diagnosis and treatment of the trouble. A pathologic process may develop gradually and still be acute. The history and symptoms given by the patient may be very vague at times. It is wise to have the patient point to the area involved before weighing complaints leading toward a diagnosis. However, it must be borne in mind that the symptoms about which he complains may be referred pain from pathology elsewhere in the body. If these complaints have acute exacerbations with no symptoms in between they are said to be intermittent.

A medical history, past and present, and including a family history is necessary. Many foot disabilities are the result of general illness or past involvements of a general nature. Pain in the feet as a result of psychosomatic illness may be etiologic of foot disability in some cases. The ideal history would be entirely in the patient's own words although few patients stick to the point and many specific questions are necessary. The examiner may compromise by writing the history objectively in the third person while the answers to his questions are woven into the description.

Upon noting the complaint, the patient's greatest symptoms and the patient's outward physical appearance, the podiatrist records the pertinent information as nearly as possible in the patient's own words. Considerable tact must be used to keep some patients on the subject of their complaint whereas others require prodding in order to gather the information desired.

Blumer (1949) suggested that a better view of the duration of a chronic ailment can be had through asking the patient, "how long is it since you felt perfectly well?", rather than "how long have you been sick?"

We do not know the initial symptoms of some of the most common chronic diseases, thus the sensitivity and intelligence of the patient plays an important part in gathering necessary information. Neurotic patients are hypersensitive and over-observant. The phlegmatic type may disregard symptoms causing acute pain.

The podiatrist must note the location, the character, the intensity, the extent of radiation of pain, the effects of exercise, emotion, posture and their relationship to various systems of the body.

It is necessary to know how and when the present complaint began and what the symptoms have been since, in order to form a diagnosis. Such information is necessary not only for medical purposes but for legal ones as well since insurance companies request this information and expect an intelligent answer. This information may reveal the etiology and may make possible removal of the continued aggravation of the pathology. Did the present complaint come about suddenly or slowly over a long period of time? Have the symptoms increased, decreased or changed in character? What sequence did they pursue? When did the symptoms occur: during summer, winter, etc? What hour of the day did the symptoms commence? If trauma is involved, note the time and place. Careful interrogation will add to the sum knowledge of the complaint.

Groups of vesicles on slightly elevated erythematous plaques distributed along one or more peripheral sensory nerves with severe pain suggest shingles or herpes zoster. This may occur in an individual who has been ill, overworked or tired.

Pulmonary embolism syndrome may be expected especially when there has been immobilizing illness, an operation or a history of vascular disease, trauma or infection of the leg. A peripheral phlebitis may be a precursor to pulmonary embolism. The patient may have frequent nosebleeds which may suggest a cardiac involvement. Shortness of breath and chest pains may indicate a cardiac or lung disorder. The general color and appearance of the patient is noted for corroboration. Nocturia may be due to a bladder disturbance. A great thirst, frequent urination, xanthoma, pruritis, furuncles, carbuncles, pustules or gangrene may suggest diabetes.

Constipation suggests intestinal stasis. A history of eating improperly cooked pork or bear meat may cause muscular aches and vomitus with other symptoms of trichinosis. Dizziness and frequent headaches suggest high blood pressure. Allergic reactions affecting the skin of the feet are common in individuals who suffer from hay fever and asthma. Many people are sensitized to drugs and foods. Redness and indurated swellings of the joints of the feet accompanied by exfoliation of the epidermis is not uncommon after antibiotic therapy for a systemic infection. Sharp shooting lightening-like pains in the extremities may be a neuritis of syphilitic origin.

Hyperidrosis and late afternoon elevations in temperature with persistent cough and loss of weight suggest tuberculosis. Respiratory infections, sore throats, tooth infections, prostatitis, middle ear and gallbladder lesions may lead to painful manifestations in the extremities.

Viruses change the cells within which they grow and multiply, resulting in hyperplasia or necrosis.

The podiatrist must recognize the symptoms of the common cold, influenza, dengue, measles, herpes zoster (shingles) and acute polio as they relate to the local foot complaints. The infectious diseases produce symptoms in the extremities involving skin reactions, myalgias, thrombophlebitis, arthritis, polyneuritis and cutaneous hyperesthesia.

Medical and Surgical History

The medical history should list all pertinent information including typical childhood diseases, scarlet fever, rheumatic heart and all other diseases and infections. A record should be kept of the patient's inoculations. Listing all allergies, especially drug allergies, is a necessity.

Pregnancy. Varicose veins, phlebitis and leg, hip and low back pains along with a calcium deficiency often bring pregnant women to a podiatrist's office.

In treating a pregnant woman or a woman with other children, the number of living children the patient has and a record of previous stillbirths should be noted. Stillbirths may be indicative of syphilis or a pelvic disorder, either of which can cause a variety of foot disturbances.

The pregnant woman should do considerable walking during and after the period of pregnancy. The marked increase in body weight during pregnancy is a strain on the pedal extremities. However, even greater damage to physiologic function is incurred by the pregnant woman who becomes sedentary or recumbent during this period.

The feet should be closely observed during the puerperium and postpartum. Many plantar warts that appear during the first trimester disappear after delivery. An examination of foot functions and posture with evaluation of their effect on body posture is necessary to appreciate some physiologic changes. Complaints of foot pains such as strained plantar fascia, cramps, fatigue and muscle soreness are quite common. Backaches, pain in the thighs and on the medial aspect of the knees are the results of faulty foot posture rather than simply relaxation of the pelvis joints. Swelling of the lower legs must be differentiated. Deep varicosities, lymphatic stasis, thrombophlebitis, cardiac, kidney disturbances, and pressure of the fetus in the lower pelvic region may result in edema.

Wearing low-heeled shoes or flat, weight-bearing inner soles and slippers will cause symptoms of pulling sensations behind the knees.

The heads of the gastrocnemius are pulled through the lowered position of the heel with resultant strain. Symptoms of biomechanical dysfunction are most commonly found after the fifth month of pregnancy. Body mechanics are altered through the addition of weight and ill-fitting footgear. Pain may be referred to the internal lateral ligaments of the knee due to pronation beyond normal range. Leg musculature may become atrophic and flabby. During the puerperium, muscular weakness becomes rapid and progressive. After parturition the patient may complain of weakness of the feet and legs. Dull aches and coldness of the feet may persist due to incomplete recuperation from physiologic changes. The stretched ligaments and joint capsules together with the elongated muscles require several months to return to normal. In treating podiatric complaints of pregnant or postparturient women, heat and violent exercises should be avoided. Oxford shoes with freedom for toes, firm fit in heel and arch, rigid shank, extended counter, Thomas heel or heel height of comfort, all leather, Goodyear welt construction should be worn. Elastic stockings with open toe, closed heel and of mid-thigh length may alleviate symptoms. If hyperidrosis exists, a foot powder of choice should be used.

Venereal Diseases and Related Factors. Ask the patient if he has a venereal infection when the symptoms lead you to suspect such a disease. Never accept a denial until all suspicious diseases are investigated by a laboratory examination. If a patient is known to have syphilis find out the date of infection. A history of inadequate treatment must be noted.

Gonorrhea is the most common venereal disease. Infections of the urinary tract and prostatitis may be the result of a gonorrheal infection with frequent involvement of the joints in the foot by a gonorrheal arthritis. A chronic inflammatory dermatosis with infection of the genital tract and of the joints may be noted in patients with gonorrhea. Symmetric eruptions of horny hyperkeratotic nodules, crusts and pustules on the palms and soles are characteristic.

If the patient is known to have syphilis or if you suspect it is present, try to elicit a history of a saucer-shaped chancre with raised, clearly demarcated, indurated margins on the genital organs. These chancres have a bloody serous discharge and usually clear up with or without treatment in 3 to 5 weeks.

Macular, papular or erythematous lesions affecting the palms and soles may occur in the secondary stages of syphilis. Nails of the toes may lose their luster and syphilitic onychia may be present.

The tertiary stages are characterized by gummatous lesions or general paresis, mental degeneration, delusions of grandeur, tabes dorsalis, exaggerated reflexes, loss of position sense and equilibrium with Argyll-Robertson pupil and perforating ulcers.

In a female patient it is necessary to know the number of miscarriages, if any, to establish background for a possible diagnosis. The underlying pathology may be syphilis or Rh factor. Repeated miscarriages followed by stillbirths and finally by viable children may suggest syphilis. The child is infected *in utero* and may at birth present a saber shin and saddle nose. Notched teeth may be noted with growth and development. If the patient is a male, ask if his wife has had miscarriages. If the patient's wife has syphilis, the male patient may be infected through sexual contact. This information is of diagnostic importance.

Other related factors causing podiatric complaints should be determined. Ask a female patient if the menstrual periods are regular, if the flow is normal, and what the duration is. Is the menopause causing undue difficulty?

Disturbances in the feet may be due to a pelvic disorder. One foot may get cold and clammy as a result of low pelvic tumors and edemas. Pressure on arteries, veins and nerves may cause pains to radiate down the extremity from an abdominal or pelvic mass.

Surgical History. Surgical history should include information on all operations and anesthetics administered, and information on accidental injuries. Hemorrhages, thrombosis or embolism point to tendencies which may be significant in subsequent illnesses. Low abdominal surgery with herniation followed by neglect results in referable damage to the pedal extremities. A history of superficial migratory phlebitis may suggest thromboangiitis obliterans.

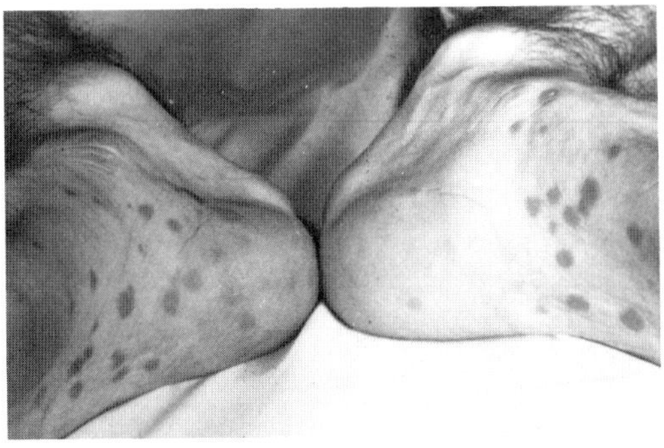

Fig. 2.1. Macular lesions, bilateral and symmetrical; syphilis questionable. Courtesy of J. F. Yale.

The Patient's Record

The above outline for an adequate history does not necessitate a thorough interrogation of the patient. It is not advisable to keep superfluous histories for minor foot involvements and certainly a laboratory study in depth is not necessary in making a simple diagnosis. Yet it is always wise to have too much information to work with than not enough.

I have some definite ideas on the type of history chart which is best for establishing an accurate diagnosis. In recent years I have tried many printed forms with great disappointment. The practitioner should be sufficiently well informed when taking a history to follow a pattern which allows great leeway in recording information. After recording the basic information of such as age, weight, sex, and so forth, the examiner asks the necessary questions as described above to establish a complete picture of the complaint.

After noting the objective and subjective symptoms and recording them on paper, all additional information is added according to date. In this way, a running history of the patient incorporating subsequent contributory information and findings may be kept. At this time a tentative impression may be made and at each visit additional information and complaints as of that date are also recorded. Each patient's set of history sheets is kept in a separate folder together with his laboratory reports which can also be referred to according to date. Regardless of the number of visits, this file adds to the total understanding of the patient's present complaint. Consultation sheets are attached also and the date of consultation is noted in regular order on the examination sheet.

The problem-oriented medical record developed by Dr. Lawrence Weed, University of Vermont, and the subject of a book written by Dr. H. Cross and J. Bjorn is receiving widespread acceptance. If mastered, it may well supplant the "source-oriented" medical record now in use that consists of an array of unrelated facts difficult to correlate from the charts.

A well-organized "problem-oriented" record will save the doctor time and patience in locating comprehensive material on a specific problem. Present methods of keeping patient records may force the podiatrist to wade through reams of vital data, charts, laboratory findings and unrelated radiographs and reports to find that the patient had previously complained of the symptom now at hand. This type of record is divided into four broad categories.

1. *Establishment of a Data Base.* This includes the sum of the patient's complaints, sociologic and psychologic history, a podiatric examination, a medical history and surgical history of the patient and laboratory data.

2. *Formulation of All Problems.* A list of all problems is recorded and given a number. Each problem is followed by a brief comment on the subjective and objective symptoms, e.g., 1) painful swollen left hallux joint; 2) deep keratotic verrucoid lesion, plantar surface, fourth metatarsal head, right foot.

The list of problems over a period of years will be numbered. Referral to these problems is made easy by using the specific number for each problem as the chart increases in size over the years.

3. *Plans for Each Problem.* Here the podiatrist continues to provide further information. He also records anticipated treatment of each problem and numbers the treatments to correspond with the problem. The patient is advised of the significance of each problem and this action is recorded by the problem number. Thus, each problem has its own treatment plan based on all findings.

4. *Follow-Up on Each Problem.* This consists of progress notes that are dated, titled and numbered by problem.

Dr. Lawrence Weed looks upon the problem-oriented record progress notes as the most important part of this structured record for which he uses the acronym SOAP: Subjective, patient's evaluation of treatment results; Objective, results noticed by the doctor; Assessment, doctor's evaluation of the treatment; Plans, reviewing of plans and formulating new plans to enhance treatment of each problem.

3

Examination and Primary Observations

The examiner must have a keen sense of responsibility toward his patient. His ability to observe through use of all his senses will reflect in the successful treatment of the patient's symptoms. A good rule to follow is to allow several minutes of examination for each minute of treatment.

Color of Skin. Abnormal changes in skin color often occur in occlusive vascular disease and must be differentiated from vitiligo and other disorders of the skin. Metabolic and endocrine conditions must be considered. Bilateral color differences in extremities and toes are very significant. Observation of a normal extremity demonstrates pallor on elevation with rapid return to normal on dependency.

A marked rubor on dependency with cyanosis occurring usually below the ankle and affecting an entire foot or part of the foot is significant of chronic arterial insufficiency. Edema, redness and heat may occur with anidrosis after a too rapid warming of cold feet. Lividity of the toes is common in healthy persons after exposure to cold.

Neurocirculatory asthenia occurs after pronounced effort in work or athletic endeavors and may result in a livid, cyanotic skin surface with coldness of the extremities. This same change is noted in immersion foot, trench foot and shelter foot. Small widely spaced cyanotic patches may develop. A vivid red or yellowish blue to black color may result.

Reddish or red-blue discoloration is a more or less normal change in the skin of aging persons. When it occurs in younger people it is significant of some constitutional disturbance such as acrocyanosis, Raynaud's disease or livido reticularis. Majocchi's disease is characterized by minute, sharply defined, rose or red to purple macules.

Slow return of blood following a blanching of the skin by pressure also suggests an imperfect blood supply requiring further study. Ischemic neuritis may produce this change. Recently, S. Michota (1971) developed a technique for photographing the plantar surface on weightbearing. The patient stands on a box with a heavy plate of glass or Plexiglas top. The impression created by the superimposed weight can be viewed through a large mirror tipped to 48 degrees within the box.

A marble white pallor with numbness, stiffness and pain is seen early in Raynaud's disease. A local asphyxia and subsequent ulcerations and gangrene of the digits is the sequel to this vasomotor instability. A sympathectomy or vasodilator drug may alter the pathology. Angioneurotic edema may result in large multiple swellings of the skin varying in color from a flesh pink to dark purple. It commonly involves the tissue on the medial, dorsal and lateral aspects of the feet. Antihistamine medications by the oral route can reduce the edema. If acute, i.v. injections of minimal doses of cortisone can be lifesaving.

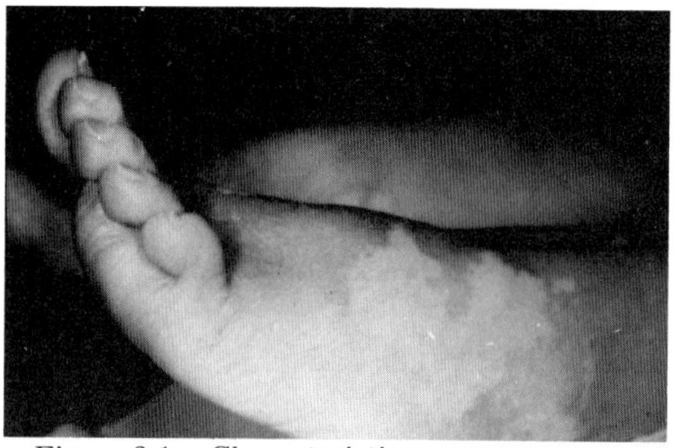

Fig. 3.1. Characteristic appearance of vitiligo. Must be differentiated from circulatory disorders which produce pallor in the extremities.

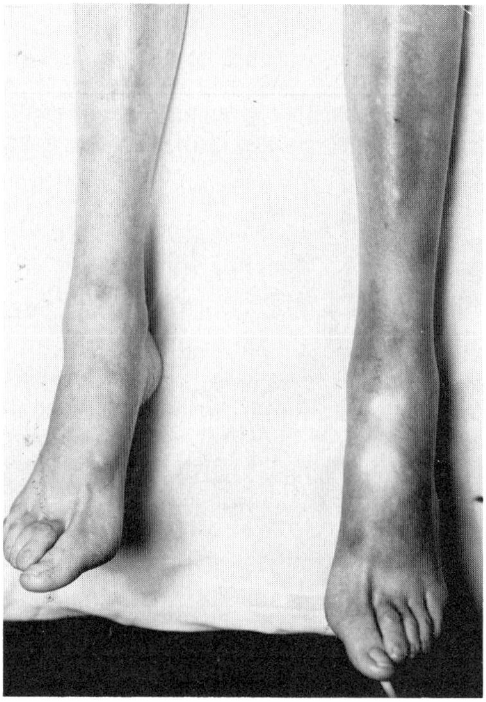

Fig. 3.2. Marked rubor with blanching on digital pressure. Courtesy of D. Mowbray.

Redness may occur from ingestion of certain sensitizing foods or medications. Treatment consists of eliminating the sensitizing agents. The use of antihistamines may be necessary.

Elevated, itchy lesions of pink to red color may occur on the sides and dorsum of the feet and backs of the hands in granuloma annulare. The lesion measures about 5 mm. and is often clear in the center. Corticosteroid topical applications should relieve symptoms of itching.

Doughy, infiltrated areas or collections of many firm bean-sized, reddish-brown or purplish nodules may be an early indication of Kaposi's sarcoma.

Erythematous lesions are seen in many eczemas and in dermatitis venenata caused by shoe polish, shoe dye, sock lining dye, leather, nylon hose and leg make-up. Dermatitis venenata is a reaction of the skin to chemical or vegetable irritants applied externally. A patch test will often prove the irritant. Removing the irritant and using medication to allay pruritis provide relief of symptoms.

Superficial reactions to extremes of temperature such as a burn or frostbite will cause notable color changes. Cold and dampness affect the local vasomotor system. A livid bluish-red color with a cushion-like swelling is the usual end result; deep fissures and bullae are common associated findings. The effects of radiant energy cause a persistent reticulated, pigmented erythema.

Colored, reddish-brown spots may be the result of the involution of indurated symmetrical cutaneous nodules in undernourished young females. They may be of tuberculous origin and the sequela of erythema induratum. A complete physical examination by an internist is necessary. Treatment includes improved dietary habits and rest.

Ill-fitting shoes and hose may cause a redness between the fourth and fifth toes in the form of an erythema intertrigo. This condition may be alleviated

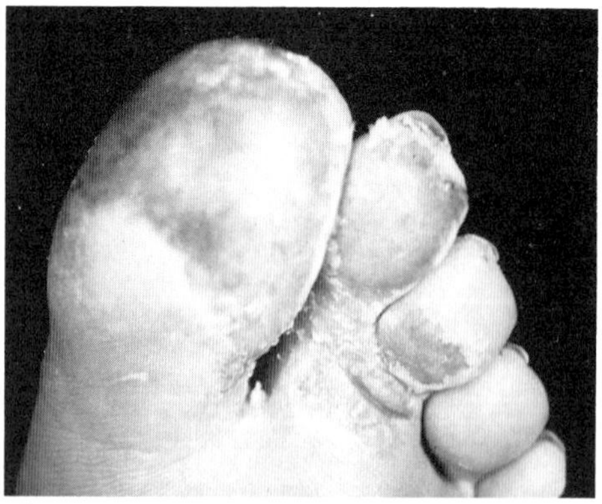

Fig. 3.3. Dermatitis venenata. Denuding of skin on plantar of toes is subject to secondary infection.

by wearing correct footgear and using a mild powder to relieve chafing.

When bright red, shiny, painful nodes which are firm, elastic, oval and tense, occur in groups on the anterior aspect of the lower third of the leg, they may indicate erythema nodosum. They subside gradually and leave a dark red and purple discoloration followed by green or brown stains. Early use of ice bags, bedrest and elevation of the legs are indicated. Supplementary diets are necessary. The nodular lesions do not disappear readily.

Dry, scaly, imbricated, silvery scales covering red patches on the extensor surfaces of the body is indicative of psoriasis. The thickened nails are dry, powdery, gray, yellow brown in color and the plate is punctate and eroded. Annointing the skin with an oil or cream, such as lanolin and cocoa butter helps remove scales. Inflammatory changes are reduced with triamcinolone acetonide cream or hydrocortisone cream ¼%. Nails are ground down and the nail grooves are curetted out. Concomitant mycotic infections of the nails are treated by local or oral medication.

Purpuric changes brought about by escape of whole blood into the tissues producing petechiae or larger ecchymoses must be evaluated. Purpura simplex may be caused by a violent strain such as a cough or fright. Henoch's purpura may be an allergic manifestation while a purpura hemorrhagica is characterized by a decrease in the number of blood platelets. Secondary purpuras may occur after acute infections and venous stasis. Careful blood studies are made to determine the cause of purpura. Purpuric lesions are best treated by good nourishment and plenty of bedrest.

Red papules the size of a pinhead, masses of capillary dilatations, covered by purplish to black hyperkeratotic caps may be an angiokeratoma resulting from trauma. Surgical excision of the red papules is indicated.

An erythema may result from occupational stress. Infection of unknown etiology may cause an erythema multiforme which is characterized by macular, papular or vesicular lesions of bright or dark red color fading to a purplish or violaceous hue. Rest is the treatment of choice. If an infection is located, treatment will depend on the location and the type of bacteria involved.

Whenever a nonspecific redness develops, the examiner must look for the possibility of a feigned irritation. Light pink, shiny plaques of angulated papules with flat tops may be the result of a "stone wall worry." The papules may be caused by lichen planus which is often seen about the ankles, soles and dorsum of the feet.

Bilateral and symmetrical plaques ranging from light to dark purple with thickening of the skin and cross-patching sometimes occur in neurodermatitis and hypopituitarism. Jaundiced individuals may present characteristic yellow color changes accompanied by severe itching.

Pallor is more significant when affecting one foot, and, when it is associated with other symptoms of vascular disease, one may look for an arterial degeneration. Blanching can be interpreted as a dimunition of blood supply to the part. Anemic individuals may have marked pallor bilaterally and symmetrically. Blood transfusions and removal of all constricting devices is helpful. Vasodilators improve peripheral circulation.

Cyanosis is due to changes in the blood of the cutaneous capillaries. The changes are due to an inadequate oxygenated hemoglobin. Cyanosis is very often evident in patients with impending gangrene and a mixture of venous and arterial blood may cause it. Cyanosis is usually indicative of occlusive vascular disease and is sometimes found in loss of tone in the vasomotor system. The great toe is a common site for early cyanosis. It is not only indicative of faulty blood flow but also of pathologic changes in the walls of the vessels. Low grade inflammations may produce cyanosis. Cardiac and pulmonary insufficiency may produce cyanosis.

Constant discoloration and cyanosis distal to the ankles may indicate acrocyanosis and may occur in Raynaud's disease following color changes of that disease. A bluish-red mottling of the skin of the feet and legs known as "livido reticularis" is present in Raynaud's disease. The mottling often extends proximally to involve the entire lower extremity and abdomen. The color changes are aggravated by cold, and ulcerations often develop at the sites of great pressure. Persistent cyanosis of an individual toe may be a manifestation of thrombosis in the distal arteries.

Vasomotor stimulators or dilators improve the functional capacity of the patient. Anti-clotting medication may improve the cyanosis and prevent gangrene. Often an injection about the posterior tibial nerve as it lies behind the medial malleolus will provide a means for relaxing arterial spasms as in a sympathectomy. The patient should dress warmly and avoid cold weather.

Pallor and coldness, or acroasphyxia, of the fingers and toes may occur after exposure to cold and are pathognomonic for Raynaud's disease. The color changes vary from pallor to redness and the temperature from cold to hot where acroasphyxia exists.

Vasodilators are helpful in relieving discomfort and altering the spasm.

In thromboangiitis obliterans it is not the temperature but the posture of the limb which causes color changes in an entire foot. In erythromelalgia heat aggravates the degree of redness which is relieved by cold. Pulses are generally strong and bounding. There is no tendency to gangrene as in acroasphyxia caused by Raynaud's and the obliterating diseases.

Erythema is not significant of heat or increased blood supply to the part but results from a vasodilatation from any number of causes. The minute vessels are damaged when the part is cold and dilated when hot. When it is warm and red inflammatory changes and drug reactions are suspected.

Redness characterized by streaking or hyperemia may result from a lymphangitis. In localized severe cases, a suppurative and phlegmonous inflammation may precede gangrene. The looseness of the subcutaneous tissue on the dorsum of the foot is conducive to edema. The toes, dorsum and lateral aspect of the foot are readily affected while the overhanging type of swelling on the medial aspect gives an appearance of pronation. The popliteal and inguinal glands may be tender and palpable. Lymphangitis may occur with infection, e.g., small puncture wound, subonychial infection, interdigital fissures, infected helomas and fungus infections of the toes.

An erythematous, butterfly-shaped area suggests systemic lupus erythematosus and the patient should be referred to an internist.

Skin redness about the toes occurs when arterial circulation is slightly impaired. The discoloration may persist on elevation although pallor is more consistent with arterial disease. An irregular reddish-brown discoloration of hemorrhagic extravasation in the skin or beneath the skin may be associated with capillary fragility. An angioneurosis, vasomotor imbalance, neurasthenia, or erythromelalgia may be the cause for marked redness, for a burning, throbbing engorgement of the veins, and for edema in anxious and neurotic patients. Vasodilators, psychotherapeutic medications, sympathectomy, and vitamins C and K may be helpful. In the presence of

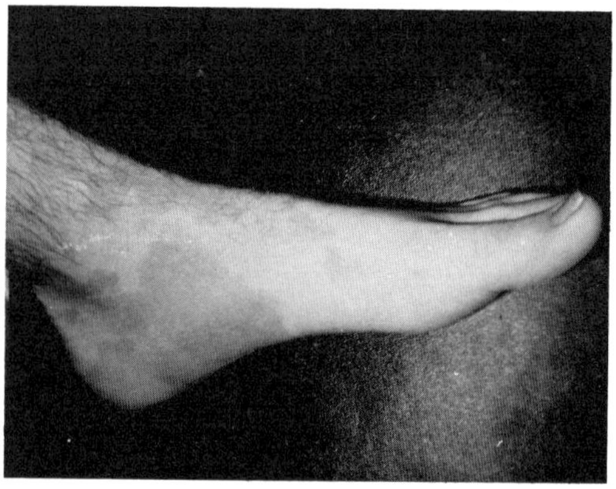

Fig. 3.4. Lupus erythematosus. Note butterfly-shaped lesions. Pattern must not be confused with extensive hyperidrosis or with lack of pigment as seen in vitiligo.

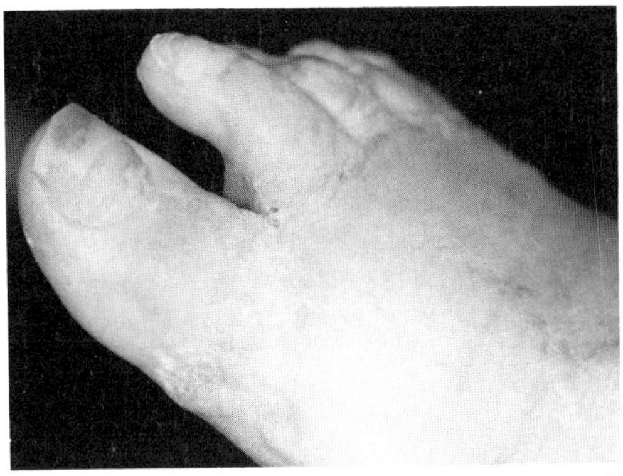

Fig. 3.5. Lupus erythematosus. Note small punctate ulcers.

infection, the proper antibiotics are mandatory.

Erythema induratum is characterized by bluish-red, deep-seated nodules in the subcutaneous tissues. The nodules range in size from 1 to 6 mm. and occur any place on the legs but most commonly on the posterior calf. The painful nodules ulcerate and heal slowly leaving the surrounding tissues indurated and a pitted, pigmentated scar may remain. Corticosteroids relieve the inflammation but the patient requires good dietary habits and plenty of rest.

Lesions of any type found on the legs or feet may help identify underlying vascular conditions. The characteristic appearances of a sinus, ulceration, dermatologic irritation, dilated veins, abnormal nails, and swelling are symptomatic of various underlying conditions.

Rose Spots. These must not be confused with dermatologic lesions of local etiology or systemic origin. Chronic venous insufficiency is seen about the ankles and is accompanied by light brown, gray to black pigmentation of the skin.

Small, painless, pinkish spots on the legs or the dorsum of the foot remain for several weeks. They ultimately become dark and pigmented. Rose spots are found in diabetics and indicate an active process taking place in the smaller vessels. These must be differentiated from phlebitic skin lesions. Fragility of minute superficial blood vessels may result in subcutaneous hemorrhage and rose spots.

Treatment of the underlying pathology is imperative. Subcutaneous hemorrhage is relieved by corticosteroïds, and vitamins B_{12} and C.

Texture of Skin. Glossy skin produced by atrophoderma neuroticum may be secondary to neuritis following severe trauma, disease of the spinal cord, gout or arthritis. De Takat has reported several cases in which the vascular supply to the sciatic nerve was affected. Vasomotor phenomena, trophic changes and causalgia are prominent. The skin becomes bluish, glossy and eczematous, and a grayness may develop resembling an atrophic scar. Skin texture is affected by contact dermatitis.

Temperature of the Foot. The temperature of the surface of the skin varies with environmental temperature, temperature of the body and with conditions of the skin and subcutaneous tissues. The temperature of the skin surface on the trunk varies between 92.3 and 98.4° F. (33.5 and 36.9° C.). Symmetrical parts normally have identical temperature.

Temperature of the foot may be determined by placing the hand on patient's foot or by using a thermocouple or skin thermometer for exact temperature. If both feet are above or below normal foot temperature, a systemic condition may be responsible. A difference in temperature between the left and the right foot indicates a local disturbance, although some variations may be caused by a systemic disorder. Excessive heat in one foot generally indicates inflammation. Coldness denotes improper circulation or nerve involvement affecting the vasomotor system. Excessively cold foot sweats are found in nervous people. Excessive cold or hot foot sweats are found in faulty foot mechanics.

Coldness may be due to room temperature and changes in environment. The examiner's hand must be warm to determine abnormal skin temperature. Instruments such as the skin thermometer and the electric thermocouple enable the podiatrist to measure skin temperature accurately. A drop in temperature with ischemia on elevation is observed in thromboangiitis obliterans. A bilateral lowering of temperature may result from a saddle embolus.

When a single digit is cold and pale the condition may be due to a vasospasm or some organic condition of the arteries. Pressure on the vessels in the lower abdomen by tumor mass or pregnancy may produce unilateral coldness. Exposure to cold may cause a vasospasm ischemia followed by dilatation and cyanosis.

Increased temperature is not always found with burning of the feet. On the contrary, if the feet are burning, the temperature of the skin is lowered. Cellulitis and phlebitis should be excluded when warmth is present along the course of an extremity. A fever of the feet, associated with deep redness is suggestive of erythromelalgia. Increase in temperature is a significant finding in infectious lesions. Atmospheric warmth may increase the temperature of the feet.

An increase in temperature may occur in furunculosis when an infection of a hair follicle or a sebaceous gland causes an extensive cellulitis terminating in pus formation. This may be due to a general debility, anemia or diabetes. *Staphylococcus aureus* may be the invading organism.

A carbuncle may develop secondary to furunculosis. Carbuncles have been seen on several occasions occurring over the dorsum of the first metatarsal-cuneiform joint caused by irritation from prominent eyelets. Bacterial sensitivity tests are done to help provide the necessary medication. Hot packs, incision, drainage, and penicillin usually resolve the infection.

An increased temperature accompanied by anorexia and chills may develop with erysipelas. The skin may burn and itch. The affected area is elevated, indurated, firm, erythematous and sharply marginated. Rest, elevation of the infected limb and systemic antibiotic treatment are essential.

A pustular eczema with all signs of infection may occur secondary to fungus infections, varicose eczema or dermatitis venenata or medicamentosa. Pustular eczema is best treated with the medication of choice following a sensitivity test.

Acute high fevers with a chill and "step-like" increases in temperature may be the result of a febrile condition in which bacteria are present in the bloodstream producing systemic symptoms of infection. This septicemia may result secondary to infectious diseases. Predisposing factors are exposure to cold and wet, fatigue, loss of sleep, chronic disease and agents which lower resistance to infection. The bacteria may enter the bloodstream through the veins and lymphatics with the most common source of infection being infected wounds, onychocryptosis, helomas and tylomas, phlegomons, carbuncles, bed

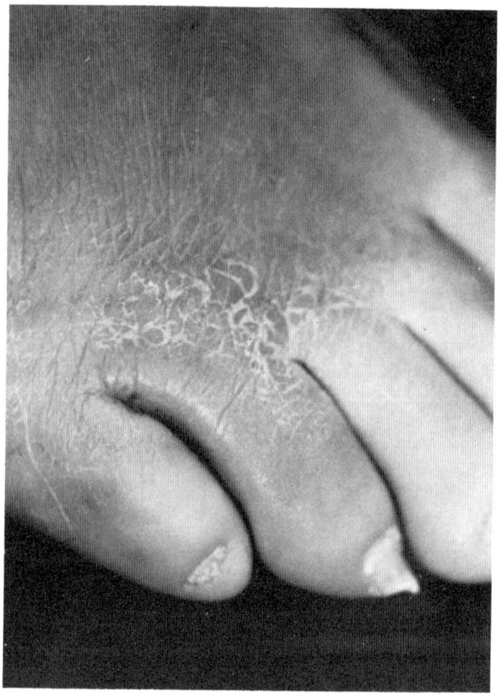

Fig. 3.6. Infection fourth and fifth toes. Note swelling, cellulitis, discoloration. Patient had inguinal lymphadenopathy.

sores and blisters. Osteomyelitis may be a sequela.

The drug of choice is based on sensitivity tests. The proper antibiotic must be prescribed in large enough doses orally or parenterally over long periods of time. Either tetracycline or erythromycin 250 to 500 mg. orally 4 times daily may be used.

Local inflammation or trauma raises skin temperature. Temperature is higher over an active part or over muscles and lower over tendons or bone. Muscular exercise increases temperature response. Removal of vasoconstrictor influence by general, spinal or local anesthesia causes a higher temperature response. Acute arthritis gives a higher response to skin surface temperature. Alcohol, thyroid and amyl nitrate raises temperature response.

Pulses of Foot and Leg. A useful practice is to grade arterial pulsations on the basis of an index of 0 to 4. *Zero* indicates complete absence of pulse; *1* indicates a marked impairment; *4* indicates normal pulsations. The examiner should not be confused by pseudopulsation in the form of pulsations from his own finger tip arteries.

The pulse of the dorsalis pedis may be felt by placing the second, third and fourth finger tips along the outer side of the extensor hallucis longus tendon behind the first metatarsal head. Occasionally it is impalpable in normal patients but this is often a sign of circulatory disturbances, especially if the dorsalis pedis pulse is not present in older people.

In cases where faulty circulation is believed to be the cause of the symptoms, the patient should be referred to a specialist in circulatory diseases for consultation.

The posterior tibial pulse is located just distal to and slightly in back of the medial malleolus. The patient should be seated when the podiatrist checks the posterior tibial pulse which may be difficult to locate in obese patients.

The popliteal pulse is difficult to find as it is palpated behind the knee in the popliteal space. With the patient prone, the examiner faces the patient's foot. With the left hand he holds the leg at the ankle in a relaxed position with slight flexion of the knee. The right hand is placed about the medial side of the extremity opposite the popliteal space and the thumb or forefinger makes repeated pressures into the space to elicit the pulsation. This pulsation can also be palpated by the second and third fingers with the knees in slight flexion and often

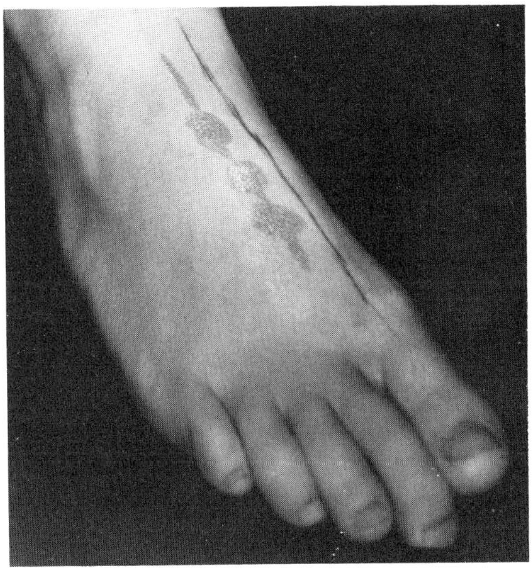

Fig. 3.7. The dorsalis pedis pulse is palpated just lateral to the extensor hallucis longus tendon by placing the second, third and fourth fingers along the course of the dorsalis pedis artery.

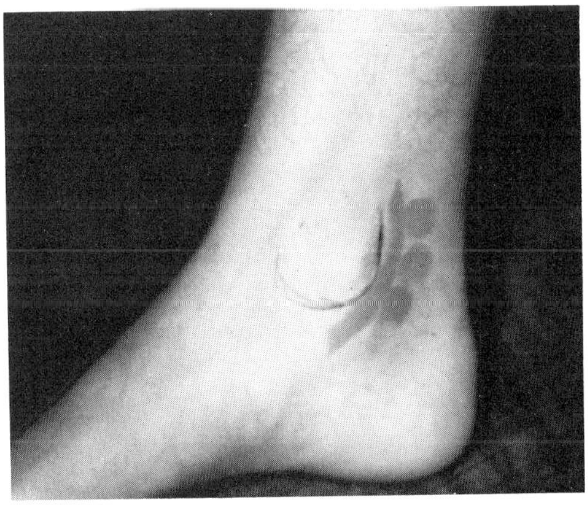

Fig. 3.8. The posterior tibial pulse which is palpated posterior to the medial malleolus.

reveals embolic occlusion or early popliteal aneurysm.

Femoral pulse is felt below Poupart's ligament line in the groin. Normally, it is full and strong. It may be diminished in embolic or thrombotic conditions of the iliac vessels of which it is a branch.

Pressure is applied with the tips of the second, third and fourth fingers in a line transverse and oblique to the axis of the limb.

Blood pressures in the upper and lower extremity are about equal in functional aortic insufficiency. In organic aortic insufficiency the systolic pressure in the lower extremity is from 50 to 100 mm or more of mercury higher than in the upper extremity. In coarctation of the aorta the blood pressure is higher in the arm than in the lower extremity. Absence of pulsations is common in thromboangiitis obliterans.

Scars. Scars which are not produced by trauma or infection may be found in individuals with impaired peripheral circulation. Small, pigmented scars which appear oval and punched out beneath the skin are commonly found in diabetics. The larger scars found usually on the crest or soft parts about the tibia, if not due to trauma, are possibly arteriosclerotic or caused by syphilis. Massive keloids may occur in Negroes following surgery, lacerations or trauma.

Total excision of the scar is helpful. Destruction by chemosurgical methods is desirable. Treatment by the internist of the diabetic is absolutely necessary.

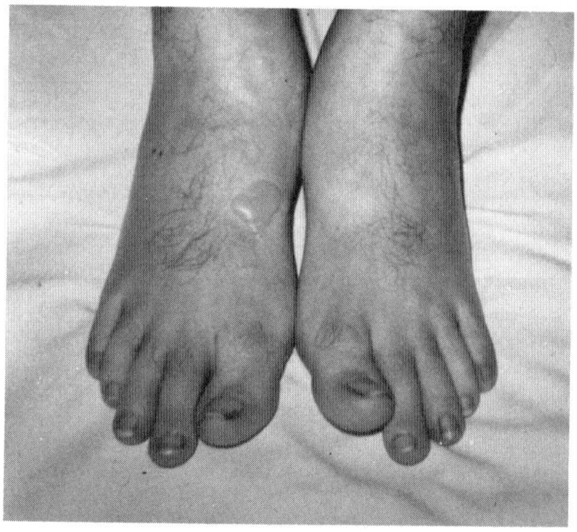

Fig. 3.9. Bullous lesion. Large bulla, dorsum right foot secondary to friction.

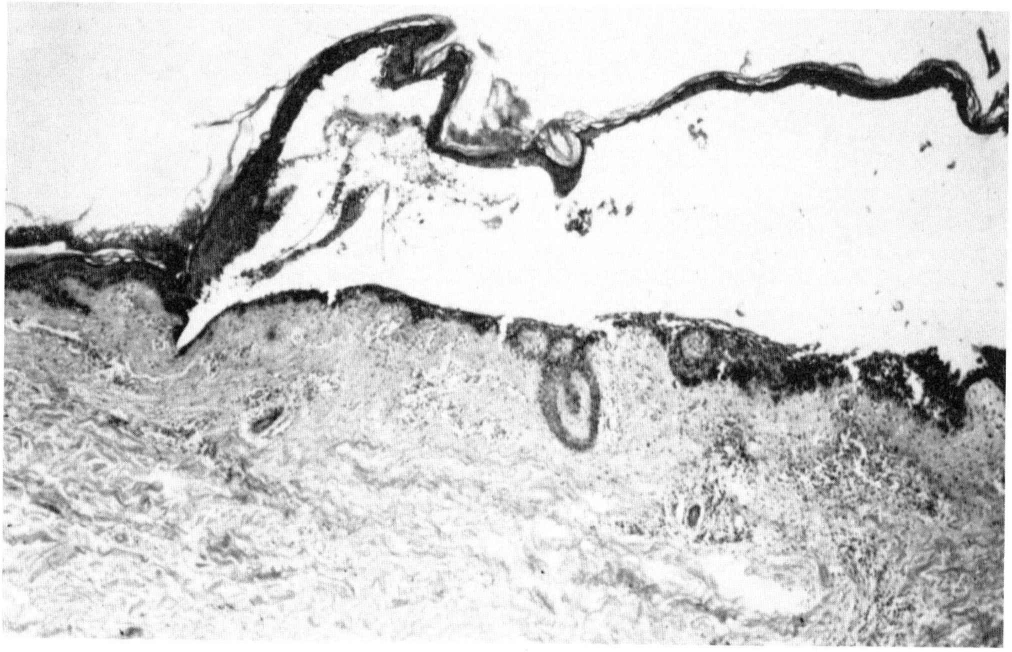

Fig. 3.10. Photomicrograph of a bullous lesion. Note both acute and chronic inflammation. Courtesy of J. F. Yale.

Blisters-Blebs. When occurring in the diabetic, blebs or bullae appear overnight without any history of injury, thermal or mechanical. Within 24 hr. the diabetic bleb becomes white and colorless. In 48 hr. the diabetic bleb fluid content becomes purple and discolored. After this the base may become gangrenous. Most gangrene starts with bleb formation when due to a change in the arteries. Blebs may occur with eczematous lesions, allergic reactions and idiosyncrasies.

Blebs must be kept clean and redressed daily. If the patient is diabetic, the lesions should be allowed to recede. Tepid soaks in 1 quart warm water and a tablespoonful of table salt is effective in providing a natural media for resolution.

The essentials of treatment are a minimum of medication, cleanliness and aseptic dressings. Bullous lesions may be caused by fungus infections, sunburn, neurodermatitis, thermal damage and separation of the dermal-epidermal juncture. The presence of fluid is the result of such skin disorders, and it accumulates by osmosis resulting from destruction of the cells.

Opening of a blister should be performed only under strict asepsis. Many believe that the bullous lesion should not be opened; however, I prefer to remove the top of a large bleb to facilitate drainage using saline soaks to dry the base. Small blebs will generally dry up with proper medication to limit inflammatory changes.

It is inadvisable to remove the top of the blister within 48 hr. of its appearance because of the marked increase in pain and susceptibility to infection. According to Cortese *et al.* (1968), "multiple aspiration of the blister fluid during the first 24 hr. or a single aspiration between 24 and 36 hr. is the optimal early management procedure."

Potassium permanganate soaks, aluminum subacetate and other astringent agents are helpful. In the presence of severe dermatoses the use of corticosteroids orally in gradually decreasing dosages aids in resolution of the problem.

Muscular Rigidity. A generalized muscular rigidity, especially in the flexor groups, may occur in Parkinson's disease. The slow and progressive disease most frequently affects males over 40. The rigidity of the arms, legs, neck and back produce the characteristic stooping or hyperextended posture. The fingers and thumb pat each other in typical pill-rolling fashion. A falling forward gait and waxen masked facial expression is characteristic of this disease.

In multiple sclerosis, a disordered gait and postural instability are prominent symptoms along with fatigue, an increase of deep reflexes, nystagmus, ataxic upper extremities, scanning speech, uncontrolled emotionalism, vague sensory disorders, and remissions. Compensatory involuntary contractions of the extensor tendons may cause an abnormal high arch with pronation to maintain postural stability.

Comparison of both extremities is essential in a differential diagnosis. Feet should be measured for length and width since both feet are rarely alike in size and a great difference in size must be accommodated. When paralysis is present, one leg shows less circumference through the calf than the other. Shortage of one extremity may produce painful symptoms in the knee, hip or back. A posture chart is blocked off with vertical and horizontal parallel lines. The patient stands erect and the position of shoulders, hips, knees and malleoli are noted in relation to the lines on the chart.

Normally a plumb line dropped from the middle of the patella will pass through the middle of the astragulus about 2 to 4 cm. in front of the ankle and at a point midway between the base of the first and second metatarsals.

Circulatory changes are notably different bilaterally in occlusive vascular disease.

In hemiplegia alterans, the involvement of the pyramidal tract creates weakness and imbalance. The paralyzed limb may drop down, the toes may dorsiflex, and the extensor tendons may contract. Tylomas usually develop under the head of the first metatarsal and the paralyzed foot is cold to touch.

Inequality of the Extremities. An extremity may be either overdeveloped or become atrophied as a result of disease, abnormal growth, trauma or mechanical dysfunction. When viewed from the front with the posture chart as a background, the standing patient presents one shoulder at a lower level than the other while the pelvis presents a tilt or shift. One patella may be lower than the other, and one elbow or arm may be closer to the body than the other elbow. Examination of the standing patient from the rear may reveal scoliosis. The inferior angles of the scapula are in different planes and the gluteofemoral fold may be at a higher level on one side. The shoe on the short side shows overriding of the upper to the outside and excessive wear at the outer aspect of the heel. In the supine position measurements taken from the anterior superior iliac spine to the lower tip of the internal malleolus will disclose the actual shortage of the affected limb. Note the position of the gluteal and inguinal folds for asymmetry.

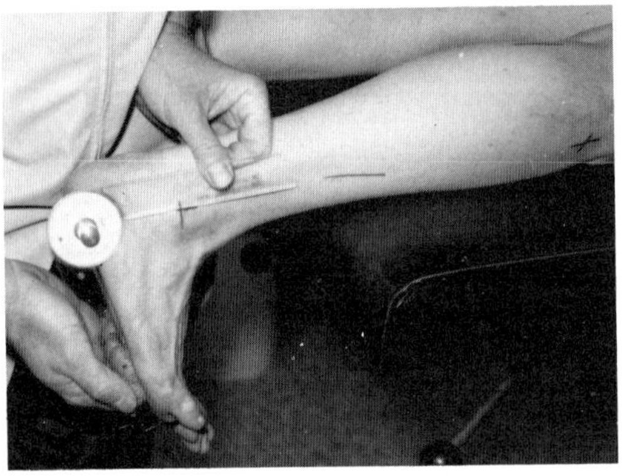

Fig. 3.11. With the knee in the extended position, the Tractograph is used to measure ankle joint dorsiflexion. Some practitioners become adept enough to use this instrument for most of the basic measurements. Marks have been made on the fibular head and fibular malleolus. The foot is dorsiflexed with the subtalar joint in a neutral position. One arm of the tractograph is held on the plantar surface and the other arm on the lateral fibular line. A 10-degree range of dorsiflexion is required for normal function. If 10 degrees is not available, an equinus condition should be considered. Courtesy of Burns Podiatric Laboratory.

Palpation. The position of an epidermal excrescence is a good sign of the underlying bone deformity present and indicates improper footgear and poorly functioning feet. Tylomas along the inner borders of the heel and the great toe may be symptoms of pes valgus while heloma on the fifth toe denotes narrow shoes, pointed shoes or shoes with an improper last. On palpatation of the talonavicular joint, first metatarsal cuneiform, cuboid and metatarsophalangeal joints, mild pressure will cause pain in weak foot conditions, arthritic changes and traumatic lesions. In biomechanical disorders of the joints, the foot may be painful on weightbearing and on motion. This condition should not be confused with infectious arthritis, rheumatoid arthritis or osteoarthritis.

The range of motion at ankle, midtarsal and metatarsophalangeal joints should be tested both actively and passively for any limitations present.

The examiner should test the anterior group of muscles for their ability to dorsiflex against resistance, the posterior group for plantar flexion against resistance, and the toes for both dorsiflexion and plantar flexion against resistance.

The calf muscles are shortened if the feet cannot be dorsally flexed more than at right angles to the leg. A shortened calf muscle is common to talipes plantaris. A pulling sensation is felt behind the straight knee when the foot is dorsiflexed on the ankle. An inability to dorsiflex may also result from a bony block.

Crepitation on movement of a joint may suggest an osteoarthritis with rubbing of spicules of bone at the joint margins. It may also be due to a tendon riding over bone. Destruction of cartilage in rheumatoid arthritis also causes crepitus. Crepitation is also felt in a tenosynovitis due to trauma or infection.

Palpation of the medial tubercle on the plantar surface of the calcaneus will elicit pain in the presence of a calcaneal spur or bursa. A periostitis often causes tenderness on palpation on the medial and lateral aspects of the calcaneus.

Infection may cause pain on palpation of the plantar surface of the heel at the origin of the plantar fascia, on palpation of the medial and lateral aspects of the heel, and on palpation at the lower third of the tendo achillis before it inserts into the mid-portion of the posterior surface of the heel.

Bursa found anterior to the tendo achillis between the bone and the tendon are painful and swollen when palpated during an acute inflammatory change. Bursa over the Achilles tendon between the tendon and the skin show the same signs with more edema when inflamed. Children may complain of apophyseal pain before firm union of the epiphysis with the body of the calcaneus.

Trophic Changes. Trophic changes of the skin should be noted. Palpation may detect scleroderma with taut skin and atrophy of underlying tissues. Ulceration between the toes may be an early trophic disturbance in thromboangiitis obliterans.

Nodules when palpated may be indicative of periarteritis nodosa, cysts or tumors, keratosis blennorrhagica, erythema induratum, lupus vulgaris, tertiary syphilis, acute rheumatoid arthritis, erythema nodosum or fibroma.

Pain on palpation together with other symptoms such as a fever and swelling may establish a diagnosis of phlebitis. When the deep veins are involved one cannot palpate the vessels. However, the superficial veins can be felt as hot, indurated, cord-like structures along the normal course of the venous anatomy. Transitory phlebitis is often associated with thromboangiitis obliterans.

Impaired circulation will disturb the growth and appearance of the nails. The nails of elderly people, arteriosclerotics and diabetics become chalky, discolored, hypertrophied and slow growing.

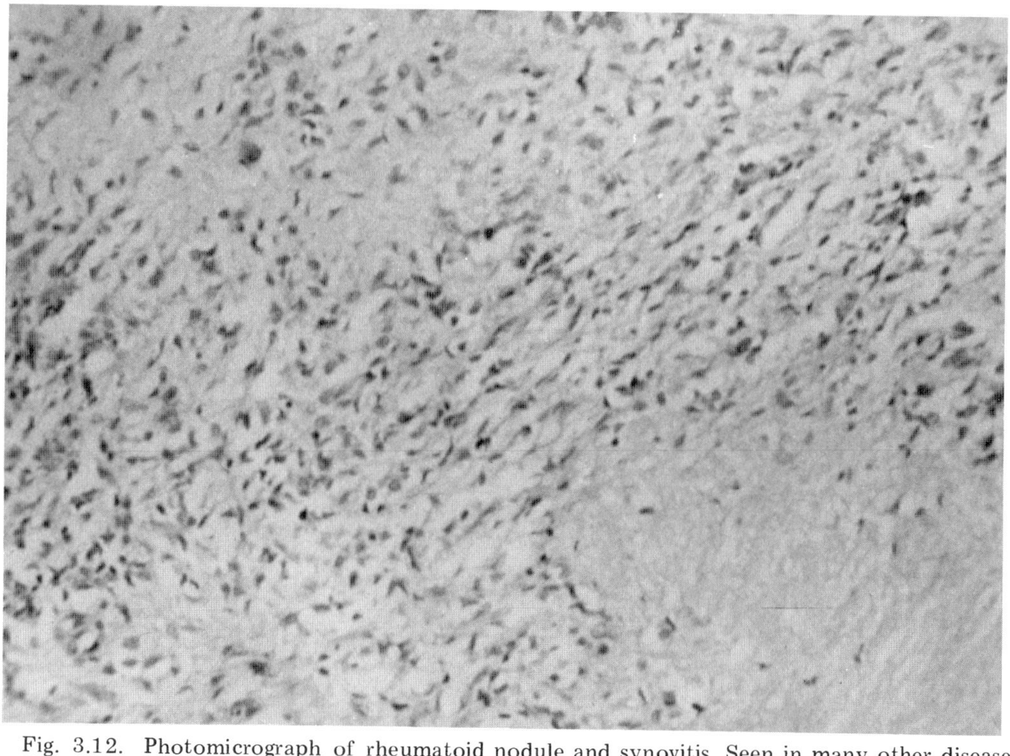

Fig. 3.12. Photomicrograph of rheumatoid nodule and synovitis. Seen in many other disease processes involving synovium.

Sclerosis. The posterior tibial and dorsalis pedis arteries, when sclerosed, can sometimes be palpated. However, the fact that one vessel is hardened does not mean that all vessels are affected. It does not mean that circulation is poor or that an occlusive vascular disorder is present. The necessary volume of blood may still be present to give a normal oscillometric index. A radiograph will often present many calcifications without subjective or objective symptoms.

Tenderness is present along the veins in acute or subacute phlebitis. When present around arteries one must consider periarteritis nodosa as a possible diagnosis. Prominent joints may present tender bursae and plantar fascia is often tender from inflammatory changes and strain. Frequent bathing of feet in strong antiseptic solutions causes tenderness of the skin and subcutaneous structures.

Enlarged lymph glands are due to infections in the extremities; general disease may cause swelling of all the glands. The inguinal and popliteal glands are usually inflamed and palpable when the foot is infected. A rapidly developing bright red nodule attaining full size in from 1 to 7 days often is noted around the nail grooves or lips. The lesion is soft and bleeds easily. It is usually caused by a staphylococcus infection of low virulence but which is capable of causing swelling of the lymph glands in the extremities.

Lymphangitis and palpable lymph glands may be found in pustular eruptions on the feet. The sequence of infection, cellulitis, lymphangitis and lymphadenopathy is characteristic.

Atrophy. One of the first signs of muscle and nerve degeneration is loss of function and atrophy of the affected muscles. Atrophy is sometimes obscured by the subcutaneous fat and is a wasting disorder characterized by a loss of physiologic function, organic substance and gross integrity. The podiatrist must utilize his powers of observation and palpation and his knowledge as to abnormal muscle function and nerve reflexes to interpret atrophic changes. Disuse of a part having a limited function will result in atrophy. Limited use may be the result of a mechanical disorder which occurs from constrictive footgear, occupational stress or lack of stress, weak foot, compensatory changes to faulty body posture, disease and paralysis.

Direct disease of the muscle itself or of the nerve tissue supplying the musculature will result in atrophy. This type of atrophy, if due to lower motor neuron disease, will show a reaction of degeneration to galvanic stimulation. Not only does atrophy affect soft tissues but it is also seen in bone. It often indicates a lesion in the anterior horn of the spinal cord or in the central or peripheral nervous system. Peripheral nerve lesions may be a cause of atrophy.

4

General Foot Discomfort

General foot discomfort can be a symptom of neurasthenia, a variety of systemic diseases, ill-fitting shoes or hose, or incipient mechanical disturbances of the feet. All the arthritides, circulatory disorders and neurologic disturbances may cause general foot discomfort. Occupational stress and environment such as metal floors, hot weight-bearing surfaces and extreme temperature changes often produce general foot discomfort. Atmospheric conditions and poorly constructed shoes also cause these difficulties. Leather in shoes is often tanned poorly, and shoes may be nailed or stitched irregularly. A single corn or other excrescence on the foot may cause the patient to limp in order to favor the painful part, thus causing other foot discomfort. This general discomfort may manifest itself as cramps, parethesias, or sharp, shooting, dull aching, burning, or tingling pain.

Cramps occur in muscles as a result of unnatural anatomic positions and impaired circulation. They are involuntary muscular contractions with severe pain and partial or complete loss of function. They may occur in debilitated patients with fevers or chronic wasting diseases. Atherosclerosis, vasospasm, varicose veins and thrombophlebitis cause cramps. They are most frequent at night and are common in pregnancy, calcium-phosphorus imbalance, faulty metabolism and profound diuresis.

Deformities of the feet, nutritional deficiency—especially vitamin B and related edema—may cause cramp-like pains in the lower extremities. Heat cramps are widespread with sudden onset affecting varying groups of muscles in individuals due to excessive loss of sweat without sodium chloride replacement.

Unnatural anatomic positions in certain occupations result in cramps, aching pains and incoordination. Moderate shortening of the posterior calf muscle and hamstring groups often induces cramps. During tetany the toes may cramp into a flexion state with the arch of the foot being domed by plantar contractures with inversion.

Treatment. Correct foot strain and pull on the calf muscles. Treat underlying infection or debilitating illness. Prescribing multiple vitamins and minerals where indicated is helpful. In the presence of sodium chloride depletion, cramps are controlled by the ingestion of salt tablets. Faulty calcium metabolism is determined through blood chemistry studies. Treatment of parathyroid dysfunction and ingestion of calcium supplements is beneficial in tetany. Calcium lactate or gluconate may be given intravenously. Peripheral vascular spasms produce avascular musculature and cramps.

Quinine capsules 3- or 5-grain b. i. d. help to releive idiopathic cramping. Nylidrin hydrochloride in 6-mg. tablets t. i. d. and cyclandelate (Cyclospasmol), 100 or 200 mg., help to relieve cramps. If the patient smokes, limiting his smoking may also effect relief. Brody and Brezak (1960), after a preliminary study of the effectiveness of small doses of quinine and aminophylline in combination on nocturnal cramps, recommend the use of these drugs for effective relief to most patients. Orphenadrine hydrochloride, 25 mg. b. i. d. or, if cramps occur at night, 50 mg. h. s., is a most effective nontoxic muscle relaxant. Occasionally, tranquilizers, such as chlordiazepoxide hydrochloride (Librium), in 5-, 10- and 25-mg. capsules or tablets, meprobamate (Miltown), in 400-mg. tablets up to 1600-mg. daily, hydroxyzine pamoate (Vistaril), in 25-, 50- and 100-mg. capsules, oral suspension or by injection are useful for short-term therapy.

Lumbar sympathectomy and vasodilator relaxants are helpful. Methocarbamol, 500-mg. tablets administered at bedtime or 1 tablet q. i. d. or 2 tablets q. 4 h., usually relieve cramps within 72 hr. Continued relief is obtained for 3 to 4 weeks after discontinuing the drug.

Pain in the legs due to polyarteritis, which often alternately attacks each leg, associated with a rash and mild pyrexia is amenable to therapy. Prednisolone, 22.5 mg. daily reduced subsequently to 5 mg. daily, has suppressed polyarteritis. Antihistamines are often helpful for short-term therapy. I have used Benadryl in 25- and 50-mg. capsules with success for muscle cramps. Benadryl is available also for intramuscular injection in concentrations of 10 mg. or 50 mg./ml. Chlor-Trimeton in 8- and 12-mg. tablets is effective, and Thephorin, 25 mg., is a helpful slow-acting antihistamine which does not cause drowsiness. Large doses of aspirin have proven helpful for relief of muscle cramps. Betamethasone, 1.5 mg. daily, has given symptomatic relief according to Golding (1970).

Intermittent claudication is a cramp due to local anoxemia resulting from deficient circulation. The patient usually complains that after walking short distances or climbing a hill he becomes tired, his muscles get sore and his calf muscles cramp. He must stop, squeeze and rub the involved muscles and rest for a few minutes before the sensation disappears. The patient is then able to walk further only to be afflicted again in a short time after mild exercise. Intermittent claudication is a common symptom in arteriosclerosis and thromboangiitis obliterans, varicosities, muscular fatigue, arterial spasm and anemia; it is often simulated in locomotor ataxia. Walking and standing do not cause intermittent claudication until muscular fatigue and failure of oxygenation of the muscles ensue.

This cramp-like symptom is brought on with muscular effort such as climbing stairs and hills, by rapid or long walks; it may also be caused by severe anemia. When the cramp comes on it usually affects the calf muscles and is so severe as to cause the patient to cease walking. The cramp may vary from a severe claudication to the sensation of a tightness in the posterior group of muscles. These cramps may develop in the feet and involve the plantar muscles, interossei or the anterior tibial as well; they should be noted carefully in order to differentiate them from an imbalance of foot posture. Sometimes the patient will complain of experiencing cramps while at rest, especially in bed at night. Such cramps cause him to get out of bed, stamp his foot, press hard on a cold floor and to kick or massage his limb in order to bring about relief. There is no relationship between this type of cramp and intermittent claudication.

Treatment. Limit as much physical effort as possible by improving foot function. Improve circulatory status by treatment of venous insufficiency and arterial diseases. Vasodilators are prescribed and daily use of whiskey in moderation is safe. Nylidrin, tolazoline hydrochloride (25-mg. tablets) and Isoxysuprine hydrochloride (10-mg. tablets) as Arliden, Priscoline and Vasodilan are proven vasodilators. The cardiopulmonary vascular system should be examined by an internist for systemic pathology. The blood is examined for blood dyscrasias capable of causing anoxia. Corrective measures are followed if necessary.

Sympathectomy may be indicated to relieve arterial spasm. A vascular surgeon may have to perform arterial transplants and by pass arterial prostheses may be necessary. Anticoagulants are prescribed by the internist who also treats metabolic and nutritional problems. Endocrine disorders are sought out and, if present, early treatment is given.

Pallor is considered a common symptom in peripheral vascular disorders, but it is not a chief complaint of a patient's condition although usually it is associated with numbness and tingling. The skin tone depends on the blood circulation. The affected area must be determined for accurate diagnosis.

Pallor may be due to an embolic occlusion in the peripheral arteries. This very often occurs at the bifurcation of the popliteal artery behind the knee. Pallor after exposure to cold or due to emotional disturbances is often a symptom of Raynaud's disease.

Treatment. Removal of thrombi from an occluded artery by a vascular surgeon may be indicated. Anticoagulants may be prescribed by the internist or vascular surgeon when necessary in embolic occlusions.

Contrast foot plunges, 2 min. in comfortably hot water followed by 1 min. in cold water is helpful. The process should be repeated for 20 to 30 min. twice daily. If the patient smokes, smoking should be limited. Burger's exercises are helpful. Vasodilators such as 100-mg. tablets of cyclandelate t. i. d. or nicotinic acid in 20- or 100-mg. tablets may alleviate this type of pain.

Vasospastic disorders in nervous individuals or patients suffering from sympathetic nervous system disease may show evidence of pallor. This condition must be differentiated from thromboangiitis obliterans which presents marked color changes on elevation. Tight garters or any constricting garment may produce pallor and should be carefully differentiated from true vasospasm. Psychotherapeutic medications may be necessary to relax hypertensive patients. Meprobamate, 200- or 400-mg. tablets; chlordiazepoxide in 5-, 10- and 25-mg. capsules; or promethazine in 12.5-mg., 25-mg. or 50-mg. tablets or in a syrup may be helpful.

Numbness and Tingling. Pressure of a tumor may cause numbness. In the feet, numbness may occur from a long standing sciatic involvement or diabetic neuropathy. Numbness is a paresthesia following nerve pressure, and, if the pressure is unremitting, it leads to a sensory nerve paralysis. Numbness may occur in circulatory involvements of a general nature or in a localized circulatory deficiency produced by malfunctioning feet or improperly fitted footgear. Numbness is common in Morton's neuralgia and in the feet of the elderly.

Vitamin deficiencies, pernicious anemia and dietary disturbances may cause numbness, and it may be an early symptom of tabes, arteriosclerosis obliterans, multiple neuritis, neurosis, multiple sclerosis and subacute combined degeneration of the spinal cord, Raynaud's disease and immersion foot or trench foot.

Cocaine addicts complain of paresthesias which they describe as being like "foreign bodies under the skin."

The beginnings of nerve degeneration is suggested when tingling sensations occur in the distal end of a divided nerve upon percussion over the area of division. Numbness and coldness of an extremity may be noted in rupture of the nucleus pulposus in the lumbar region. Dermatomes are carefully evaluated to ascertain the cord level of pathology.

Although characteristic mainly of a neuritis or some lesion in the posterior columns of the spinal cord, numbness and tingling are also characteristic in circulatory involvements. Usually numbness develops at night while the patient is asleep or when sitting for long periods of time, and it may be attributable to pressure on the extremity. Sometimes the numbness and tingling is symmetrical due to a vasospasm; frostbite or severe trauma may also cause the condition. Numbness and tingling may indicate an embolus in a large vessel of the extremity.

The sensation of numbness and tingling may suggest pernicious anemia, and it is often a symptom of causalgia. The patient suffering with a neuroma often has the neuralgic symptom early. Ill-fitting, constrictive shoes and hose may cause numbness.

Treatment. Correct circulatory and neurologic disorders by close liaison with specialists in the respective fields. Remove tumors compressing nerve trunks, e.g., neurinomas.

Have an internist examine and prescribe for systemic diseases and blood dyscrasias and deficiencies. Examine the patient carefully and treat existing local pathology. Prescribe dietary supplements. Maintain the integrity of the musculature.

Pruritis. Pruritis may be secondary to many skin diseases and may be a symptom of certain systemic diseases. It may include fungous infections, insect bites, eczema, contact dermatitis, psoriasis, lichen simplex and neurodermatitis or it may be a result of dry skin especially in elderly patients.

Diabetes, nephritis, diseases of the liver, malignant tumors, Hodgkin's disease, leukemia, tuberculosis, arteriosclerosis and a myriad of metabolic disorders can also cause pruritis.

Treatment is aimed at breaking up the scratch-itch syndrome. Ice packs or cold wet dressings may be helpful. Corticosteroid ointments or lotions four times daily may be prescribed to relieve symptoms. Menthol 0.1% to 0.25% or coal tar are added if necessary. Topical calamine lotion with or without 0.5% menthol or phenol 1% is helpful.

Tripelennamine (Pyribenzamine) 25- or 50-mg. tablets q. 4 to 6 h. for drug reaction, Chlorpheniramine maleate (Chlor-Trimeton) and Thephorin help relieve urticaria. Fifteen milligrams of phenobarbital after meals and at bedtime may be helpful in some cases. X-irradiation is used in severe cases. Soothing ointments and emulsions may be the only medication necessary. Oral use of vitamin A and a topical cream is helpful. Note that the medications listed under atopic dermatitis are also suitable for pruritis. Teldrin, 8- or 12-mg. spansules, may relieve symptoms.

Soreness is a symptom of overworked muscles, ligaments and joints and is common to abused or overworked structures before these structures acclimate themselves to the exercise required of them. Bruises, old scars and migrating phlebitis can cause soreness. With twelve muscles originating in the leg and inserting into the foot, a mechanically malfunctioning foot may cause soreness of one or more groups of leg muscles. Soreness develops from multiple minimal traumas to the foot. Skin lesions may be a direct cause of soreness in the foot.

Constant severe uninterrupted pain may suggest a malignancy if no history of recent trauma is given. Neuroma and bone infection should be differentiated by careful clinical and radiographic examination. The possibility of neuritis of infectious origin is great.

Intermittent pains suggest a neuritis or a neuralgia caused by pressure or infection. An arteritis and arterial occlusion may cause an ischemic neuritis.

Treatment. Mild massage of overworked musculature improves muscle metabolism and relieves soreness. Contrast foot baths are helpful. Whirlpool may relieve symptoms. Low voltage muscle stimulation relieves fatigue and sore muscles.

Eliminate traumatizing agents and locate and eliminate infection. Correct the cause of ischemic neuritis. Improve structural deformities to assist function and relieve strain.

Multiple therapeutic vitamins are helpful.

Pain on Arising. Difficulty in walking after getting out of bed in the morning suggests arthritis or fibrositis. These possibilities must be investigated in all painful conditions of the feet.

Traumatic lesions are usually unilateral, whereas static foot disarrangements are commonly bilateral. However, one foot usually has been affected before the other. The podiatrist must determine whether both feet are disturbing the patient. Increased pain in one extremity often causes the patient to present only that limb for treatment. Very often, however, the foot giving the most pain is not the one presenting the greater deformity, but the history should reveal that the more deformed foot was the object of severe pain at sometime. If both feet are not equally affected, the treatment varies accordingly.

Pain during rest occurs before ulceration and gangrene in thromboangiitis obliterans and consists of severe burning sensations. This is pretrophic and common with the disease.

Hereditary trophedema is a chronic edema of one or both legs, the arms or the face. It may affect a single toe or one foot and occurs most frequently in females. The nonpitting edema may cause pain if profuse; the skin is thickened with no pain or tenderness.

Causalgia due to irritation of a nerve by injury may present painful swelling, redness, sweating, trophic changes in the nails and a glossy appearance of the skin.

Treatment. Eliminate all etiologic factors. Relieve strain of weak feet and support structural defects to prevent unusual motion. Physical therapy, such as shortwave, ultrasound, infrared, sinusoidal currents and contrast baths, helps relieve pain on arising after periods of rest.

The diagnosis and treatment of the arthritides is necessary for a differential diagnosis leading to adequate treatment. Immobilization by adhesive tape or construction of appliances are often indicated to correct deforming states. If a localized joint is affected, injections of local anesthetics and a corticosteroid relieves acute pain.

Prescriptions of antirheumatics, analgesics, muscle relaxants and definitive medications for specific diagnoses are necessary to relieve pain on arising after periods of rest. Steroids, salicylates, phenylbutazone and methocarbamol (Robaxin) can be useful. In causalgic states, Edmonson and Calandcruccio (1957) prescribed 15 mg. of Dibenzyline four times daily with good results. Sympathectomy is often necessary to relieve pain. Injections of plain 1% lidocaine for a posterior tibial block are often helpful to the patient who cannot walk. Phenoxybenzamine hydrochloride, 10 mg., and Tolazoline hydrochloride in 25-mg. tablets t. i. d. serve as adrenergic blocking agents.

Sudden severe pain with no history of injury occurring at the site of bifurcation and along the course of an artery suggests general debility, malnutrition, endocarditis or valvular disease with embolus formation. The extremity below the embolus is cold, edematous and pulseless.

Treatment. This patient may require immediate vascular surgery to remove an embolus and preserve the limb. Do not traumatize the limb with massage or manipulation. The use of extremes of cold or heat will destroy the impoverished tissue leading to ulceration and gangrene.

Empirin compound with codeine phosphate up to 1 grain, and acetaminophen (Tylenol) potentiated by promethazine in a 12.5- to 25-mg. dosage may control this type of pain.

Neuritis, a nerve inflammation, is characterized by various etiologic factors and symptoms which occur in all age groups. Usually it is caused by trauma, such as fracture and luxation in which there is contusion, compression and torsion of the nerve. Compression may be due to swelling of local lymph node or to the presence of a neoplasm, aneurism or callus. The extension of an inflammatory process from contiguous tissues is often the cause of neuritis. Ischemia, which leads to degeneration of the nerve, may occur in Raynaud's disease, arteriosclerosis and obliterative endarteritis causing neuritic pains. Chronic infections such as syphilis, diphtheria, typhoid and chronic intoxications from lead or carbon dioxide may cause a neuritic syndrome.

The primary symptom of neuritis is pain which is limited to the area of distribution of the nerve. The pains may be severe and may be brought on or intensified by local movement or pressure. The disturbance of sensation—paresthesias, hyperesthesias or complete anesthesia—are characteristic symptoms of neuritis. The impaired muscle power indicates the severity of the disease and may run from a weakness of the muscle to a paralysis. Sensation is restored before the motor function is healed. The paralyzed muscle is flaccid and flabby and, unless the conducting fibers are re-established, it goes on to atrophy. Tendon reflexes are diminished or abolished. Flexion of the thigh on the hip followed by extension of the knee causes pain in sciatica (see Lasèque's sign). Deformities may result such as with equinovarus. Tarsal tunnel syndrome may occur with entrapment of the posterior tibial nerve.

An altered electrical reaction occurs in neuritis. In mild cases there is just a decreased excitability of muscle, but in severe cases, partial or total degeneration is found when muscles are tested. Trophic and secretory disturbances of the skin occur in the area affected by the neuritis; the skin is smooth or glistening and red. Later it may become rough, furrowed and brittle. Hair will fall out or may grow in excess and there may be profuse sweating. A postural list to either side may be evident in sciatica, but usually it is away from the affected side. Neuritis usually lasts 10 days to 2 weeks, but it may last for months or years. The symptoms diminish with proper treatment and removal of the cause.

Treatment. A thorough physical examination by an internist is called for to rule out or to diagnose and treat systemic diseases. A neurologic consultation is mandatory; a circulatory consultation may be indicated.

Localized foot problems are corrected. Faulty foot function is improved and sites of abnormal pressure are protected. Supportive measures are used where needed if pathomechanical problems are severe. Pressure behind the knee, about the head of the fibula, over the ankle and on the dorsum of the foot and toes is relieved.

Mild galvanism is used for its sedating effect. Billig's exercises are prescribed (Billig and Brennan, 1943). Analgesics and muscle relaxants are prescribed. The strength and frequency of medication depends on the extent of the neuritis, its acute or chronic nature, and the degree of pain.

Hypersensitivity of Superficial Nerves of the Skin. Podiatrists' observations have led to the consideration of irritation of the peripheral nerve endings as a pathology in itself. Irritation of the peripheral nerve endings develops as a peripheral neuritis often complicated by pressure neuritis. The condition most frequently is found in high strung, middle-aged, neurotic women. The predisposing factors are often increase in weight, anemia, psychic phenomena, vasomotor instability and environmental anxieties.

Patients experience such symptoms as not being able to tolerate even minor pressure or friction from ill-fitting footgear; heavy shoes and improperly tanned leather cannot be tolerated; the feet burn and are hot and sensitive; the patient is often awakened at night with burning, hot, painful feet which are relieved only slightly by cold air and cold water foot soaks.

These patients are very nervous and many other biomechanical disturbances develop concomitantly with minor foot disorders. The shoes seldom fit and color changes in the toes are observed with metatarsalgic symptoms and circulatory and neurologic manifestations. The patient is generally apprehensive.

The condition must be differentiated from Raynaud's disease, vasomotor instability, frostbite, allergic disease and metabolic disturbances.

Treatment. Place the patient at ease and concentrate on good rapport. Improve the patient's general health and refer him to an internist for treatment of blood dyscrasia or psychomotor instability. Large doses of vitamin B_{12} are helpful (1000 μg. i.m. weekly). Warm sitz baths may also be beneficial.

Prescribe mild sedatives—e.g., sodium butabarbital (Butisol sodium) 1/4 to 1/2 grain 3 to 4 times daily or meprobamate 200-400 mg, or promethazine (Phenergan) 12.5-25 mg. 3 to 4 times a day.

Periarticular Fibrositis. This syndrome commonly affects the feet and is primarily characterized by soreness and stiffness, pain on arising after long or short periods of rest or following exercise.

On arising in the morning, the patient's first few steps are with a limp. The limp gradually disappears only to come back after prolonged weightbearing. Objectively the joints are neither stiff nor unusually painful. In the early stages, there is no deformity of the joints, swelling, or other physical findings. The fibrous connective tissues about the joints are involved. Usually a history of injury or faulty functions of the affected joints is elicited from the complaining patient.

The talocrural, first metatarsophalangeal, talonavicular, first metatarsal cuneiform and second metatarsophalangeal joints are most commonly affected.

Treatment. Bedrest or functional adhesive immobilization is indicated. Physical therapy is helpful. Corticosteroid solutions in minimal doses of 0.3 to 0.5 ml. injected into affected joints are beneficial. Analgesics and muscle relaxants should be taken. Pentazocine hydrochloride (Talwin), by injection or in 50-mg. tablets q. 4 h. p. r. n. relieves pain. Traco-gesic tablets, Zactirin, or aspirin help to maintain comfort. Carisoprodol (Rela) 350 mg., methocarbamol 500 mg. or chlorzoxazone may be used as muscle relaxants.

Restless Leg Syndrome. This common complaint of an unpleasant burning or crawling sensation in the extremities may be caused by emotional strains or long periods of inactivity. It is more prevalent in women and is often experienced by persons who travel for many hours with the feet in a dependent position as on an extended plane trip. Elevation of the lower extremities, hot and cold foot plunges and alleviation of emotional stress bring relief in most cases. The possibility of local or systemic pathology must be evaluated if symptoms persist.

5

Pain as a Symptom

Subjective Symptoms

The presence of pain associated with podiatric complaint is of definite importance in making a diagnosis. If the type of pain is accurately described the podiatrist should have a reliable indication of possible pathologies. Many general afflictions are characterized by certain sensations affecting the lower extremities. I shall discuss the implications of the presence of different types of pain and their relationship to local and general involvements.

Pain is defined as distress or suffering; it is a form of communication. It advises us of the presence of what purports to be a harmful situation.

The cause of pain in the foot ranges from ill-fitting footgear or improper weight distribution to trauma or disease. Individuals with pernicious anemia or degeneration of the brain and spinal cord may have difficulty in interpreting painful stimuli. Circulatory diseases and peripheral nerve lesions also affect reception of stimuli; but many podiatric complaints involve characteristic pain and discomfort.

Mechanical factors such as pressure from inflammatory exudates and swelling results in painful irritation of local sensory nerves. A prolonged contraction of a hollow organ such as spasm of blood vessels results in pain of a severe nature. Pressure from a neoplasm may cause degeneration of surrounding organs or tissue, while hemorrhage into body tissue increases density causing great pain. Ill-fitting clothing (shoes, hose and garters) may cause pain. Faulty foot posture may result in excessive weight bearing on a metatarsal or on the medial or lateral aspect of heels. Stress in joints as a result of poor foot function may cause degenerative lipping, spurs or osteophytes. Destruction of joint cartilage causing pain may result.

Ischemia of a part as a result of emboli lodging in small arteries causes ischemic neuritis. The impoverished tissues and nerves are painful and often cause focal gangrene. Bacterial toxins result in increased temperature and infected tissue with heat, redness and pain.

Acroparesthesia may be slow or acute in onset, bilateral and characterized by "pins and needles" sensations of fingers and toes in females.

Anesthesia is a state in which there is an entire or almost complete absence of sensations. Loss of pain and temperature sensations is often noted in immersion foot. Anesthesia may be noted in a central nervous system disorder. A severed nerve, or spinal cord tumor or myelitis may produce anesthesia, or it may be caused by toxic agents such as cocaine, phenol, arsenic and belladonna affecting the nervous system. Injection of procaine hydrochloride, lidocaine or other local anesthetics results in the loss of sensation for short periods of time.

Anesthesia includes hypoalgesia, tactile hypoesthesia, loss of temperature sense, loss of sense of muscular activity, absence of vibratory sensation and loss of joint sense. Anesthesia may occur in distal parts in the neural form of leprosy.

Analgesia is manifest when sensation of pain alone is absent. It may be present in tabes dorsalis along the distribution of the peroneal nerve. It may be brought about through the central nervous system and originate from within or outside the brain. Voluntary analgesia is commonly seen in neurotic individuals who practice autosuggestion.

In functional nervous disease and especially hysteria the patient with hysterical anesthesia of an extremity will be unable to move the affected part when the eyes are closed. When eyes are open, however, and attention is directed to the involved limb, volitional movement can be made, thus simulating a loss of muscle sense.

Classification of Pain

Subjective Pain

Subjective pain has no physical cause; it is the product of mental action arising from a disturbance in the coordinating centers of the sensory areas in the brain.

Hysterical pain is characterized by rapid changes in location, degree and severity. Pain may disappear by autosuggestion with the will of the patient. Pain appears for the same reason and is generally as severe as pain caused by a physical pathology. Emotionalism incites pain and may leave the patient exhausted. Hypnosis pain is a subjective pain. It is possible to bring forgotten pain sensations to consciousness through hypnosis and through the same mechanism eliminate emotional or organic pain.

Objective Pain

Objective pain is excited by an agent which is foreign or abnormal to an area.

Central nervous system objective pain may be due to a lesion in the optic thalamus which is a relay center of the brain or it may come from any structure within the sensory system.

Peripheral objective pain is due to a disturbance of an axon, ganglia cells, or receptors. Its cause may be organic and due to changes in structure, as in intrinsic inflammation, new growth, displacement of parts and abnormal muscular contractions.

Extrinsic peripheral objective pain may be due to displacement with pressure on adjacent organs or stretching of ligaments. Excessive use of an organ may also result in this type of pain.

Propagation of pain is the phenomenon of pain experienced in areas other than that in which the pain originated.

Referred pain is the result of irritation which occurs along the course of nerve fibers and pain is felt in the peripheral distribution of the affected nerve, e.g., imbalanced feet can cause pain in the knee; osteoma in the tibia may cause pain in the groin; pain in the ankle may be due to a tumor in Scarpa's triangle; pain in the extremity at certain dermatomes caused by a ruptured disc suggests the level of the lesion.

Burns and decreased alkalinity of the blood causes excruciating pain. Electrical shock and other strong stimuli may result in great pain. Extremes of heat and cold with barometric variance is a factor to be considered in arthritis and painful helomas. Intermittent claudication occurs in circulatory disorders and usually manifests itself as a cramp.

"Real pain then is a form of communication. It is an intelligence report from a portion of our body. It advises us of the presence of what purports to be a harmful situation" (Rubin, J. A. P. A., 1955).

Perception of pain. Tenderness is a painful condition produced by pressure; contusion may cause tenderness of connective tissue. Frequently, nails, helomas and bony prominences are irritated by ill-fitting shoes.

Hyperalgesia is an abnormal sensitivity to pain. It is commonly observed after trauma or in individuals with neurocirculatory disease. It is also common in the aged and in neurotic patients and women of menopausal age. The lightest brush of the finger over the hyperalgesic area causes extreme sensations of tenderness. Hysterical hyperalgesia is common over joints. In hysteria the sensation does not follow the distribution of peripheral nerves. Hyperalgesia is severe in gout and vasospastic disorders.

Tabes dorsalis, multiple neuritis and subacute combined degeneration of the spinal cord present early hyperalgesia. Alcoholic polyneuritis may cause pain and tenderness, increased temperature, loss of deep reflexes and paralysis. An ischemic neuritis, especially around the toe nails may cause severe pain.

Paresthesia is a symptom simulating pain. It is a perverted sensation (prickling, itching, sensations of heat and cold, tingling and numbness) not strong enough to give the pain sensation. One may also have decreased sensation with severely painful paresthesia.

It may occur in neurasthenics with marked perversions in type and location of the sensation. Numbness, tingling and weakness may occur in transverse myelitis. The symptoms vary with the severity of the pathology which exists. Paresthesias occur more often in females.

A feeling of walking on cotton balls with numbness of the feet is felt in peripheral neuropathy and tabes dorsalis. A traumatic neuritis often manifests itself as a pins and needles sensation.

Arsenic, alcoholic and diabetic neuritis and anemias cause the extremities to feel "dead," with numbness, tingling and burning. Some cases of neuritis are characteristically motor or sensory.

Early symptoms of cerebral episodes are felt as paresthesia in the affected extremity. Arteriosclerosis, pernicious anemia, acroparesthesia and Raynaud's disease present symptoms of paresthesia. Paresthesias are seen in immersion foot.

Besides the primary symptoms, multiple sclerosis may present a heaviness of the limbs.

Projected pain is the sensation of pain in a part which has no feeling or in an amputated limb. Patients with projected pain may have "pain sensations" in extremities which have been amputated. This is also known as "phantom pain." Pain may also be due to a neuroma on the amputated stump.

Description and Causes of Pain

The patient's ability to describe or to explain with similes the type of pain is important to proper diagnosis. Pain may be continuous, intermittent or remittent. Diurnal pain may be noted in involvements of the locomotor apparatus. Nocturnal pain is common in peripheral vascular problems.

Peripheral neuropathy. Entrapment of peripheral nerves may cause a unilateral foot pain that manifests as a burning and tingling. Peripheral neuropathy must be differentiated from compressions in the lower back due to a degenerative disc, tumors or compression secondary to severe injury anywhere along a nerve trunk. When a nerve is entrapped there is generally an acute tenderness proximal to the site with numbness distal to the compression. It is all too easy to pass off local pain or pain far removed from the site of a structural foot disturbance as being of local origin. Strain, ligamentous stress and articular pathology may be obvious but the source of pain may be due to peripheral nerve entrapment.

Nerve entrapment may occur anywhere along its course, especially where constriction develops from anatomic distortions or trauma. Inflammation due to pressure on the nerve and its intrinsic blood supply may cause rest pain. Tenderness is noted at the site of entrapment and slightly above and below this site along the nerve trunk.

Kopell and Thompson (1960) state that diagnosis can be confused by the presence of symptomatic low back derangement, diffuse nerve trunk tenderness, atypical pain distributions, secondary autonomic nervous system hyperfunction and by the presence of foot and ankle injuries causing pain and disability.

Entrapment of the peroneal nerve as it

passes around the fibular neck may produce pain on inversion and plantarflexion of the foot and ankle. If the entrapment continues, the lateral aspect of the leg and dorsolateral aspect of the foot become painful and often numb.

The posterior tibial nerve may become entrapped with neuropathy developing in the ankle and foot. The calcaneal branch may give symptoms of a bruised heel, and the medial and lateral plantar nerves will direct symptoms to the muscles on the sole of the foot, the adjacent joints and cutaneous sensation of the sole and toes.

The digital nerves are traumatized by the transverse intermetatarsal ligament. The distal edge of the ligament often keeps the digital nerve from assuming a position of safety between the metatarsals resulting in trauma from the metatarsal head. All intermetatarsal and digital spaces may be affected even though neuroma in the third space is the most common. Pain may be burning, lancinating, sharp and shooting or even vague.

Relief brought about by injection of a local anesthetic, corticosteroids or vitamin B_{12} is considered a confirmatory diagnosis of neuropathy. However, often the structural pathology must be corrected by manipulation, stretching exercises and mechanical devices for lasting relief. Surgical intervention may be necessary to relieve the entrapped nerve. It is essential to recognize and differentiate these problems.

Fatigue, including debility, asthenia, exhaustion, weakness, languor and lassitude, frequently arises from overstrained muscles. When foot posture is faulty and function is impaired, fatigue becomes an important symptom. Weakness may result from overstrain, disuse of certain groups of muscles, general illness, prolonged rest in bed, high heels and ill-fitting shoes and hose, or occupational stress. Fatigue is an early symptom of peripheral vascular disease and usually appears months before organic occlusive vascular disease. It may be a symptom of neurologic disturbance, anemia, tuberculosis or other debilitating diseases. Emotional stress, overwork, warm and humid weather, diarrhea, and abuse of alcohol, tea, coffee and tobacco may reduce the ability of the patient to withstand normal everyday muscular effort.

Dull aches may arise from muscles which are fatigued as a result of improper usage. Arthritic changes in joints and reactions to changes in climate may cause dull aches in the feet and legs. Long hours of standing and a history of injuries with resultant bone changes may cause dull aches. Vagueness of the complaint is often evident in neuroses requiring sedation for relief of the discomfort.

Sharp pains may follow the course of nerves as a result of nerve impingement or they may occur in the joints limited in function due to degenerative joint disease. Painful joints in static foot conditions are due to the pull of ligaments on the periosteal attachments to the bone. Sudden trauma such as a sprain, a direct blow on an exposed bony prominence or pressure on toes may cause sharp pains. Multiple sharp, shooting pains of unknown etiology may be evidence of syphilis. Neuritis is also suggested in the presence of shooting pains. The presence of foreign bodies in the foot will cause pain on weightbearing. Verrucoid tissue may cause sharp pain on weightbearing following a short period of rest.

Lancinating pain in the leg may occur in locomotor ataxia and occasionally in cerebrospinal syphilis. The examiner must ascertain whether the pain is shooting up or down the extremity in order to establish the etiology. Locomotor ataxia is usually bilateral with evidence of syphilis.

Embolism and thrombosis of the peripheral arteries are diagnosed early on the basis of sudden intense pain in the limb. Tenderness is noted at the site of thrombus; the affected limb is cold, white and tender. Gangrene follows embolism and thrombosis of the lower extremities where there is insufficient collateral circulation.

Throbbing sensations may result from

infection (e.g., heloma, tyloma, furuncle, infected nail lip). Pressure on blood vessels by constricting garters or bandages may cause throbbing. The podiatrist usually finds this symptom in heloma and onychotic infections. Throbbing is common as the end result of verruca treatment when liquefaction necrosis of the growth occurs. Phlebitic changes or inflammation will result in throbbing sensations. Abcess formation or acute osteomyelitis may cause throbbing.

Burning sensations, when not due to paresthesia, are attributed to abnormal pressure on blood vessels and cutaneous nerve endings which respond to mechanical treatment. These sensations are found where tylomas are present. Epidermophytosis, especially the interdigital type with its fissures, may produce burning sensations. When the skin is too dry or is hyperidrotic, or when hose are too harsh on sensitive feet, burning sensations may occur. Improperly tanned leathers in footgear may also produce burning of the feet. The author has observed burning symptoms in the feet of anemic patients and occasionally in the feet of patients with hyperthyroidism. The aged will often complain of burning sensations as a result of circulatory instability. Erythromelalgia and vasomotor disturbances cause burning sensations. A pressure neuritis from contraction of the fascia lata may cause pain, muscular spasm, tingling and numbness. The peripheral nerves are involved in these symptoms according to Billig and Brennan (1943). Occupations resulting in chemical contact often cause burning of the sensitized tissues.

Stiffness of muscles may be a spasticity which follows work in which the muscles have been forced to function improperly or to excess; trauma may also cause stiffness of muscles. Moderate use of muscles in an activity that is new often brings on symptoms of stiffness. It may also occur as a result of poor circulatory response to muscular effort. When a muscle is hypertonic and stretched, it may cause irregular and jerky movements. Spasms of the muscles are seen early in tuberculosis and rheumatoid arthritis.

Joint stiffness may be the result of chronic arthritis or adhesions as the result of static foot disability. Trauma to a joint may result in a traumatic degenerative arthritis with possible joint mice, lipping, osteophytes and spur formation limiting normal range of motion. The metatarsophalangeal joints are usually affected. This may be caused by stubbing the great toe, a misstep, dropping an object on the metatarsophalangeal joint, or from improperly fitted shoes which are either too short or too narrow. Rheumatoid arthritis osteoarthritis, gout and many general involvements cause joint stiffness. Repair after infectious changes may cause joint stiffness.

The judgment of the foot specialist is essential to proper utilization of medication to relieve the symptoms of pain. Systemic diseases are properly diagnosed and consultation with an internist is necessary to provide continuity of comprehensive care for the sick patient. Depending on the history, the complaint, onset and duration of the symptoms, the analgesic medications discussed below are useful in relieving the painful foot as described above. Special situations, such as treatment of infections, require specific medications which will be discussed in other chapters.

Drugs Used for Relief of Pain

Dibucaine hydrochloride, Nupercainal, in ointment or cream and Quotane as a lotion may be applied to the skin to relieve painful abrasions. A 1 to 40 dilution of aluminum acetate and a 1 to 16 dilution of a Dalibour solution help reduce inflammation and swelling of trauma and superficial skin problems.

Articular, periarticular and fibrocytic inflammations are often relieved by local injections of dexamethasone (Decadron), betamethasone (Celestone) or triamcinolone acetonide (Aristocort, Kenalog).

Tablets for oral use are also available for their systemic effect. They should be used with caution and only upon proper study of the problem and consultation with the internist to rule out contraindications and interaction with other drugs prescribed for the patient.

Short and long acting barbiturates may be used with analgesics to control pains with neurasthenic overtones. Tranquilizers and psychotherapeutic agents are helpful to relieve anxiety associated with pain and as a preoperative and postoperative aid to recovery. Salicylates by themselves or in combination with other pain ameliorators may be the most efficacious and problem-free treatment for moderately painful symptoms. Indomethacin (Indocin) in 25-mg. or 50-mg. capsules, propoxyphene hydrochloride (Darvon) in 32-mg. or 65-mg. capsules taken q. 4 to 6 h. and acetaminophen (Tylenol) in 325-mg. tablets are effective pain relievers. Acetaminophen is also supplied as an elixir and in drops to accommodate the needs of the patient who is sensitive to aspirin.

Where pain is severe or intractable, narcotic analgesics such as APC with codeine (or Empirin compound with codeine) or acetaminophen with codeine (Tylenol with codeine) (8-mg., 15-mg., 30-mg. or 60-mg.) will aid in proper control.

Pentazocine (Talwin) in 50-mg. tablets for oral use, or 1-ml. ampules (30-mg.), 1½-ml. ampules (45-mg.), 2-ml. ampules (60-mg.) or 10-ml. multiple dose vials (30-mg./ml.) is used for severe pain and has proven effective in many situations that might otherwise have required a narcotic. The oral tablet dose is 1 to 2 tablets q. 4 h. Its injectable form as pentazocine lactate intramuscularly is especially useful in lieu of a narcotic pain reliever. Other drugs used by podiatrists to relieve pain are ethoheptazine (Zactirin) 100-mg., meprobamate and ethoheptazine citrate with aspirin (Equagesic) 1 to 2 tablets q. 6 h., mefenamic acid (Ponstel capsules) 250-mg. for short term analgetic activity, and chlormezanone with aspirin (Trancopal) 300-mg. in tablet form. Empirin compound with codeine (or ASA compound with codeine phosphate) in 15-mg. and 30-mg. strengths seems to be most useful. Phenaphen with codeine No. 2 (15-mg.), No. 3 (30-mg.) or No. 4 (60-mg.) taken 1 capsule q. 4 h. p. r. n. for pain is highly effective.

Promethazine (Phenergan) in 12.5- mg. or 25-mg. strength is useful to potentiate the action of analgesics.

When pain is due to muscle spasm, orphenadrine citrate (Norflex), 1 tablet twice daily, relieves rigidity and pain.

In the presence of pain, especially following foot surgery, the patient should have complete rest. Dalmane (flurazepam hydrochloride) in a 30-mg. capsule on retiring is helpful to adults in assuring a good night's sleep. A 15-mg. capsule is more desirable for the elderly. Methyprylon (Noludar) 300-mg. capsules provides 5 to 8 hr. of sleep at night. Doriden tablets, 0.5 g., taken at night for sleep do not produce a morning hangover.

Diazepam (Valium) is useful for relief of tension, anxiety and muscle spasm associated with foot pathology. It is supplied in 2-mg., 5-mg. and 10-mg. tablets, and may be prescribed in 2 mg. and 5-mg. doses three times daily for spasms and associated pain.

Intractable pain often requires the use of class A narcotics such as meperedine hydrochloride (Demerol) 50-mg. or 100-mg. tablets, or parenteral administration q. 6 to 8 h. p. r. n. for pain. Oxycodone hydrochloride (Percodan), 1 tablet q. 6 h. with milk is helpful in relieving severe pain. Injection of such hard narcotics as morphine sulfate brings rapid relief of pain. As in the use of all drugs, the patient's general physical status is important when calculating dosage, and narcotics should be used in lieu of the stronger analgesics and potentiating agents only when absolutely necessary.

6

Evaluation of Neurogenic Disorders

Neurologic Tests

A great challenge to the skill of the podiatrist is his ability to differentiate the neurologic syndrome from that of circulatory and biomechanical problems. Of great importance is the evaluation of the findings of neurologic testing. The podiatrist must ascertain whether the problem is an upper or lower motor lesion or combinations of each. Recognized techniques and observation is imperative for proper evaluation.

A wisp of cotton, a brush, a common pin, test tubes filled with hot and cold water, a small flashlight, galvanic or sinusoidal current, percussion hammer, and a tuning fork are the necessary equipment to carry out an examination for sensory and motor involvements.

The nervous system controls sensory discrimination, motor activity and reflex responses and the reflex response serves as the connecting link between the sensory and motor nerves.

It is possible for man to maintain an upright posture and stance when his sensory receptors function well. This is dependent on the integrity of the labyrinth of the ear, the retina of the eye, the proprioceptors of the neck muscles and the muscles and joints of the trunk and lower extremities.

Sensory Discrimination

This function is divided into exteroceptive impulses which give an impression of the outer world (e.g., through sight and hearing) and proprioceptive impulses associated with position and tension of muscles and tendons, and particularly impulses from within the body. These propriocepetive impulses never reach consciousness but receive proper reflex response. Gait and posture are dependent on their function.

Other sensory impulses are carried by mixed nerves in the form of superficial sensibility produced by impulses from the skin and as deep sensibility consisting of impulses from muscles, tendons, joints and bone. The mixed nerves carrying these impulses also supply the motor fibers to the muscles.

Superficial Sensibility. Nerves supplying the skin provide sensations of touch (pressure), pain and temperature and make possible the distinction of single or multiple stimuli. Tests for touch, pain and temperature sensitivity should be carried out with the patient's eyes closed and his attention focused on what the examiner is testing. The most sensitive points of the skin seem to be at the base of hairs and on the soles and palms.

Touch. The quality of touch perception maybe tested by either a wisp of cotton or a camel's hair brush to stroke the skin. The hair follicles are receptors and therefore should be avoided. Allowances are made for interpretation of the results on the thicker skin of the palms and soles.

Discriminitive sensation is tested by having the patient discriminate between

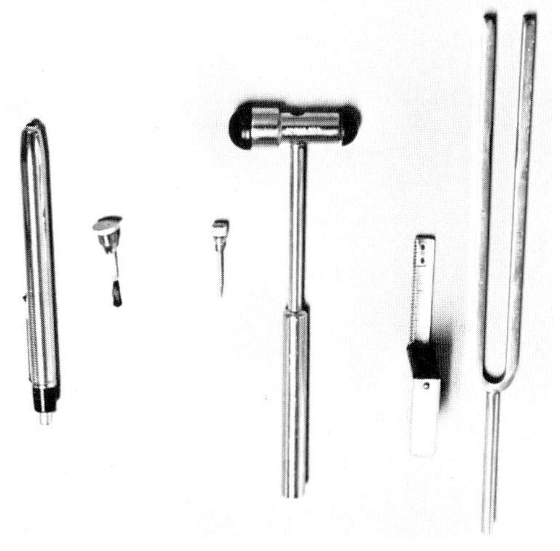

Fig. 6.1. Neurologic examination equipment. *Left to right:* flashlight for pupillary reflexes and examination of body orifices; brush for touch sensation; sharp, pointed object for pain perception; percussion hammer for reflexes; tape measure for mensuration; tuning fork for vibratory sensations.

the pressure of one or two fingers held about ¼ in. apart. Damage to sensory mechanism above the level of the thalamus will show evidence of an inability to discriminate. An absence of position sense in ataxia may be found with an inability to discriminate. A few seconds of light pressure is made on the normal side to allow the patient to discriminate from one point or two points of pressure. The abnormal side is then tested. Dermographism or wheal formation at the site of irritation suggests a neurocirculatory lesion.

Pain. The ability to discern painful stimuli may be determined by alternately touching the skin with the pointed and dull ends of a common pin while the patient's eyes are closed. An area of sensory distribution of a nerve root is known as a dermatome, and outlining the dermatome may be an area of increased sensitivity. A thorough knowledge of the sensory distribution of nerves enables the examiner to locate the level of a spinal lesion.

In some cases, e.g., tabes dorsalis, the patient feels the touch sensation produced by the stimulus but does not immediately perceive pain. The pain may be felt seconds after the prick of the pin since conduction of pain sense is apparently delayed in tabes. A double sensation is often experienced with the single prick of the pin.

In many disturbances of sensory perception, the border of hypoesthesia is not sharp but is gradually impaired. One must note whether the loss of sensation is bilateral and symmetrical or whether mixed sensations affect the same area. Other types of sensations may be due to either a segmental loss of sensation or involvement of a particular peripheral nerve supplying the part. Perspiration, temperature and color of the skin must be noted in confirming evidence of the pathologic findings. Careful examination must be made to clarify the evaluations of intensity of the pin prick and the site of irritation.

Temperature sense is checked by applying test tubes filled with hot and cold water to the part being evaluated. This procedure tests the patient's ability to localize the site of application as well as to distinguish hot and cold stimuli. The area manifesting loss of heat sensation is usually larger than an area with loss of cold sensation.

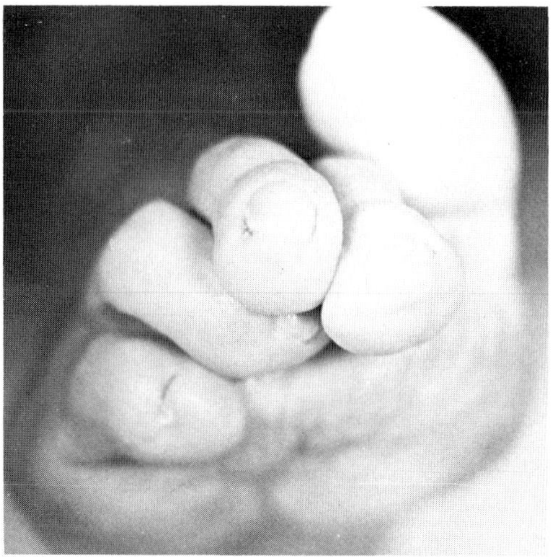

Fig. 6.2. Underlapping, overlapping toes secondary to contractures caused by upper motor neuron lesion.

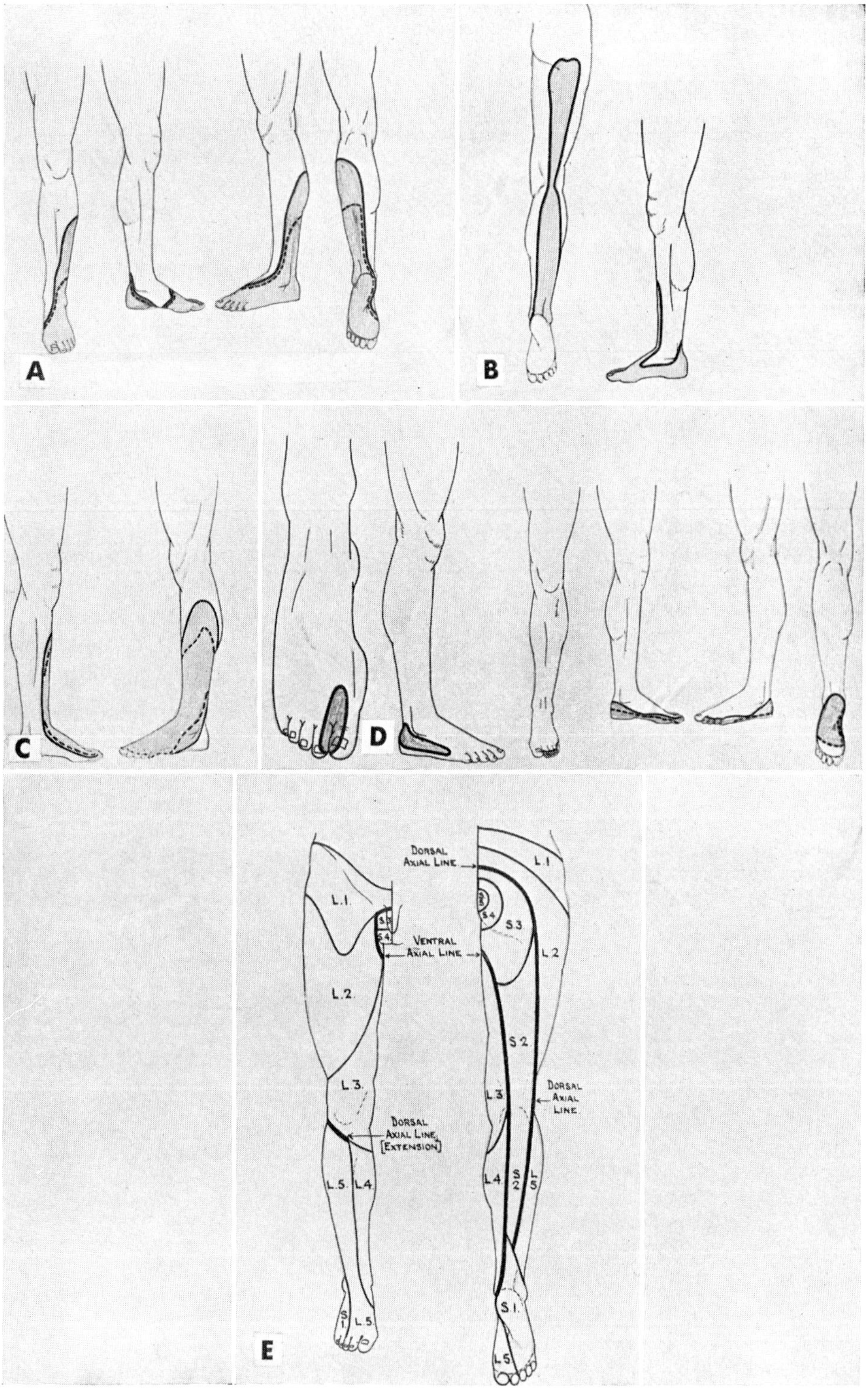

Fig. 6.3. Dermatomes in extremities.

Deep Sensibility. There are several methods of evaluating deep sensibility.

One test of deep sensibility is to have the patient differentiate between light touch and deep pressure on the skin. The results are obvious when squeezing the tendo achillis. Abadie's sign is present when, in locomotor ataxia, pressure on the tendo achillis does not produce pain. Normally the patient complains of pain and withdraws his foot.

Vibratory Sensations. The sensation from bone is limited to perception of pain and pressure and, most importantly, vibration. Vibration is tested by placing a vibrating tuning fork directly over a bony prominence. One must make sure that the patient feels the vibration or humming and not just pressure.

Skeletal changes with age or the value of therapeutic approaches may be calculated by measuring the vibrating of a bone to sound.

Diminished or absent vibratory sensation is caused by injury or trophic disturbances of the peripheral nerves or the posterior columns or roots of the spinal cord. These lesions may occur in diabetes, arteriosclerosis, pernicious anemia, tabes dorsalis and multiple sclerosis.

When combined with an Argyll-Robertson pupil and a positive serology the diagnosis is evident. Very often the bones may show evidence of syphilitic density, gummatous lesions, Charcot's joint or neurotrophic degeneration with loss of deep sensibility.

Position sense is checked by passively moving the toes in a firm and definite manner, demanding that the patient describe or reproduce the motion. In severe cases of deep sensibility disturbances, patients cannot tell whether a part is flexed or extended. It is necessary to differentiate the reaction in both extremities. In spinal disease the maximum loss of position sense is in the toes and fingers. It is wise to evaluate all findings in an effort to rule out the possibility of suggestion, malingering or hysteria.

If rombergism is suspected, the patient is requested to stand with his eyes closed and his feet parallel and close together. Romberg's sign is present if the patient begins to sway, losing all sense of direction and balance. The sensation disappears when the eyes are opened. A positive Romberg sign is found in locomotor ataxia, cerebrospinal disease, alcoholic neuritis, pernicious anemia and diseases of the columns of Goll and Burdach.

Faulty equilibrium may result from degeneration of the dorsal roots and tracts. Afferent activity in the cerebellum may be disturbed. When loss of equilibrium is positive the examiner might suspect tertiary syphilis with neurologic manifestations.

Finger-to-Nose Test. The patient stands with eyes closed, feet parallel and close together and arms outstretched. He brings the index finger first of one hand, then of the other to his nose. Incoordination is demonstrated by rhythmical tremor at right angles to the line of movement in the finger-to-nose test. The heel-to-knee test may be used to evalualte cerebellar disease as the finger-to-nose test. When the object is overshot and rhythmical tremors are present, a cerebellar ataxia is suspected and if the tremors are irregular and unsteady a sensory ataxia is considered.

The André-Thomas sign or spring-like phenomena is noted in the finger-to-nose test when the patient appears to touch the nose several times as if on a rebound. This same sign is observed when the patient raises his hand above his head. When requested to let it drop down on his head a rebound will occur in cerebellar diseases.

Another sensory symptom is seen in Lasègue's sign with the thigh flexed, when extension of the knee is accompanied by pain due to stretching of the nerve roots. Inflammation of the sciatic nerve or the perineural tissues caused either by pressure or pathology, will present a positive Lasègue's sign.

Motor Function

The strength of various muscles upon voluntary movement is examined by directing the patient to flex and extend a particular joint against resistance. The strength of these movements, observation of the patient's gait and familiarity with the patient's complete history contribute to an accurate diagnosis.

Early examination for motor function should include notation of posture, tremors and spasm of the extremities while at rest. This examination of the lower limbs is accomplished by asking the patient to raise first one, then the other limb from the examining table while lying in a face downward position. The patient flexes the leg at the knee to a vertical position and is instructed to maintain this posture. Failure to hold the limbs in this position is called Barre's sign. It is not, however, an indication of a specific type of motor defect.

The functions of each joint are tested for power of movement. A simple method for recording these functions is the use of a four point scale in which 0 = no contraction, 1 = feeble contraction, 2 = ability to counteract weight of gravity, 3 = fair, but movement weaker than normal, and 4 = estimated full power of movement.

Ataxia. Due to a loss of power of coordination, the voluntary muscular movements are awkward. Swaying and irregular movements when standing or walking may be evident. Jerky and uncoordinated motions when walking, and a loss of position sense of the hands and feet are all a part of the ataxic syndrome. In Fournier's test for ataxic gait, the patient is seated comfortably and he is commanded to rise on a given signal and begin walking quickly toward the examiner and stop at a given signal. He may be commanded to rise from the comfortable sitting position, walk and turn around at a given signal. During the execution of the above commands, the doctor should note any slight waverings, unsteadiness, staggering and associated abnormal movements. Owing to a loss of deep sensibility, the patient will experience difficulty in quick coordinated actions if ataxia is present. Advanced pernicious anemia is characterized by an ataxic gait.

Tremors. This is a slow, rapid, or moderate trembling or oscillation of parts of the body. Trembling of a part while at rest is known as passive tremor. Passive tremor may be seen in Parkinson's disease or it may be a functional weakness of the musculature.

Intention tremor is trembling occurring when one is about to begin a muscular motion or is in the act of performing a voluntary function. This type of tremor often occurs in multiple sclerosis. A rapid and fine functional tremor may be seen in the fingers of an outstretched hand of one with an exophthalmic goiter.

Abuses of alcohol, tobacco, mercury, lead and other toxic substances may cause tremor. Very often in elderly persons there is a tremor of the head resembling the passive tremor.

Postural Tonus. An increase in tone causes the muscle to feel firm and thick; greatly increased tone causes the muscle to contract and shorten resulting in deformity. The evidence of such a spasticity is an increased activity of the tendon reflexes. Postural tone is established by noting any undue resistance of muscles to passive lengthening. In corticospinal lesions the resistance met is of the spastic type affecting the extensors of the knee and plantar flexors of the ankle and which gives way with continued passive stretch. This phenomena remains the same from hour to hour but varies from day to day. It is known as a hypertonicity of the muscles and should be differentiated from muscular rigidity. The former has an elastic resistance to passive movement and is a result of an involvement of the pyramidal tract. The muscular rigidity has a lead pipe-like resistance to movement, the tendon reflexes are diminished, and the Babinski and ankle clonus are absent.

Rigidity may be due to widespread pyramidal and extrapyramidal involvements and may be associated with pain on manipulation. Either hysteria or a local lesion should be considered. If a passive movement is limited by firm fixation, the muscle is probably contracted permanently. Arthritic changes may limit passive motion and should be differentiated from pyramidal disease.

Hypotonicity is a decrease in muscular tone. Muscles have unusual extensibility and are abnormally flaccid. The paralyses found with hypotonia are of the flaccid variety. Here there is a loss of tendon reflexes which is indicative of either a lower motor neuron disturbance such as occurs in infantile paralysis or a peripheral nerve lesion.

Atrophy. An examination to determine the normal muscle volume is very important in diagnosing nerve lesions. When muscles remain inactive for long periods of time atrophy results. This may occur in severe, acquired pes valgus conditions where certain muscles have been inactive for years. When a joint is painful it may become fixed resulting in inactivity and atrophy of the muscles moving the joint.

Atrophied muscles will react to direct stimulation of percussion but irritability is definitely decreased. When a motor nerve is cut or poisoned the peripheral end degenerates in a few days and is not affected by electrical stimulation. This occurs because the striated muscles under the control of the nerve involved are removed from nervous control; with the nerves destroyed, the muscle can no longer be stimulated to perform a normal function.

Fibrillations may occur as flickering involuntary contractions of muscle fibers.

Excitability of muscles may be diminished or increased. In response to a tap on muscle substance with percussion hammer, normal muscles present a local jerk in the fasciculi struck. Flickering may occur for a few seconds in an emaciated person, but is of no value as a diagnostic sign. Atrophic muscles show slight evidence of contraction. A percussion myotonia is a sustained local contraction lasting a minute or longer in particular muscular dystrophies.

A muscle without the nerve supplying it still reacts to the break of galvanic current but with a slow type of contraction. This reaction is present in degeneration of the anterior horn of the cord or any lower motor neuron lesion.

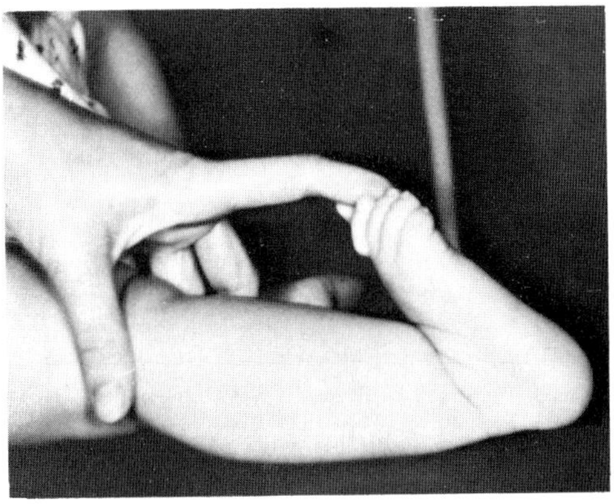

Fig. 6.4. Hypermobile foot showing passive dorsiflexion.

Reflex Action

Reflexes give the examiner an objective group of symptoms with which to analyze his case. If the examiner is trained to understand the reflex arc and a few simple techniques, successful elicitation and interpretation of reflexes is assured. The reflexes serve as sensitive indicators of the state of the nervous center and its pathways. The most important reflective stimulus for muscle consists of a stretching of muscle tissue upon receiving a sudden and brief concussion resulting in a quick, longitudinal pull. This is a "muscle stretch reflex" (Wartenberg, 1945) and is the so-called deep or tendon reflex. A slowly applied blow or stroke of the part is ineffective.

Reflex strength varies with the individual muscle or muscles and from one person to another. The reflex may become apparent only when there is functional or organic increase in muscle tone. Pyramidal lesions will excite and increase reflexes. The presence of the "muscle stretch" must not be construed as pathologic. A latent normal response may be exaggerated in the presence of pathology and may indicate pyramidal lesions. Many methods are used to reinforce a reflex action. Among these are a cough, pulling apart clasped fingers and the patient squeezing the examiner's hand and diversion of attention to other interests in the office environment. A slight stretching of the muscle to be tapped reinforces the reflex response.

In regeneration of nerves the most distal parts are the last to regain function. Muscle tone returns first, atrophy of muscle diminishes, voluntary movements return, and, finally, the electrical reactions become normal. Unequal reflexes on the two sides between superficial and deep reflexes are more valuable in diagnosis than slight deviation from a hypothetical standard. Right and left reflexes may be evaluated using the simple code: hyperactive reflex = ++, absent reflex = 0, and diminished reflex = dim.

Deep Muscle Reflexes. There are five deep muscle reflexes the podiatrist should test.

Patellar Reflex. It is not possible to define a normal knee jerk as they may vary with individuals and at different times in the same individual. Absence of the jerk or inequality of the jerk on two sides is suggestive of organic abnormality. The knee jerk may be exaggerated, diminished or lost. The presence of neurasthenia or chronic diseases such as arteriosclerosis may cause failure of pyramidal inhibition of the response to patellar tendon tapping resulting in functional exaggeration of the reflex.

The knee jerk examination must be supplemented by examination of other reflexes. Exaggerated knee jerks which are equal on both sides and associated with a normal plantar response are not considered the result of organic loss of control of the reflex arc. However, if the plantar reflex is of the extensor type and the patellar response is exaggerated, organic changes in the motor area of the brain or in the pyramidal tracts are indicated.

When the pyramidal tract is affected equally on both sides, the patellar response in both legs is exaggerated. In hemiplegia, only the affected side is exaggerated since only one pyramidal tract is involved. The presence of a well sustained patellar clonus indicates organic disease in the pyramidal tracts. Acute febrile and debilitating disease decreases activity of the knee jerk in children.

The knee jerk reflex is lost only in organic disease such as involvement of the quadriceps extensor muscles or of the afferent pathway or the reflex arc. Diseases affecting the anterior horn cells such as myelitis involving the third and fourth lumbar segments of the spinal cord may result in loss of the knee jerk reflex. Peripheral neuritis affecting the efferent fibers may be noted when the knee jerk reflex is absent.

Complete transverse myelitis affecting the spinal cord in the dorsal region, frequently the result of severe fracture dislocation of the vertebral column, results very early in loss of the patellar reflex. A transverse myelitis at a level capable of deactivating the patellar reflex may not disturb the reflex arc of a deep muscle reflex below the level of damage in the cord.

When intracranial pressure is present, the knee jerk may vary with the ebb of the intracranial pressure. The knee jerk may be lost in diabetes mellitus and associated peripheral neuritis.

Absence of the tendon reflex is seen in locomotor ataxia, in some spinal or cerebral diseases, and in spinal cord tumors. In spinal cord tumors, absence of the tendon reflex is unilateral.

Achilles Reflex. The ball of the foot is pushed slightly against the examiner's hand while the Achilles tendon is tapped eliciting a deep muscle reflex. The foot extends at the ankle during the "muscle stretch" with this reinforcement.

The best position for eliciting the ankle jerk is with the patient lying down, the knee slightly flexed, the thigh rotated externally and the ankle slightly inverted. The plantar response can also be tested in this manner, but if the results are questionable the leg should be fully extended.

In cases of pyramidal lesion, tapping of the patellar tendon may cause contraction in the plantar flexors of the foot and toes and sometimes of the hip extensors in addition to contraction of the quadriceps muscle. Such a reaction to a single concussion is called a reflex of spinal automotism and is not a deep muscle reflex.

Plantar Muscle Reflex. The foot must be warm as in all other reflexes and the plantar muscles lightly stretched by exerting pressure in dorsiflexion. The stroke must be sharp and relaxed, brief and sudden with a dull, blunt or pointed object directed from the lateral plantar aspect of the heel upward to the plantar surfaces of the four lesser toes. Flexion and fanning of the lesser toes with extension of the great toe will occur in pyramidal tract lesions.

The plantar muscle reflex is considered the most valuable of all physical responses in the nervous sytem. The normal response is a slow deliberate plantar flexion of the great toe. The stimulation is not painful except in pyramidal tract disease.

All dorsal foot reflexes act by the same mechanism as the plantar reflexes because of stretching of the plantar muscles by concussion. The plantar reflex can be produced by tapping the flexor muscles at many points of the sole.

Patellar Clonus. The leg is extended, the patella grasped between the thumb and the forefinger and the patella is briskly pushed down one or more times. A clonus is seen when there is a rhythmic jerking of the patella. When only a few jerks result, a clonus is said to be exhaustible and if the jerking continues as long as the patella is held it is said to be inexhaustible. This is most marked as a sign of lateral cerebrospinal tract disease and disseminated sclerosis.

Ankle Clonus. The reflex center is located in the fifth lumbar and the first sacral segments of the cord. The leg is held in one hand, the foot is grasped with the other and briskly dorsiflexed one or more times. A clonic repetition of the ankle jerk in the form of an exaggerated tremor results. Both the ankle and patella clonus possess the same significance.

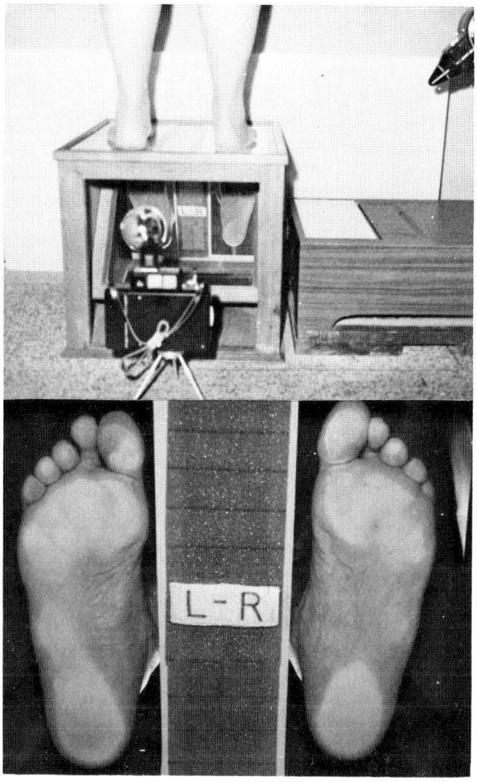

Fig. 6.5. *Upper*, phalangeal stance reflex. Reflecting mirror and Polaroid camera with flash attachment. *Lower*, asymmetrical foot prints, excessive toe activity in flexion. Courtesy of S. V. Michota and F. A. Michota.

In old spinal cord injuries, ankle clonus is present when the plantar response has again become flexor and it appears later than other signs in progressive lesions of the cord. False ankle clonus sometimes occurs in nervous people, but in these cases the gait is not spastic.

Percussion of the tibialis anticus muscle induces dorsal flexion and supination of the foot. When the response is extremely pronounced, it indicates an organic disease of the central nervous system.

Leichtenstren pointed out that in cerebrospinal meningitis tapping of the bones of an extremity revealed evidence of increased irritability.

Superficial Reflexes. The Babinski reflex is a superficial reflex. It is negative if, when the outer sole of the foot is stroked upward and inward, there is normal plantar flexion of the toes. It is positive when this action causes fanning of all the lesser toes and dorsal flexion of the great toes.

The diagnostic significance of the Babinski reflex varies depending on age and whether or not temporary incapacitation or disease is present. A physiologic Babinski can be elicited in infants up to 6-months-old and sometimes in children up to 2- to 4-years-old. A temporary Babinski reflex may be found during normal sleep or during morphine, chloroform or scopolamine narcosis, or in epileptic seizures.

A pathologic Babinski reflex may be the result of a pyramidal tract lesion at any part of the pyramidal tract or cortico-spinal pathway. A positive Babinski sign may be seen in any lesion of the pyramidal tracts either in the brain or spinal cord.

Additional Tests of Inerest to the Podiatrist. There are five other tests which the podiatrist should be able to use when indicated.

Lasègue's Sign. This is significant in diseases of the sciatic nerve. The thigh is flexed on the abdomen and the leg extended at the knee. This maneuver causes stretching of the nerve root. When there is disease of the nerve, pain and resistance on the part of the patient will result.

Patrick's Test. This test indicates hip joint disease. When the patient is supine, the thigh and knee are flexed and the external malleolus is placed on the patella of the opposite leg. On depressing the knee, pain is noted if arthritis of the hip is present.

Pupillary Reflexes. Normally a light thrown upon the retina of the eye causes the pupil of the eye which is being tested to contract. Light thrown upon the opposite eye causes the pupil to contract. When the eye is shaded the pupil dilates. When looking at near objects the pupil accommodates by contracting and at a distance the pupil dilates.

Argyll-Robertson Reflexes. The pupillary reflex does not react to light but reacts to accommodation. The Argyll-Robertson reflex may be found in syphilitics manifesting local symptoms in the foot.

Hirschberg's reflex is seen in pyramidal tract disease and organic hemiplegia and is elicited by tickling the sole of the foot at the base of the great toe. It is characterized by adduction of the foot.

Many times a mild, permanent hyperextension of the great toe is noted on the affected side of a unilateral pyramidal tract disturbance. This sign may be seen before the Babinski reflex.

Differential Diagnosis of Paralysis

There are basically two types of motor paralysis, one caused by an upper motor neuron lesion and the other caused by a lower motor neuron lesion. The upper motor neuron lesion causes a characteristic spastic paralysis and the lower motor neuron lesion causes a flaccid paralysis. An evaluation of the reflexes, signs and symptoms of disease and characteristic syndromes will help differentiate neurologic disorders from other diseases of the extremities.

The exact location of a lesion in the brain or spinal cord is left to the neurologist for interpretation. It will suffice for the doctor to know whether the lesion is peripheral, of lower motor neuron origin, or of a cerebral spinal origin.

Peripheral paralysis may be due to nerve trauma or pressure, poliomyelitis nutritional disorders or poisoning.

Cerebral, upper motor neuron, lesions are caused by injuries to the motor pathways, abnormal pressures on cerebral centers by hemorrhage, tumors or emboli.

Differential Diagnosis of Foot Drop

Poliomyelitis. The onset of the general disease is usually in childhood but may affect adults. There is a marked atrophy of muscles and symptoms of a lower motor neuron lesion rapidly develop. Sometimes the muscle or group of muscles affected are flaccid for only a few months and then return to normal. When the attack is in childhood, there is usually a shortness in the limb due to a lagging of bony growth caused by faulty nutrition. A foot drop generally develops resulting in faulty weight distribution. Excrescences may develop under the first or fifth metatarsal heads and corns are common on the dorsum of the toes and along the lateral border of the fifth toe nail. Toes are dorsiflexed and extensor tendons contracted.

Multiple Neuritis. (Synonyms: acute febrile neuritis, alcoholic neuritis, diphtheritic neuritis, diabetic neuritis, infective neuritis, plumbic or lead neuritis and arsenical neuritis.)

This disease demonstrates a bilateral foot drop due to a weakness of the dorsal flexors. In walking, the toes catch on the ground giving the characteristic steppage gait. A wrist drop may also be present. Symmetrical pains in the extremities, numbness and tingling are also characteristic. The degree of weakness of the muscle is out of proportion to the minimal atrophy.

Deep Peroneal Nerve Injuries. Trauma involving the head of the fibula causes a tendency toward the development of talipes equinus varus with a flexor contraction of the toes. A history of an operation in that area with prolonged use of bandages or splints is common. Anesthesia of the outer side and dorsum of the foot is present. Sensory perception is diminished and a numb, dead feeling is noted. When present for a long time, abnormal pressure of weight bearing results in development of tylomas under the fifth metatarsal head. A digiti quinti varus is common and digiti flexus of the lesser toes is usual.

Paralysis often occurs in elderly individuals who habitually cross one leg over the opposite knee. Wedged between the ipsilateral fibula and the external condyle of the heterolateral femur and heterolateral patella, the repeated pressure traumatizes the peroneal nerve.

Patients convalescing from a severe illness, hyperthyroidism and mental depression are particularly susceptible to this lesion. Minor operations on the foot and postinjection therapy for varicosities have been reported as etiologic.

Complete Transverse Myelitis. The foot drop occurs in complete transverse myelitis bilaterally. There is a loss of deep reflexes and very often a history of syphilis or trauma to vertebrae. This disorder also presents an anesthesia or impairment of sensation at definite levels below the paralysis. The extensor muscles are affected resulting in a flaccid paralysis and bilateral drop foot.

Peroneal Muscle Atrophy. Onset of drop foot caused by peroneal muscle atrophy occurs before the age of 25. The condition tends to be familial and pursues a slow progressive course with an atrophy of the small muscles of the feet. Similar atrophy occurs in the hands. Peroneal muscular atrophy may result from trauma, alienation of the muscle in polio, disuse, alcoholism, neuritis and acute febrile disease.

Treatment. Treatment instituted must depend on whether experience indicates that corrective forces can be exerted with some reasonable assurance of results. In a flaccid paralysis such as may develop with a polio or peripheral nerve injury, it is essential to try to coordinate the mind and body in bringing about active motion in the affected part during the early stages. At all times a firm shoe should be fitted to the affected part. It is essential that a knee-length brace be utilized on the affected extremity either by a double bar or a posterior bar inserted into the shoe to maintain the foot in a functional position without dropping. In a peripheral neuritis, proper medical treatment should be instituted to offset the damaging effect of pathology on the peripheral nerve. This must be aided by the utilization of a foot drop appliance in gait. While at rest, maintenance of the foot at right angles to the leg is essential. An early attempt should be made to maintain the length of the tendo achillis. If this tendon is allowed to shorten, the tendon could be lengthened only by surgical intervention.

Patients with ataxic gait must be referred to the neurologist to establish the etiology and provide systemic care. Podiatrists can maintain the foot at right angles to the leg by utilizing knee-length braces. In gaits of various types, the prime approach to the treatment is an attempt to maintain the foot at right angles to the leg and to add sufficient support through use of proper orthotics to maintain confidence and improvement of gait.

Cooperative treatment by the internist, neurologist, orthopedic surgeon, psychiatrist, physiatrist and podiatrist usually relieves pain and restores some function.

Gait

In patients with a normal gait, the weight of the body is supported by one foot while the other is advanced. The heel of the weight bearing foot touches the ground first; the toes touch last as the heel raises. Repeated alternations of this pattern result in a smooth and rhythmical locomotive process.

Variations in gait may have a hereditary basis involving skeletal muscular or nervous system peculiarities, or they may simply be acquired through imitation of a parent. Abnormal gaits are the result of wearing improper footgear, trauma, arthritis, motor neuron lesions, congenital or hereditary disorders, muscular dystrophies, atrophy and faulty adipose distribution.

A slow exaggerated gait with staggering toward support may be evidence of loss of confidence in the patient's legs. A long-term illness, cerebral pathology or peripheral neuropathy may cause this gait.

A spraddle-legged gait in children is really compensatory to give the child a broader base for balance in his early days of progression. The infant learning to walk usually spreads his legs apart, lifts his elbows up in wing-like fashion and adopts a spraddle-legged gait.

The hemiplegic has a short phase of support on the paralyzed side with a slow, spastic propulsion resulting in a long progression on the same side. The patient holds the leg stiff and the progressive phase of walking is in circumduction; the arms also move more than normally. Sometimes the affected limb is dragged because of the secondary muscular involvement in the paretic, the knee is stiffer and the foot scrapes the ground.

In tabes dorsalis the progressive phase is long because of the time element required in observation by the patient of how high he is raising his feet and how hard he places them down. The tabetic must watch his step to see where he is going.

In drop foot or steppage gait the toes strike the ground first followed by a slapping down of the heel. This type of gait is very common and usually the result of a flaccid paralysis. Infantile paralysis, peripheral neuritis, trauma to the external popliteal, and muscular dystrophy may result in a foot drop; an alcoholic neuritis predisposes to drop foot. The tendo achillis may be shortened; the patient is unable to stand on his heels. Flexion of the leg on the thigh is increased while the foot is raised high when walking.

An ataxic gait is a jerky, unsteady support and progression in which the patient may reel and lose his balance. A test for ataxia is to have the patient walk sideways with eyes closed and then, with open eyes, walk forward, backward and sideways. The ataxia will manifest itself at all times. If it disappears with the eyes closed, the ataxia may be due to hysterics.

The spastic gait is a slow, stiff-legged gait with legs extended and feet shuf-

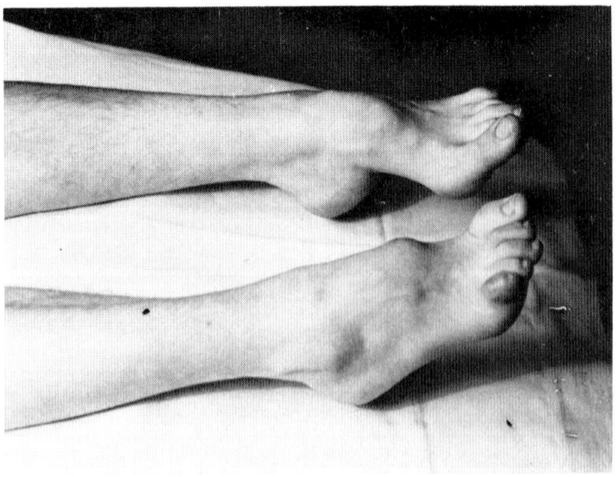

Fig. 6.6. Talipes equinus varus.

fling. This is due to an upper motor neuron lesion. It may be noted in hemiplegics.

Scissors gait is characterized by crossed leg progression with spastic shuffling; the hips and knees are flexed and the legs have a tendency to cross in gait. This gait is seen in patients suffering chronic muscular disease.

Short steps may be seen in cerebral arteriosclerosis. The patient appears to hesitate with each step before shifting to the opposite foot.

Waddling gaits give the impression of being very top heavy with a resultant sway above the hips. This gait occurs in patients with muscular dystrophies, spinal muscular atrophy or bilateral dislocation of the hips and in the very tall and obese patient.

Festination is seen in parkinsonism. It is characterized by a falling forward of the body resulting in the center of gravity being forward of the midline. In an effort to maintain balance the patient progresses faster and faster resulting in either a fall or bump into an object.

Hysterical gaits and loss of confidence may be suspected when the gait is marked by hesitating foot movements followed by sudden shuffling and grotesque balancing movements.

Cerebellar Gait. In the absence of rigidity and spasticity, lack of swinging of an arm while walking may be seen in cerebellar disease of the same side. The patient with a disorder of the cerebellum may present with an unsteady gait, loss of balance with the eyes closed, an unsteady route when bringing the finger to the nose and a positive Romberg's sign.

7

Interpretation of Laboratory Findings and Nutritional Disorders

Careful evaluation of the podiatric patient requires knowledge of his general health and the possibility of systemic diseases with symptoms in the feet. Laboratory analysis of blood and urine is often desirable and is mandatory where foot surgery is planned. An accurate laboratory report protects the patient and aids the podiatrist by confirming his initial appraisal of the condition and by revealing additional data. I recommend that preoperative examinations be conducted by a certified laboratory technician. A laboratory report becomes an authoritative part of the patient's record and can be helpful in medico-legal problems should they arise.

The podiatrist orders the appropriate tests for the suspected pathology as well as urinalysis and blood studies. Specimens may be sent for biopsy and other tissue examination. The podiatrist may aspirate a lesion for abnormal fluids and take smears for Gram staining. He may send specimens of synovial fluid or joint fluid for examination and may request complete microbiologic studies when indicated.

Urinalysis

Urine should be passed into a clean receptacle and kept in a cool place until examination. The first specimen in the morning is usually best for study. Urine taken a few hours after a heavy meal may contain many abnormal products of metabolism. Urine is examined routinely for color, specific gravity and pH; odor and the presence of sugar, albumin, blood, casts, epithelial cells, pus, crystals and bacteria are indicators of disease. Table I presents analytical data on the chemical composition of urine.

Blood Tests

Blood examinations for routine office procedures may include a hematocrit, hemoglobin evaluation, red count, white count and differential. Sedimentation rate, clotting time, bleeding time and prothrombin time are also determined. Determination of blood glucose, urea nitrogen, uric acid, blood calcium, inorganic phosphate and alkaline phosphatase, sodium, potassium, chlorides, total protein and the ratio of albumin to globulin may be necessary for the diagnosis of certain foot disorders.

Coagulation Time. Blood coagulates normally in 3 to 6 min. in a capillary tube. Lee White coagulation time in 10- x 75-mm. test tubes is 5 to 14 min.

Bleeding time is how long it takes for a drop of blood to clot, close the puncture in the skin and stop bleeding. Normal bleeding time is about 2 to 5 min. (Duke's).

Table I[a]
Normal Chemical Composition of Urine

	Amount in 24 hr.	Concentration in g. per 100 ml.[b]	Chief variations in disease	Podiatric considerations
Volume	1000—1500 ml.		High in chronic nephritis. Low in acute renal failure, water depletion, intestinal obstruction, fevers, etc.	Differential diagnosis of edema in the lower extremities. The volume excreted is important in the presence of acute foot infections and in diabetes.
Specificity gravity	1.012—1.020		Low and tending to constancy in chronic renal insufficiency; high in water depletion, intestinal obstruction, cardiac failure, fevers, etc.	A specific gravity over 1.030 should arouse suspicion of diabetes when differentiating ulcers, circulatory signs and neuropathic foot symptoms.
Urea Urea nitrogen	15—35 g. 6—18 g.	1.0—2.5 0.4—1.2	Total high in fevers; concentration low in chronic nephritis, high in the nephrotic syndrome, intestinal obstruction, fevers, etc.	Increase noted in the presence of extensive fulminating foot infections with fever.
Chlorides (as NaCl)	5—15 g. (i.e., about 80—240 mEq.)	0.3—1.5 (i.e., 50—250 mEq. per liter	Concentration low in chronic renal insufficiency, but total normal; concentration and especially, total, low in intestinal obstruction and other conditions involving persistent vomiting, during the following severe trauma, and in pneumonia.	Useful in the differential diagnosis of edema. Chlorides may be depleted by persistant vomiting due to interaction of medication or sensitivity to drugs prescribed preoperatively or following surgical trauma.
Ketosteroids	Men 10—25 mg./day Women 5—15 mg./day		Both low in Addison's disease; hypopituitarism and myxedema, high in hyperadrenalism. Ketosteroids high in interstitial tumor of testes.	Of clinical interest in disorders of growth and development of the feet. The relationship of endocrine dysfunction to anhidrosis, dry and fissured skin may be evaluated.
Ketogenic steroids	Men 8—20 mg./day Women 6—18 mg./day			

[a] Adapted from *Stedman's Medical Dictionary*, Ed. 21, Baltimore: The Williams & Wilkins Company. Modified from C. P. Stewart and D. Dunlop, *Clinical Chemistry in Practical Medicine*, Ed. 3, Edinburgh, E. & S. Livingstone, Ltd., 1962.
[b] Unless other units are stated.

A low prothrombin concentration alters coagulability of the blood. Normal prothrombin time is 85 to 100%. Partial thromboplastin time is 30 to 45 sec.

Hemoglobin values in males are about 14 to 18 g and in females 12 to 16 g. An anemia may readily become a complicating factor in the treatment of circulatory involvements, nail and skin lesions and structural and postural instabilities.

Blood Counts. The number of red cells increases in high altitudes, after muscular exercise, in emotional states and in high environmental temperature.

A decreased red count to a low 1 to 1.5 million, depending on when studies are performed, and a low hemoglobin with a decrease in reticulocytes are often seen in pernicious anemia. When the count is below 4 million with differences in size and shape, it is usually due to an anemia. Red cell survival time is shortened. Smears should be examined for macrocytic red blood cells.

A white cell count below 5,000 indicates leucopenia above 10,000 leucocytosis. A count of 12,000 to 13,000 or more is indicative of inflammatory or infectious changes. A count of more than 40,000 white blood cells is seldom found except in leukemia.

An increase in eosinophiles is suggestive of parasitic infection; a decrease is a sign of severe toxemia.

An increase in basophiles may suggest sarcoma when the clinical picture and confirmatory radiographs support this finding.

Blood Chemistry. The podiatrist may be confronted with symptoms that relate to abnormal physiologic functions or positive diseases involving the foot. He may find it necessary to evaluate for syphilis by ordering a V.D.R.L. screening procedure and the fluorescent treponemal antibody test. Where bone and joint disorders create symptoms, blood calcium, serum inorganic phosphorus, serum alkaline phosphatase and sedimentation tests may be helpful in diagnosis. Urea nitrogen is helpful in determining the degree of protein catabolism in destructive disorders of the feet. A host of laboratory tests are available to the internist and the podiatrist working as a team to improve the patient's health. Some common tests are given in Table II.

The blood sedimentation rate test is an invaluable adjunct to the diagnosis and prognosis of disease. It gives additional, corroborative evidence in the differentiation of functional from organic disease; infected from non-active inflammatory lesions; benign from malignant tumors. The rate of sedimentation is more rapid in women than in men. There is an increase in the rate during pregnancy after the first few months. In children, excitement causes some increase. Generally, clinical improvement is followed by decreased sedimentation rates. In podiatry, the sedimentation test has its greatest value in the differential diagnosis of the arthritides affecting the feet.

A rheumatoid arthritis will have a highly abnormal rate of sedimentation by comparison with degenerative joint disease in which the sedimentation rate, except in the presence of infectious complications, is normal.

Thyroid Function Tests

Chemical tests such as protein-bound iodine and butanol extractional iodine have been the most popular tests for thyroid function. However, radioassay is now replacing chemical methods.

In hyperthyroidism the skin may be warm and perspiring. Among other symptoms of a systemic nature in hypothyroidism, there is decreased sweating, the skin is dry and cold and the skin, hair and nails are coarse and grow slowly. Thyroid function tests are necessary for a differential diagnosis.

Tissue and fluids from skin lesions may be examined under the microscope to evaluate the type of pathology or type of bacteria if any, affecting the part. Mycology medium may be inoculated for colony growth of fungi.

Biopsy

Wherever pathologic tissues present a problem in interpretation it is best to biopsy. This procedure can be readily performed in a pathology laboratory. A small portion of the diseased tissue is removed, stained and examined. At the hospital operating table a frozen section sent for evaluation helps determine the presence of malignancy.

Aspirated Fluids

Aspiration is the drawing off of fluid of an excretion, secretion, pus or tissue. In tuberculosis, aspiration of abscess cavities in the affected bones of the foot determines the presence or absence of acid-fast bacilli and possible osteomyelitis. The pus or fluid may be thick or contain tissue debris. It is necessary to use a heavy-gauge needle for aspiration to avoid blockage. Histologic examination of the fluid withdrawn from a foot joint is a necessary procedure in the diagnostic interpretation of the pathology present.

Pap smear techniques may be applied to cytologic preparations from most fluids. Fluid from a draining wound in the foot may be subjected to a Pap smear examination.

Synovial fluid may contain blood which is not readily absorbed in the joint. This blood may precipitate fibrin, become firm, and undergo chondrification or degenerative calcifications. Degenerative joint disease may result.

Aspiration may be conducted on neoplastic tissues to differentiate the benign from the malignant. This method can be done in the podiatrist's office or in the emergency rooms or laboratory of a hospital following infiltrative local anesthesia. Using sterile technique, the overlying tissue is punctured by a surgical knife. An 18-gauge needle is inserted through the skin wound to the tumor mass. As the needle enters the mass the plunger is withdrawn to create suction on the tissues being forced into the needle. Care must be exercised in removal of the tissue and it is often wise to hold the plunger in the suction (withdrawn) position while three or more insertions are made into the suspected neoplasm. The tissue removed may be placed on a slide. If the specimen is sufficiently large, it may be impregnated in paraffin, hardened and sectioned for staining and microscopic examination by the pathologist.

Spinal Fluid Examination

Spinal fluid examinations are necessary and conducted by the pathologist to evaluate the cellular changes in poliomyelitis, syphilis and meningitis. Pressure within the spinal cord by tumor masses are reflected frequently in neurologic symptoms in the extremities. Myelograms and electroencephalograms are also performed by a skilled medical or osteopathic specialist.

All tests and examinations not readily done as general office procedure should be sent to medical laboratories. The laboratory report plus the clinical findings should assist in making the diagnosis. If the condition is out of the field of podiatry the patient is referred to the medical specialist for treatment.

Bacterial Sensitivity Tests

Infected or slow-healing wounds may be examined for bacterial flora. The colony growth is subjected to antibiotic disks to ascertain the sensitivity of the organism to specific antibiotics.

Nutritional Disorders and Deficiences

Anemia

The extremities are readily affected by anemic disturbances of a systemic origin. Neurologic, circulatory and gastrointestinal disturbances caused by anemia may produce symptoms in the feet.

Edema of the ankles is frequently seen in severe chronic secondary anemia.

Table II[a]
Normal Chemical Composition of Adult Blood and Cerebrospinal Fluid

Constituent	Fluid	Normal range	Units	Chief variations in disease	Podiatric considerations
Calcium	Serum	9.0—11.4 (4.5-5.7)[b] 9.6—11.2 (4.8-5.7)[c] 9.0—10.5 (4.5-5.3)[d]	mg./100 ml figs. in parentheses give mEq./liter	Low in parathyroid tetany, spasmophilia, osteomalacia, severe renal failure; high in hyperparathyroidism	Low blood calcium may be etiologic of cramps and spasms in the feet and legs. Bowing of long bones may be related. Multiple fibrocystic changes in bone may be due to hyperparathyroidism.
Chloride	Blood Plasma[e]	77—90	mEq./liter	Often low in disturbances of acid-base equilibrium and in other conditions involving salt depletion	Chlorides in plasma are increased in some cases of marked edema of the extremities
	CSF	123—128	mEq./liter	Sometimes low in meningitis, especially tuberculous	
Cholesterol Total	Plasma[e]	130—240	mg./100 ml.	High in the nephrotic syndrome, diabetes mellitus, myxedema; low in pernicious anemia,thyrotoxicosis	High plasma cholesterol believed to stimulate development of arteriosclerosis. Useful in differentiating diabetic and arteriosclerotic ulcers from those caused by pernicious anemia
Free	Plasma[e]	60—190	mg./100 ml.	High in various liver diseases	
Creatinine	Plasma[e]	0.6—1.2	mg./100 ml.	High in terminal chronic renal failure	Low values assume importance where pronounced muscular atrophy exists
Glucose	Blood (fasting)	60—95	mg./100 ml.	High in diabetes mellitus, hyperthroidism, excitement	Diabetic foot lesions. Infections, dry skin, fissures, slow healing wounds. Diabetic neuropathy
	CSF	45—70	mg./100 ml.	Low in bacterial meningitis; high in diabetes mellitus	
Nonprotein nitrogen	Blood Plasma[e]	25—50 22—35	mg./100 ml. mg./100 ml.	High in acute and *advanced* chronic renal failure, cardiac failure,intestinal obstruction, fevers, water (and salt) depletion; low in pregnancy	Useful in the differential diagnosis of pedal edema

Phosphatase Acid	Serum	1—4	King-Armstrong units/100 ml.	High in Prostatic carcinoma, especially with metastases invading blood and lymph channels	If values are high and secondary swelling in the extremity is present, the patient should be referred to an internist
Alkaline	Serum	3—12	King-Armstrong units/100 ml.	High in rickets, osteomalacia, hyperparathyroidism, Paget's disease, obstructive jaundice, etc.	Necessary in differential diagnosis of demineralization bending deformities of long bones and abnormal metaphyseal-epiphyseal growth in the feet
Phosphate, inorganic	Plasma[e]	2.5—4.5 1.5—2.7	mg./100 ml. mEq./100 ml.	High in terminal chronic nephritis and in "renal rickets"; low in rickets and in hyperparathyroidism	Inorganic phosphates may be low in multiple bone cysts secondary to hyperparathyroidism
Potassium	Serum	3.5—5.5	mEq./100 ml.	High in Addisonian crisis	Low potassium and chlorides may be induced by diuretics taken to relieve edema of the extremities.
Uric acid	Plasma[e]	2—4	mg./100 ml.	High in gout, advanced renal failure, eclampsia, leukemia	Increased blood uric acid accompanied by clinical symptoms, of gout may develop with prolonged use of diuretics. A thiazide induced hyperuricemia has been a common finding in patients suffering acute foot pain

[a] Adapted from *Stedman's Medical Dictionary*, Ed. 21, Baltimore: The Williams & Wilkins Company, 1966. Modified from C. P. Stewart and D. Dunlop, *Clinical Chemistry in Practical Medicine*, Ed. 6, Edinburgh, E. & S. Livingstone, Ltd. 1962.

[b] Oxalate precipitation.

[c] Flame photometry.

[d] EDTA titration.

[e] Plasma or serum; in other cases the fluid specified is essential or greatly to be preferred.

Diminution in red blood cells and hemoglobin may result from a chronic infection, inability to digest and absorb food, or frequent hemorrhages. The patient feels faint and complains of a "swimming head." Appetite is lost, pulse is rapid and soft. A pallor is noted and dyspnea produced by lack of oxygen-carrying cells is present.

Edema of the feet is common in pernicious anemia. Usually associated with it is a tingling and numbness of the feet and hands indicating a loss of deep sensibility. Spasticity, indicative of a posterior or lateral column sclerosis, may be evident. The onset is insidious and usually occurs in patients over 40 years old. Weakness, dyspnea, lemon-yellow pallor and gastrointestinal disturbances are the usual symptoms. The red cell count is low, color index 1+ and volume index 1+. A neuroanemic syndrome of sensory and motor disturbances coexists in pernicious anemia.

The patient suffering from pernicious anemia may have presenting complaints of chilliness, extreme fatigue and utter exhaustion, edema of the legs and ankles; the tongue is sore and atrophic. The bones are tender to deep pressure.

In chronic hemolytic icterus the long bones show very few changes. Vertical striations may be present in the medulla in hemolytic icterus as well as erythroblastic anemia. All long bones are weakened by calcium absorption resulting in a broader diameter to sustain weight.

Vitamin Deficiency Disorders

Tissue changes resulting from vitamin deficiencies are varied and widespread and produce many types of clinical symptoms.

Vitamin A is essential to growth, normal function of the eye and maintenance of certain specialized tissues. The skin and related structures are affected when deficiency exists. Unusual susceptibility to infection and hyperkeratosis are often early signs of pathology. Sensible perspiration may be absent and skin becomes dry, firm and covered by pigmented papular patches. Vitamin A is believed to act as an epithelial stimulant. Nails have been observed as brittle and splitting in hypovitaminosis. In a series of cases of gangrene and in vascular disease a hypovitaminosis of vitamin A was consistent. Vitamin A taken orally or by injection into plantar warts has shown evidence of being effective treatment.

Vitamin B. The following disturbances have been attributed to deficiency of vitamin B complexes: lesions of the peripheral nerves, characterized by peripheral neuritis, heart muscle lesions, characterized by cardiac insufficiency; and possibly pellagra, acrodynia and combined systemic disease. The lower extremities are most often involved with changes in the sensory and motor mechanism. Polyneuritis from chronic alcoholism is common. Thiamin hydrochloride deficiency seems to have a predilection for producing tenderness of the anterior lower one-third of the tibia.

The chief pathology of hypovitaminosis B is beriberi and peripheral neuritis which is manifest by a heaviness of the legs, tenderness and weakness of the calf muscles, burning of the soles of the feet, numbness, diminished or absent Achilles and patellar reflexes, toe drop, hyperesthesia and anesthesia, and trophic skin lesion. Many times clumsiness, stiffness and sensitivity to cold are improved by administration of vitamin B. Diabetic neuropathies are often treated successfully by vitamin B therapy. The vitamin B group is extensive and should be used selectively.

Dixon and Mastin (1957) recommend the use of the active alcoholic analog of pantothenic acid, a B-complex vitamin, to stimulate epithelization and granulative ulcerations due to diabetes, arteriosclerosis and trauma.

Vitamin C. Scurvy is due to lack of vitamin C. Some of the pathologic changes seen in hypovitaminosis caused by vitamin C deficiency are increased capillary permeability, cutaneous hemorrhages, fragility of bones and secondary anemias. Marked hemorrhage may be noted subcutaneously, under periosteum, in the gums, muscles and urine. Pain on pressure over the affected parts is great. The symptoms are readily remedied by dietary supplements of ascorbic acid or orange juice. Wound healing is accelerated by large doses of this vitamin. Vargas (1961) reported marked improvement of leg aches, burning feet and cramps when he prescribed hesperidin and vitamin C. The usual dosage was 200 mg. of each, t. i. d.

Vitamin D. This vitamin is basically associated with bone growth and development. Vitamin D promotes absorption of calcium and phosphorus from the intestines, reduces loss of calcium and phosphorus in the feces and restores a normal calcium phosphorus relationship in the blood. Vitamin D plays an important role in maintaining foot muscle nerve irritability. It aids in hastening the coagulability of blood. When vitamin D is required for therapy, administration of calciferol and a special diet is indicated.

Vitamin E. Muscular dystrophies, amyotrophic lateral sclerosis have been thought to be due to vitamin E deficiency. Neuromuscular symptoms such as weakness, cramps, burning and aching sensations in calf muscles and in the soles of the feet have been observed in cases of malnutrition involving a lack of vitamin E. Alpha tocopherol is useful in hypertensive heart disease. Tocopherols are destroyed in the presence of unsaturated fatty acids. Schreiber (1955) states that wounds, cuts, burns and ulcers "respond dramatically" to vitamin E unction.

Vitamin K. Excessive spontaneous hemorrhages in the skin and muscles may be due to vitamin K deficiency.

Deficiency of Protein and Fat

This painful foot syndrome was first noted in the Far East during the Japanese evacuation. It was believed to be the result of deficiency of protein, fat and vitamins. When the deficiency factors are not adequately corrected, the patient becomes progressively worse and prolonged severe deficiency may result in death.

The syndrome is characterized by hyperesthesia, increased skin temperature, vasomotor changes of the vessels of the feet, general body wasting and severe burning and aching of the feet. The syndrome is not an angioneurosis and it is said not to be associated with neuropathic diatheses.

8

Podiatric Manifestations of Circulatory Disorders

Diagnosis of circulatory disorders is based on such subjective and objective complaints of the patient as cramps, coldness, fatigue and numbness as well as objective signs of rubor, cyanosis or pallor with diminished pulsations and dystrophic alterations of the skin and nails. It is not the purpose of this text to study in depth the diagnosis and treatment of peripheral vascular disease, but rather to convey the important role of podiatry in the team approach to the prevention and treatment of debilitating sequelae of circulatory disease.

The presence or absence of pulses is not in itself a good indicator of circulatory instability. Pulsations may be present in patients suffering impending gangrene, while a congenital anomaly or arterial replacements may result in absence of pulsations as adequate circulation is supplied by compensating vessels.

The stethoscope, sphygmometer, clinical thermometer and oscillometer are used to evaluate circulatory complaints. More sophisticated equipment such as a podiatry digital plethysmograph may be needed for diagnosis of borderline cases requiring surgical intervention.

If, after thorough examination and careful consideration of the symptoms, the podiatrist believes vascular disease is involved, he should refer the patient to a peripheral vascular consultant for further study and treatment and a cooperative attack on the problem is made by the consultant and the podiatrist.

Bartels and Rullo (1958) recommend that all patients showing evidence of peripheral vascular disease should be thoroughly tested for abnormal glucose tolerance since in a study of 100 patients with symptoms of claudication, paresthesia, rest pain, gangrene, absence of pulsations in the extremities, radiologic evidence of arterial insufficiency, rubor, slow venous filling time, blanching on elevation and ulceration, 43% showed abnormal glucose tolerance tests indicating possible diabetes.

DeWeese (1960) developed a test for arteriosclerosis in patients complaining of fatigue, aching and severe leg cramps with palpable pedal pulses at rest. He had patients run in place at the rate of 140 to 160 steps a minute until claudication occurred and he then showed that pulses disappeared with the activity. DeWeese explained the phenomena as a "shunting of the insufficient blood supply to smaller, vasodilated arteries so that weakened pulsations are observed in the larger arteries."

Observing color changes, temperature alterations and dorsalis pedis, posterior tibial, popliteal and femoral pulsations may be followed by corroborative testing when indicated.

Diagnostic Tests for Circulatory Disorders

Calorimetry is the study of heat loss and skin temperatures. It has been calculated that when the vasoconstrictor impulses are blocked, there is a resulting rise in temperature which may reach 33.5 to 35° C.

Local anesthesia in the form of an infiltration of 5 to 10 ml. of novocaine in a 1% solution into or near the posterior tibial nerve as it lies below the medial malleolus serves well in evaluating the effect of the sympathetic nervous system to the toes. The effect of this local anesthetic is a sharp rise in temperature of the toes as well as paresthesia, numbness and motor changes. Hyperemia of the plantar surface of the foot may develop early and usually subsides readily.

The thermocouple is useful in distinguishing between organic obliterative disease and spastic states as it compares the temperature of two limbs at frequent intervals. It is an important diagnostic aid in peripheral vascular diseases and also in determining progress and prognosis in therapy where peripheral vascular diseases occur. The thermocouple is simple to use and any number of successive readings may be taken without lag or calculations of any kind.

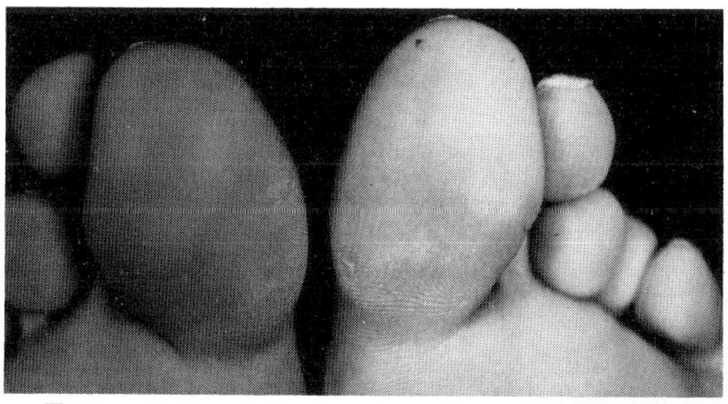

Fig. 8.1. Arteriosclerosis. Note color changes in right hallux.

The podiatry digital plethysmograph provides the podiatrist with data on the vascular system which enables him to: differentiate between vasomotor disease and organic arterial disease, evaluate presurgical vascular conditions, detect certain cardiac irregularities, study circulation of small arteries in the digits, locate areas of obstruction in large vessel disease, determine small artery disease, assess continuity of sympathetic system, and detail the extent of collateral circulation.

The pneumoplethysmograph was originally developed by Windsor and Burch (1963). Lorenzo E. Johnson (1970) assisted in the development of a pneumoplethysmographic device especially suitable for podiatrists.

The findings of Landis and Gibbon have been observed by Kramer (1940)

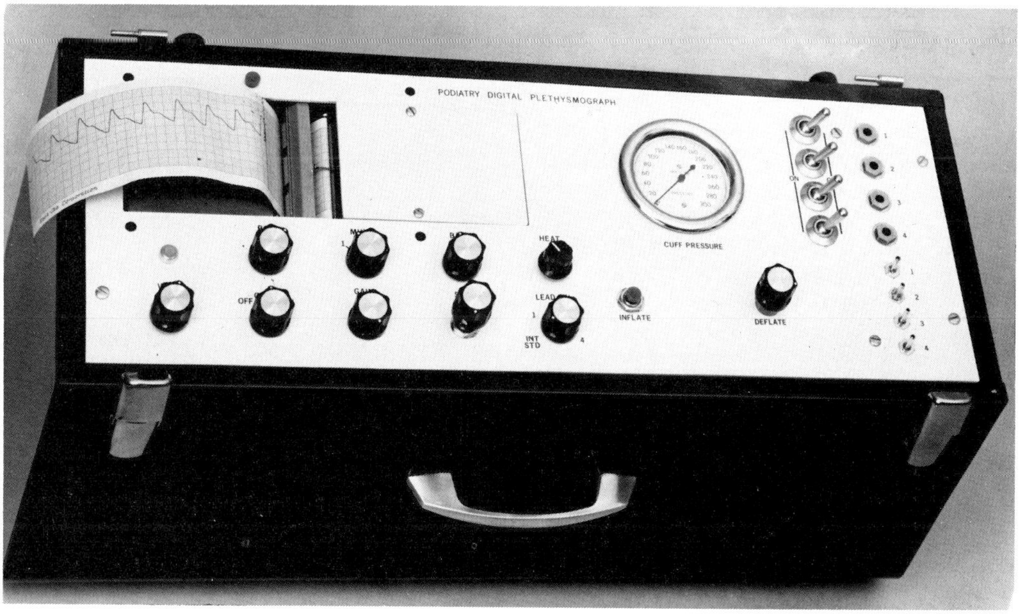

Fig. 8.2. Podiatry plethysmograph.

who has noted excellent results with the following technique for reflex dilatation. They discovered that by immersing the forearms in warm water for 1 hr, reflex vasodilatation can be produced in the lower extremities in the same manner as it is produced by local infiltration. When the temperature rises from 33.5° to 34.5°C., the condition of the circulatory disturbance is vasospastic and the spasm is overcome. When it remains unchanged after immersion, an occlusive vascular disease must be suspected.

Histamine Flare Test. Lewis (1936) studied the reaction of capillaries to various stimuli and discovered that when histamine was inoculated, dilatation of capillaries at the site of injection followed by a zone of erythema about the injection area due to relaxation of arterioles occurred. This is known as the "flare." Wheal formation from outpouring of plasma through the capillary wall usually follows.

The test is performed in the following manner. With the patient completely relaxed in a warm, well-lighted room, 1 drop of a 1:1000 solution of histamine acid phosphate with 0.5% Chloretone as a preservative is placed on the dorsum of the foot, above the lateral ankle and below the knee. Using a fine needle, multiple inoculations are made in these areas. Extreme care must be taken to avoid bleeding.

The reaction takes place from 2½ to 5 min. after inoculation and is accompanied by itching and wheal formation. A circulatory disease may be suspected when the test fails to produce a wheal within 10 min.

Roentgenography. A diagnosis of sclerotic vessels may be confirmed by x-rays. Yale (1957) found that many lateral roentgenograms of the foot taken to confirm a possible calcaneal spur have instead disclosed a sclerosis of the medial calcaneal branch of the posterior tibial artery. The high percentage of such sclerosed vessels in patients 20 to 40 years of age who have no other evidence of circulatory changes in the feet demonstrates the need for the radiograph as a diagnostic adjunct in circulatory involvements. The presence of calcified larger vessels does not necessarily indicate the state of the arterioles. Often the nutritional state of the bones themselves indicates the presence of a circulatory fault by disclosing a general demineralization in bones of the feet. Increased circulation may cause demineralization.

Trophic osteitis or Sudeck's syndrome is a neurocirculatory disturbance. In thrombosis of the vessels, x-ray does not reveal calcifications unless arteriosclerosis exists. Phleboliths and calcified veins suggesting degenerative pathology may be visible on the radiograph. Where infection is present, the circulatory stasis within the Volkman and Haversian canals may result in failure of resorption with subsequent condensation of the affected part.

Arteriography is useful in observing collateral circulation and the behavior of

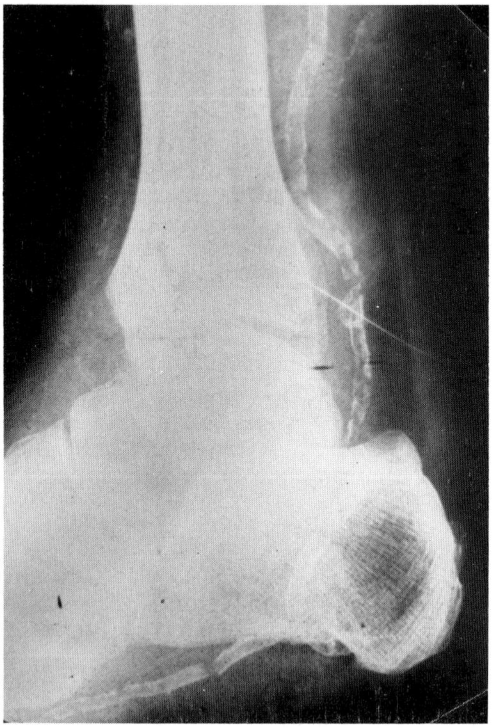

Fig. 8.3. Arteriosclerosis posterior tibial artery. Calcification of posterior tibial artery represented by calcification of arterial wall. Courtesy of *Clinical Foot Roentgenology*, Baltimore: The Williams & Wilkins Company, 1966.

vessels in spasms and claudication and in determining a favorable site for amputation and arterial implants. Radio-opaque substances injected into the arterial tree allow for prompt visualization of defects and occlusions. Abnormal irritability of the vessel injected may result in spasm and local symptoms of pain, redness and increased temperature. This may persist for a few days when some of the solution is injected into the wall of the vessel or outside the vessel. The arteriogram is of great assistance in determining suspected congenital absence of an artery.

Occlusions of the vessel lumen are readily observed. When an artery is partially occluded, a large collateral vessel arises just proximal to the occlusion. This vessel usually passes at right angles to the main artery and then turns abruptly to run a parallel course. This can be visualized in arteriography. Arteriography should be used only by highly qualified radiologists and peripheral vascular surgeons.

Measurement of Plantar Ischemia. Samuel noted that when the patient is in a reclining position and the legs are elevated to a 90-degree angle, and are flexed and extended 40 to 60 times, pallor will occur around the toes and soles of feet within 1 min. if occlusive vascular disorders are present.

Claudication Time. Many times a patient cannot tell how long or how far he can walk before the onset of intermittent claudication. In a test devised by Barker *et al.*, the patient, after a rest, is instructed to walk 120 steps/min. until claudication ensues.

Kisch Test. The reclining patient is asked to flex the thigh on the abdomen and the leg at the knee at the same time. This is followed by extension of the extremity. This action is repeated 30 times/min. Plantar ischemia and claudication time are noted.

Venous Filling Time. Collens and Wilensky studied the filling time of veins in recumbent patients by having patients elevate their limbs until the veins had been drained off and then having them lower the limbs to a dependent position. Observing the medial and lateral marginal veins, they found that the filling time is normally 6 to 10 sec. A slower filling indicates an occlusive vascular disorder. Kramer (1940) and his coworkers found that such other factors as venous disorders may influence the slowness of return. The slow venous filling time may affect only one toe or it may affect the whole foot or the entire foot and leg. A patchy return of color may indicate irregular arterial occlusion or arteriolar spasm.

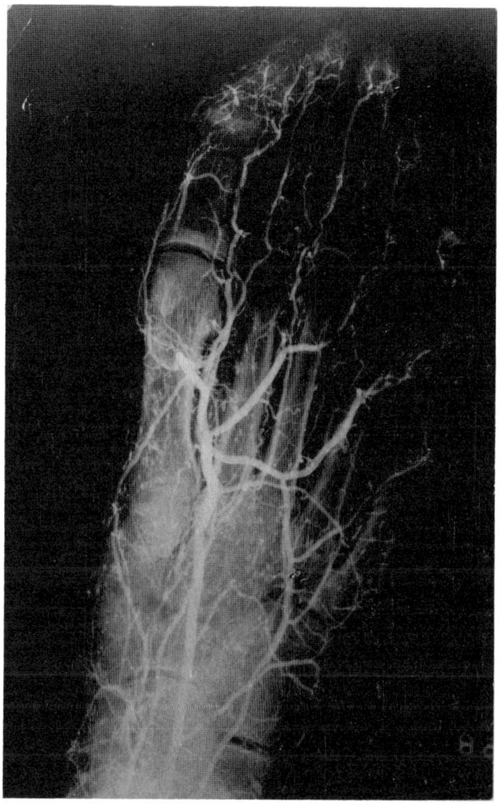

Fig. 8.4. Arteriogram of the foot showing dorsalis pedis, intermetatarsal and digital vessels. Courtesy of *Clinical Foot Roentgenology*, Baltimore: The Williams & Wilkins Company, 1966.

Homan's Sign. The symptoms of deep thrombophlebitis may evade the most careful examiner but in most cases light compression of the calf muscles in the affected limb will elicit pain when deep thrombophlebitis is the cause of symptoms. This sign must be differentiated from simple strain or myositis of the belly of the gastrocnemius or soleus. A tear or rupture of the thin string-like plantaris muscle must also be ruled out. Skin inflammation also limits the reliability of Homan's sign.

Oscillometry. The oscillometer registers the volume of pulsation in the extremity. The number of units over which the needle passes with each systole of the heart is called the index.

Since it was introduced in this country by Samuels in 1927, podiatrists have used the oscillometer in an effort to be more exacting in their interpretations of a patient's circulatory status. The normal oscillometric index in the lower extremity is 8 to 15 at midthigh, 4 to 10 below the knee, 3 to 8 at midleg, 1 to 5 above the ankle, and traces to 1 in the foot.

The value of oscillometry in the diagnosis of circulatory disease has been questioned. Kramer believes that the oscillometer is not the most reliable guide for determining the effect of treatment. In organic vascular disease, collateral circulation and improved nutrition after ganglionectomy are not readily registered.

A differential of occlusive disease from vasospastic diorders is not substantiated by oscillometry. Nor are the causes and mechanisms of circulatory disease disclosed with this technique. Clinical judgment is necessary. Goldy (1956) described the value of recording with an oscillograph oscillations of both extremities simultaneously. The oscillations, recorded on graph paper, become part of the patient's permanent record.

The following factors influence the reliability of oscillometric readings. A loose-fitting cuff takes up too much buffer of the oscillometer capsule and gives a false reading. An edematous leg similarly acts as a buffer. The temperature of the room in which the extremity is exposed can also influence the reading. A cold room produces sufficient vasoconstriction to reduce the oscillometric reading. Fever, which causes diffuse vasodilatation, also influence the reading in the oscillometer. Lowenberg (1958) noted that patients with apparently healthy limbs who complained of the pain on use of the oscillometer cuff were subsequently proven to have phlebitis.

The Pratt modification of Trendelenburg's test is used in locating incompetent communicating branches. The patient's limb is raised and the leg and thigh are gently massaged from the distal end in order to empty all superficial veins. With the leg still in the raised position, an Ace bandage is applied from the toes to high on the thigh. The patient is instructed to stand. The bandage is now slowly unwound while the uncovered areas are carefully observed. An incompetent valve will be evidenced by the sudden appearance of a saccule, or "blow out," caused by back pressure developing against the wall of the superficial vein where blood from the deep system is regurgitating into the superficial vein because of nonpatent valves in the communicating branch.

Pratt's Early Sign of Femoral Thrombosis. In over 80% of pathologic clotting, three dilated veins appear over the tibia. Pratt believes this to be the earliest sign of deep vein thrombosis. The clotting in the calf progresses to the popliteal vein thus occluding the vessel and resulting in swelling, tenderness and cyanosis with possible extension causing a pulmonary embolism.

Perthes' Test. All cases with varicosities of the superficial veins must be tested to ascertain the competency of the communicating deep systems and valves of the veins. The deep veins must be patent before surgery is attempted on the superficial veins. Very often in a deep thrombosis the superficial veins dilate due to an inability of the deep veins to conduct blood away from the extremity.

A tourniquet is applied to the upper thigh with the patient standing to constrict the superficial veins. The patient walks around the room or flexes and extends the extremity vigorously several times. The superficial veins should collapse during the exercise and fill up from above when the tourniquet is released.

When the deep veins are not patent the superficial veins remain dilated during this test and the test is negative. Injection of the superficial veins is then contraindicated.

Venous Disorders

Varicose veins are common and easily diagnosed. They are tortuous dilitations of the peripheral veins with a bluish or blue-brown-red discoloration of the skin, edema and often a complicating inflammation and ulcer. Transitory phlebitis may be a feature of thromboangiitis obliterans.

Increased blood pressure, low abdominal pressure on the veins, weakened leg musculature, and venous cusp degeneration may be the direct causes of varicose veins. Imbalanced feet, obesity, occupations requiring long periods of standing, trauma, constricting garters, rubber panties, and pregnancy are predisposing factors. Phlebitis may incite the formation of varicosities or be a secondary complication of varicose veins.

Varicosities usually appear between the ages of 25 and 50 and occur more often in females than in males. There are hereditary predispositions in some families. The patient complains of a heavy feeling in the extremities followed by a dull ache and often severe pain. Fatigue is common and very often a symptom of fullness or swelling is noted. The edema which occurs after long periods of standing may be unilateral and reach its greatest severity toward the end of the day. The swelling is generally diminished in the morning or upon arising after periods of rest.

Complicating phlebitis may occur after trauma, operative surgery or following septic diseases. The vessels are cord-like and indurated, and redness, heat, swelling and severe pain are noted around the affected part. The long saphenous vein is involved more commonly than the short saphenous vein. Phlebitis is most commonly found around the ankle and extends upward. The femoral vein is often affected with venous thrombosis as an etiologic factor. The skin frequently becomes red or cyanotic in venous thrombosis.

A varicose eczema with dry scaly patches or scales and crusts with underlying oozing excoriations may complicate varicose veins. The superficial vessels break down and cause itching, burning and pain. Excoriations may result in ulcerations with secondary infections. Lymphangitis and septicemia can result from faulty care and uncleanliness; osteomyelitis is an infrequent complication.

Phleboliths may develop in chronic venous insufficiency and are visible on radiograph. They show up as rounded calcareous bodies of increased density. A calcified vein reveals streaks in the vein walls and must be differentiated from arteriosclerosis in which the vein looks tube-like.

Thrombosis of the peripheral veins may be consequent upon some preexisting disease. Thrombi may be septic or bland. The femoral vessels are most commonly involved and there are irregular intervals of chills and associated

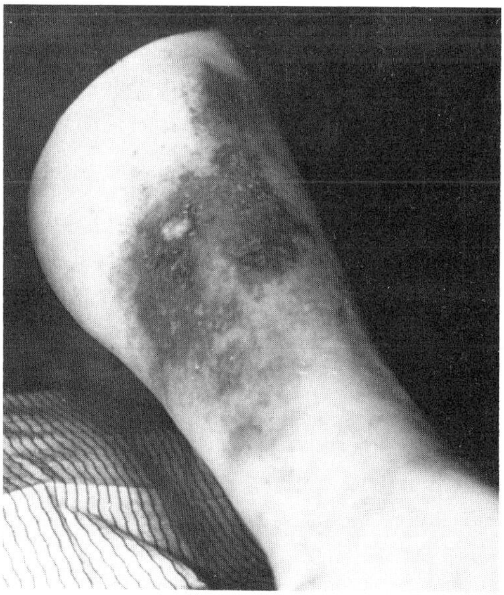

Fig. 8.5. Varicose eczema secondary to ruptured and distended veins. Note extensive skin pigmentation.

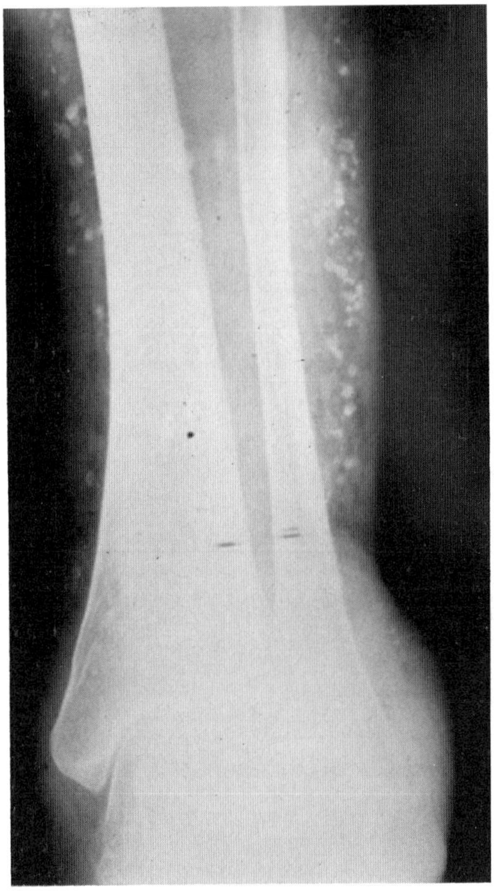

Fig. 8.6. Phleboliths. Rounded calcareous deposits in superficial veins may break down and cause ulcerations. Courtesy of *Clinical Foot Roentgenology*, Baltimore: The Williams & Wilkins Company, 1966.

moderate temperatures. In severe septic cases the temperature may rise as high as 105° F.

A deep thrombosed vein is cord-like; a dull ache, tingling, numbness and vague feeling of discomfort is noted. Edema begins in the most distal parts and extends upward; the skin becomes pale, cold and shiny.

Brennan (1965) noted that on an annual basis there are at least 400,000 victims of postsurgical thromboembolic disease causing 18,000 deaths. Anesthesia resulting in voluntary muscle flaccidity is an important factor. The flaccidity impairs the pumping action of the leg musculature resulting in a sluggish venous return producing a phlebothrombotic nidus.

Thrombophlebitis and phlebothrombosis must be differentiated from varicose veins. Phlebothrombosis presents a thrombus that is loosely attached to the vein wall. It may appear after surgery or it may occur during pregnancy or postpartum. Minimal swelling does not reflect the seriousness of the problem which often ends in pulmonary embolism and critical illness. Chronic venous insufficiency generally follows thrombophlebitis and phlebothrombosis.

Treatment. Compression bandages and/or elastic stockings may relieve symptoms.

Periodic elevation of the extremities decreases pressure against the expanded vein wall. In the event of an acute inflammatory episode elevation and the use of an ice bag over the affected parts are recommended. Sometimes hot wet compresses are effective. The pain is relieved by systemic analgesics and the infection is controlled by antibiotics.

Thrombosis is treated with anticoagulants under an internist's supervision. Saphenous ligation and tying off superficial veins or stripping by a vascular surgeon may be necessary. Occlusion of sacculated veins by injections of sclerosing agents may be effective in controlling further degeneration.

Elliot (1956) states that injection therapy, high ligation, multiple ligation, and high ligation with retrograde injection-are inadequate as primary forms of treatment of varicose veins because of recurrence and such complications as deep vein thrombosis.

Ulcerations are treated by venous "heart" dressings, gelatin boots, compression bandages, bed rest and elevation, suitable antibiotic and enzymatic debriding medications, systemic antibiotics and high protein diets to decrease capillary fragility.

Varicose eczema is treated with antipruritic anti-inflammatory corticosteroid preparations, emollients for dry, scaling skin, and mildly astringent applications where weeping exists. Occlusive gelatin compression dressings relieve the physiologic dysfunction.

The use of physiologic saline soaks in the acute stages followed by occlusive gelatin flexible castings often relieves the dermatologic symptoms and aids in repair of ulcerations.

Gertner (1956) reported the successful treatment of 20 cases of superficial thrombophlebitis by injection of a suspension of 0.5 ml. of hydrocortisone suspension and 1.0 ml. tetracaine solution directly into the painful indurated thrombotic process.

Owens (1961) recommends the use of adenylic acid therapy as adenosine-5-monophosphate in the form of its sodium salt to relieve edema, inflammation, pain and pruritis resulting from thrombophlebitis. A series of intramuscular injections given daily for 3 days and then on alternate days for a total of 10 injections is suggested for mild to moderate cases. One milliliter of 20 mg./ml. is the usual daily dose followed by 1 or 2 injections weekly to maintain relief after symptoms subside.

Arteriovenous fistula occurs as a result of communication of artery and vein due to trauma and may also be of congenital origin. The patient may be aware of a murmur in the region of a penetrating wound. The foot is a common site for such an injury. Ischemia results in atrophy and gangrene of the distal portions of the toes at an early date. Later the circulation improves to the point of increased temperatures and increased physical development of the affected side.

Varicose veins are evident in congenital arteriovenous fistula and port wine cavernous hemangioma may be present in 50% of such cases. Increased perspiration, hair growth, enlargement of the limb, skin warmth and an oxygen saturation of venous blood is present in the affected limb. Surgical excision of the defect and very often vascular grafts are required to correct arteriovenous fistulas. Early consultation with a vascular surgeon is indicated.

Edema

Pearlman (1957) offered the following definition of edema. "Edema is a condition in which the volume of extracellular water on the outside of the circulating intravascular compartment is increased. Normally there is a constant equal, well-regulated exchange of water and electrolytes through the capillary wall from the circulation into the interstitial spaces and returning to the circulation." Generally the maintenance of fluid balance depends on the concentration of serum proteins, the amount of protein in the interstitial tissues, hydrostatic pressure in the capillaries, tissue tension, and the flow of lymph.

Helfand (1959) noted that an "increase in capillary blood pressure, hypoproteinemia, increased capillary permeability, venous or lymphatic obstruction, or a defect in the water balance of the body will be found in the presence of edema."

Edema may be symmetrical or asymmetrical. Swellings are classified according to etiology. Asymmetrical edema may be caused by congenital anomalies, varicosities, sprain, cellulitis, gout, drugs, artificial ligatures, pressure from ill-fitting footgear, poor posture and pantyhose constriction.

Symmetrical types of edema are classified according to the following etiology: Congestive heart failure, pernicious anemia, chronic kidney disease, secondary anemia, wasting diseases (carcinoma, tuberculosis), diabetes, obstruction of inferior vena cava, prolonged convalescence, Milroy's disease, myxedema and menstrual edema.

Sensitivity to certain foods or chemicals may cause wheals accompanied by

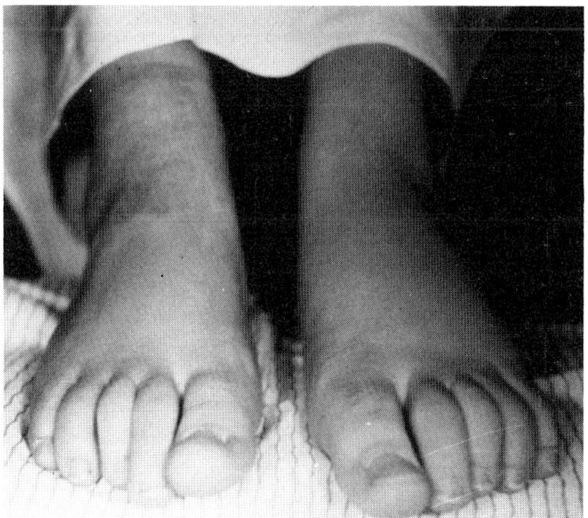

Fig. 8.7. Asymmetrical cellulitis; edema with deep rubor in left foot.

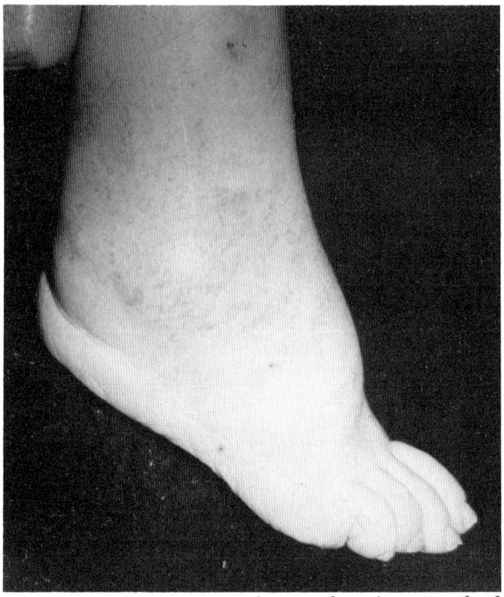

Fig. 8.8. Cardiac edema showing marked swelling and distention of superficial veins".

swelling. Wheals in symmetrical edema may be uniformly rose red to purple with a white periphery. They also may be flat or elevated conical papules surrounded by vesicles. Often they are linear and several inches long.

Drug edema may occur from such drugs as aspirin, bromides, iodides, diphtheria antitoxin, mercurials, sulfa drugs, penicillin and others which cause urticarial lesions accompanied by edema.

Lymphatic Obstruction. An obstruction in the removal of the lymph fluid may be caused by inflammation, the pressure of tumors, parasites and tumors of the lymphatics. Lymphangitis with occlusion of lymph vessels causes an excessive accumulation of proteins in the interstitial fluid. Growth of fibroblasts and production of scars is stimulated. Moist, warm macerated skin with fissures and vesicles between the toes may cause repeated attacks of lymphangitis and lymphatic obstruction. Dermatomycotic infections often reoccur. Young and DeWolfe (1960) report on 25 consecutive cases of recurrent lymphangitis with dermatophytosis.

Onset in these cases is sudden; severe symptoms of pain develop over a period of a few hours and are attended by chills and fever up to 106°F. The chills and fever last from a few hours to 3 days. Headache, fatigue, malaise, nausea and vomiting are common. The extremity becomes swollen and tender. Acute symptoms may persist from 4 to 14 days, but swelling will persist until inflammation subsides.

Treatment consists of bed rest and elevation of the part, local antifungal applications and systemic antibiotics for secondary infection. Inflammation is reduced with oral or parenteral anti-inflammatory or antifungal agents. The use of anticoagulants and often dissection of vascular growths or aspiration of thrombi from the lymphatics may be necessary to maintain flow of lymph in the larger vessels.

True elephantiasis, caused by *Acanthocheilonema perstans* (*Filaria sanguinis hominis*), is rare in the United States. Pseudoelephantiasis is due to longstanding lymphatic obstruction of other etiologies. The skin becomes roughened, thickened and fibrous. A deep thrombosis, an operation which interferes with the lymphatics, or postfracture complications may cause pseudoelephantiasis.

Edema of Inflammation. Edema may be caused by increased capillary permeability resulting from inflammation which occurs when fluid accumulates in the tissues. An infected toe, a suppurating wound or an infected mycotic lesion may be present. Edema of inflammation is not influenced by gravity because of the increased fibrin in the soft tissues. The lymphatics are obstructed by clots or leukocytes and are compressed by the exudate.

Treatment. Infection must be controlled with local and oral antifungal agents and such antibiotic medication as griseofulvin and proteolytic enzymes when necessary to decrease capillary permeability. Resolution of thrombi and fibrin accumulations decreases the edema.

Cardiac Edema. Cardiac edema is a congestive swelling caused by passive venous congestion secondary to myocardial insufficiency. The diminished circulation causes increased venous pressure resulting in increased capillary pressure and permeability. Such myocardial insufficiency may result from long-standing valvular abnormality.

Edema is a very important sign of cardiac failure. It usually begins in the feet and legs and spreads upward at a time when the circulatory system is decompensated. As the cardiac problem worsens, the edema, which at first is slight and appears only toward the end of the day, becomes greater and more extensive. The failure of circulation in the extremities is due to insufficient cardiac strength and overly distended veins. Pulmonary engorgement produces intrathoracic pressure and impaired respiration and cardiac function. At first dyspnea subsides after rest but later it is noted even at rest. A pitting edema is noted over the shoe tips in the early stages. The degree of cyanosis generally depends on the amount of myocardial damage. The podiatrist is often the first doctor to see and recognize this problem. Immediate referral to an internist for treatment is indicated.

Renal Edema. Since renal edema resembles cardiac edema, the swelling is not too difficult to differentiate. However, the fluid is less influenced by gravity. Decreased blood protein causes decreased osmotic pressure in the blood. Osmotic pressure in the tissues remains high and edema results. The edema is present in the morning on arising. The podiatrist may note the early changes in renal edema while treating the complications of pressure produced by the swelling.

Treatment. Maintaining a high blood protein to increase osmotic pressure in the blood may be helpful in decreasing osmotic pressure in the tissues. Consultation with a urologist or internist is indicated since local treatment is unproductive. A differential diagnosis of the etiology is essential if complications are to be avoided.

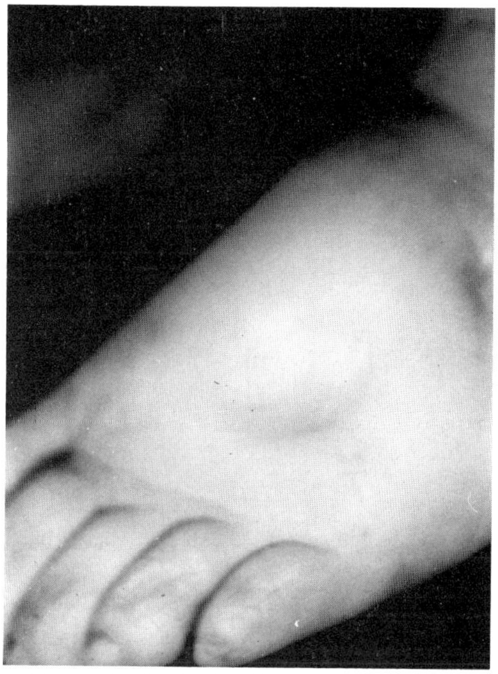

Fig. 8.9. Marked pitting edema which is usually bilateral and of systemic origin. This case was the result of renal pathology.

In famine edema blood proteins are low because of an abnormal diet. This results in decreased osmotic pressure leading to a loss of fluids which pass to the tissues. The presence of local inflammations and infections in corns, calluses and nail grooves is not uncommon.

Treatment. Increase of blood protein is necessary to maintain fluids within the blood vessels. Nutritional supplements are indicated as prescribed by the internist. All pressure on the toes and heels is to be avoided.

Milroy's disease is a chronic familial and hereditary condition occurring as edema of the legs without obstruction or constitutional etiology. The swelling may be unilateral or bilateral with a solid type of edema. Milroy's disease occurs more frequently in females and is first observed early in childhood. The swollen and nonswollen parts are differentiated at the joints such as the ankle or knee. In reducing calluses and corns in patients with Milroy's disease, the podiatrist must exercise extreme care to avoid secondary infections and ulcers.

Treatment. Since the etiology is unknown, the best approach to treatment is even compression of the affected extremity by elastic bandages or stockings extending from behind the metatarsophalangeal joints upward to midthigh. Shoe fitting problems become critical and allowance should be made for the edema.

Myxedema commonly occurs in women but also occurs in males with hypothroidism. The edema is bilateral with noticeably dry, thick skin. The patient is mentally dull, has precocious development of hair on the face with thinning or loss of hair elsewhere on the body. The edema is solid and of the non-pitting variety around the ankles. Skin around the heels and toes may be dry, fissured and ulcerated.

Treatment Treatment by an internist is necessary to reverse the symptoms. There is no physiologic advantage to the use of compression bandages in this condition as prescribed for Milroy's disease. The dry skin is treated with emollients, the fissures and ulcers by the use of tincture of benzoin compound and protective bandages. A plastic heel cup may protect the heel from undue stress.

Menstrual edema is a normal finding in healthy premenopausal females. Both ankles may become swollen 1 to 3 days before menstruation, the shoes are tight and the patient has an increased body weight caused by excess water retention. The swelling may cause pressure and pain in the feet which resolve naturally as the edema subsides.

Treatment. Rest and elevation of the extremities and the use of mild diuretics beginning about 7 days prior to the onset of the menstrual flow help minimize edema. Consultation with a gynecologist should be suggested.

Pregnancy Edema. Over 50% of pregnant women show evidence of edema. In many instances the patient is toxic or presents nephritic symptoms. The edema may manifest itself as an elastic puffiness which does not pit. When the edema is generalized and is accompanied by albuminuria and hypertension, toxemia, renal or hepatic disease is possible and the patient should be referred to the obstetrician for treatment. Mechanical factors such as tight garters, muscular weakness, obstruction of circulation by pressure from an enlarged uterus and varicose veins may be etiologic. Abnormal foot function and faulty foot structure may contribute to edema in pregnancy and should be treated. Elastic stockings to support venous flow is beneficial.

Sprain. In sprain there is a history of trauma which results in early edema and pain. Venous thrombosis caused by the trauma may cause swelling. Marked connective tissue inflammation may result in a fibrosis with development of a firm, indurated edema at the site of the injury. Fracture must be ruled out to facilitate repair.

Treatment. The most common sprain affects the lateral ankle joint. Treatment of choice is adhesive tape immobilization in a neutral right-angled position. The use of an ice bag is mandatory with acute sprain. Oral enzymes aid in absorbing and dispersing fluids. Hyaluronidase injections act as a medium for dispersion. Analgesics commensurate with the degree of pain reduce discomfort.

Cellulitis. Acute cellulitis is easily recognized by all the signs of infection: redness, swelling, heat and pain. Infections result in cellulitis around the ankle with associated edema of the affected parts. In a study by Travis (1965), 10% of the admissions to a military hospital were for foot infections. A high percentage of these involved cellulitis secondary to infection by *Staphylococcus aureas.*

Treatment. Treatment of the etiologic cause of cellulitis is necessary. This may include treating severe trauma or secondary infections. There should be no pressure on the cellulitic tissue. Warm, moist dressing, elevation, incision, drainage and proper antibiotics are essential.

Phlegmasia Alba Dolens Thrombophlebitis. Thrombophlebitis of the iliac and femoral veins may be a mild or a deep phlebitis with marked swelling of the leg and ankle. The disease often complicates serious febrile disease, abortion, pelvic operation, childbirth and fracture. The patient is usually young with a history of having been confined to bed for several days.

Many cases are called to our attention wherein ill-fitting footgear, circular garters and abnormal pressure from occupational stress cause edema. Removal of local pressure relieves the stasis which in some cases extends up to the knees. Hosiery with elastic tops pressing just below the knee causing pressure on the saphenous veins may produce afternoon and night edema which subsides during the day. Tight shoes, straps or short-vamped pumps may cause swelling of the feet and toes from pressure on the dorsal superficial veins. One-strap shoes accompanied by an open throat of such shoes causes pressure on the dorsal venous arch producing local and generalized swelling of the limb.

Obliterative Arterial Disease

Calcification of the arteries in the feet may be of the tunica media type (Mönckeberg's) with few symptoms of an obliterating disease. Intermittent claudication, decreased skin temperature, absent or feeble pulsations and such color as marked pallor and cyanosis in elderly people are the early signs of arteriosclerosis obliterans. Gangrene is a common sequela. Jahsman (1956) points out that claudication pain in hip or thigh muscles with or without leg pain arouses suspicion of segmental occlusion of the femoral or iliac arteries with or without more distal occlusive arterial disease. Important studies on arterial disease have been made by DeBakey *et al.* (1957) and Pepin and Lauritsen (1962).

Treatment. Cranly (1956) presents the following criteria for grading the severity of obliterative arterial disease of the lower extremities.

Decrease in amplitude of the dorsalis pedis and posterior tibial pulsations indicates grade one disease. Treatment consists of good foot hygiene, avoidance of extremes of heat and cold and use of tobacco. Vasodilating drugs are helpful and surgery is not usually desirable.

Absence of the dorsalis pedis and posterior tibial pulses is characteristic of grade two disease. Treatment involves lumbar sympathectomy and/or use of vasodilators such as cyclandelate (Cyclospasmol), nylidrin HCl (Arlidin) in 6-mg. tablets and niacin in 25- to 100-mg. tablets. Nylidrin HCl in combination with vitamin E has been helpful in relieving symptoms. Quinine sulfate or Benadryl taken at bedtime can relieve cramps. Cyclospasmol is a peripheral spasmolytic and vasodilator available in 200-mg. capsules and 100-mg. tablets. The dosage is 400 to 800 mg./day taken in two to

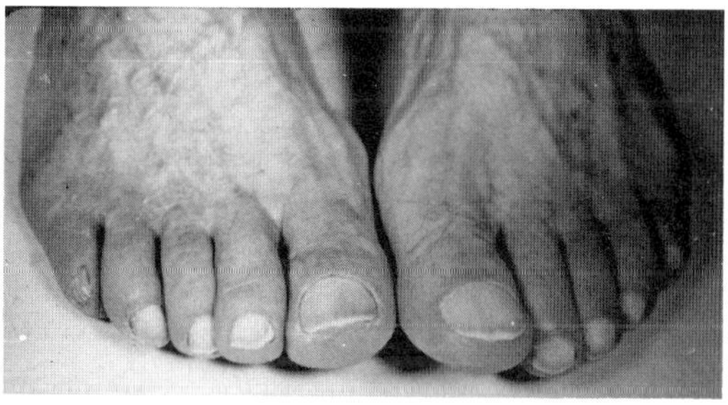

Fig. 8.10. Endarteritis obliterans showing change ranging from rubor to cyanosis. Absence of hair on right hallux indicates greater circulatory distress.

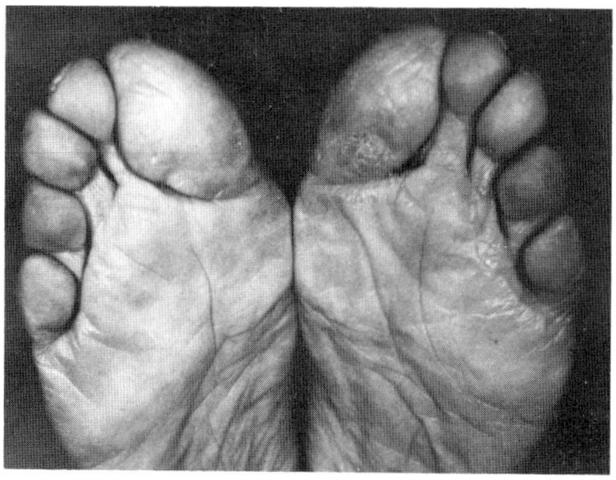

Fig. 8.11. Arteriosclerosis obliterans showing cyanosis in left foot and pallor in right foot.

four doses. Definitive angiography is helpful in approaching the surgical treatment of occlusive vascular disease.

Absence of the dorsalis pedis, posterior tibial and popliteal pulses characterizes grade three disease. If vessels are judged suitable for by-pass grafts in thigh or leg, this may be the treatment of choice. Lumbar sympathectomy and long-term use of vasodilating drugs, good foot hygiene and avoidance of infection, and Buerger exercises may be indicated.

Grade four disease is indicated when there is rest pain and rubor on dependency. A femoral artery block may have to be removed. Vasodilators do not help in this stage. Quinine sulfate capsules 2 to 5 grains h. s. for leg cramps may be beneficial.

In grade five disease there is continuous pain, petechial hemorrages on the dorsum of the foot and gangrene. Amputation is the treatment of choice in this advanced disease.

Raynaud's Disease

Raynaud's disease may occur in both males and females. The hand and/or toes may undergo color changes precipitated by cold and emotional stress. These changes vary from pallor to cyanosis and a deep redness of the toes. Slight swelling, paresthesias and excessive perspiration may be seen early. The tips of the toes undergo necrosis; scleroderma is considered pathognomonic.

This is a vasospastic disorder occurring in cold-sensitive people. However, vasospastic changes on exposure to cold may also occur in arteriosclerosis and thromboangiitis obliterans. A peripheral vascular specialist should be consulted early.

Treatment. Sympathectomy is helpful when Raynaud's is the primary disease. Treatment of local manifestations is imperative to prevent infection. Excess sweating and mycotic infections can be reduced with dilute potassium permanganate soaks. Protection of the toes and weight-bearing areas from trauma prevents serious breakdown of tissue. The feet should not be exposed unnecessarily to increased temperatures or to cold. Smoking should be prohibited. Vasodilators must be used with caution since they can congest the area and create undue pressure on the embarrassed circulatory supply. Tolazoline (Priscoline) taken 25 mg. 4 to 6 times daily may be beneficial. Posterior tibial nerve blocks often produce a helpful reflex dilatation.

Thromboangiitis Obliterans

Thromboangiitus affects men under 50 and is a generalized disease often involving the viscera, blood vessels, heart, lungs, kidney and brain. Pain in the legs, intermittent claudication and migratory phlebitis with absent or diminished pul-

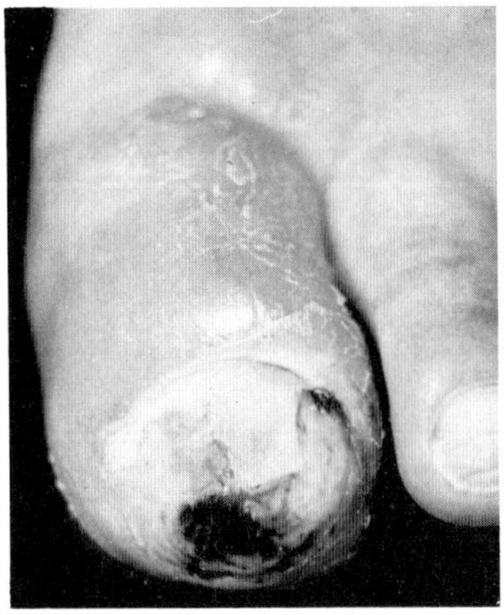

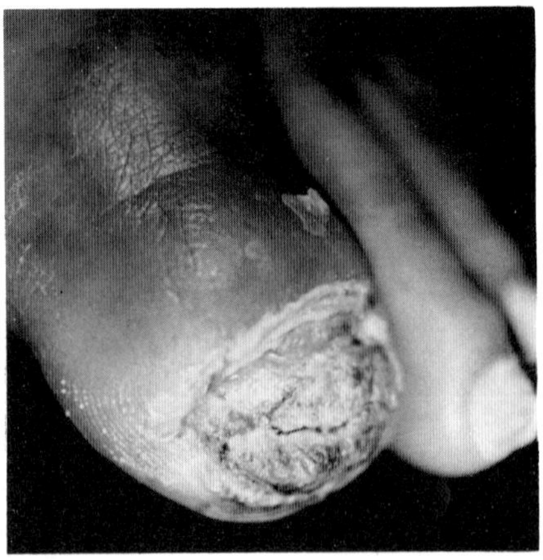

Fig. 8.12. Thromboangiitis obliterans. Gangrene at distal end of hallux although part of nail is viable. Note cellulitis proximal to nail plates.

Fig. 8.13. Same as Fig. 8.12. showing progressive destruction of distal phalangeal tuft.

sations are pathognomonic. Marked rubor on dependency and pallor on elevation is noted. Ulcers followed by necrosis and gangrene of the feet is a common sequela to this systemic obliterating arterial disease.

Immersion Foot

Immersion of the feet for long periods of time in water, mud or damp shoes in temperatures above freezing may cause a variety of severe and disabling symptoms. The colder the water, the more rapid the onset of ischemia and vasospasticity. The condition is aggravated by time, constrictive shoes and hose, dehydration and nutritional deficiencies, a decrease in systemic temperature, trauma and inactivity.

Numbness and coldness accompanied by anesthesia in localized patches, cyanosis or pallor with petechial hemorrhage is noted early. Later, the feet burn and get hot with redness. Swelling, paresthesia and intense pain followed by bullous lesions and secondary infections may occur at this time. The sequela to this pathology is a late vasospasticity. The skin temperature subsides and vascular tone improves. The pain may persist and the tendons contract with flexion deformities. Gangrene may occur.

Treatment. A comfortable body temperature should be maintained. Hose and shoes should be changed frequently. The feet should be well-powdered and kept dry and warm.

If symptoms have developed, the feet should be kept dry and warm and the legs elevated. Blisters should not be broken. The feet should be exposed to room temperature and dried by cooling with a fan to reduce tissue metabolism. A hexachlorophene solution is used to bathe skin lesions and maintain a diminished bacterial flora. Bacterial sensitivity tests are made where open lesions are present. The antibiotic of choice for the bacteria present is given. The patient should not smoke. Anticoagulants should be used where thrombosis is present. Extreme cold should be avoided. A warm climate is recommended.

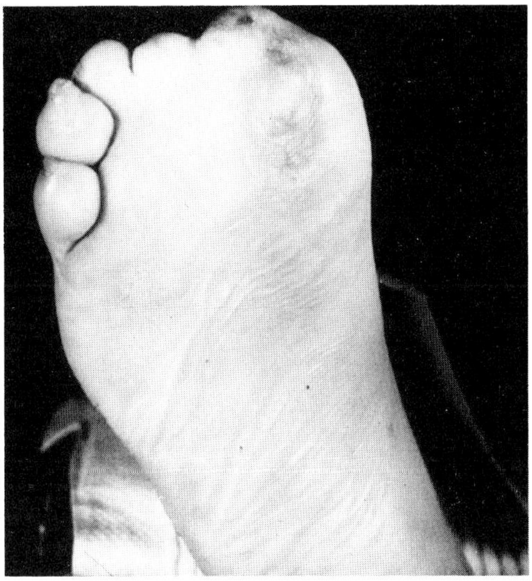

Fig. 8.14. Amputation of toes following gangrene due to frostbite. Skin graft plantar surface of first metatarsal head.

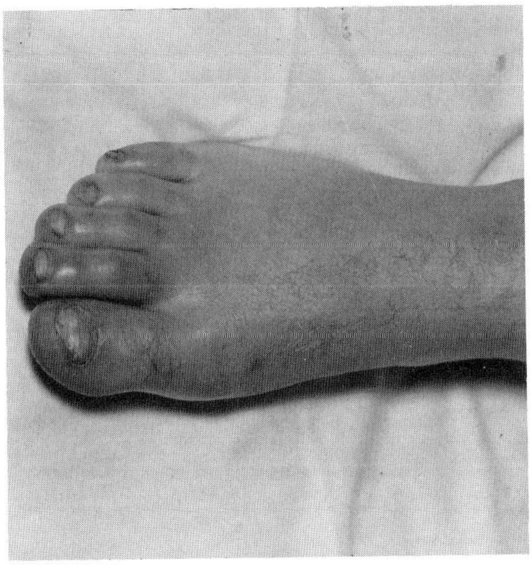

Fig. 8.15. Immersion foot. Hyperemia and edema. Courtesy of Armed Forces Institute of Pathology, #3550.

Ainhum

Ainhum, a condition of unknown etiology which is most frequently observed in Negroes, is characterized by a firm, constrictive, fibrous band on the undersurface of the fifth toe. Eventually the entire toe is involved. The condition must be differentiated from helomas and

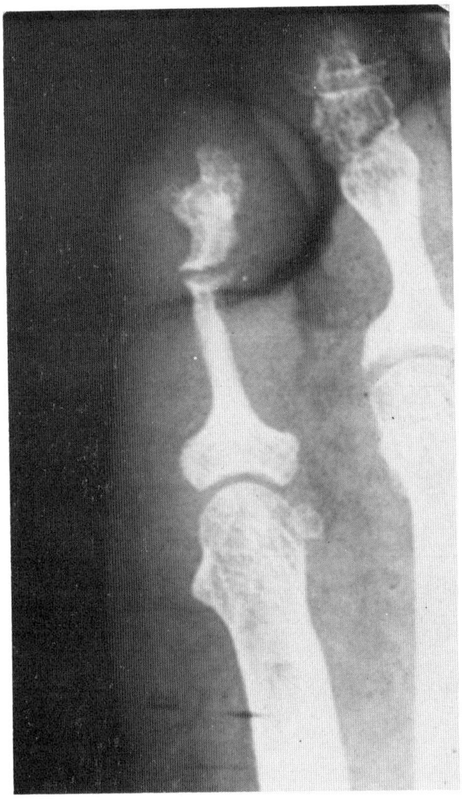

Fig. 8.16. Ainhum. Courtesy of *Clinical Foot Roentgenology*, Baltimore: The Williams & Wilkins Co., 1966.

tylomas. The end of the toe becomes bulbous and painful and the clinically visible band may become calloused and indurated. The circulation is gradually cut off resulting in ischemia followed by dry gangrene. Repair proximal to the site of the constrictive band is usually good following removal of the distal end of the toe.

Constricted digits with a starfish keratosis of the dorsum of the hands and feet accompanied by hyperkeratosis of the palms and soles may be due to "keratoma hereditaria mutilans" Gibbs (1966) and must be differentiated from ainhum if proper treatment is to be instituted.

Treatment consists of prescribing analgesics and watchful waiting for a line of demarcation. Amputation may be necessary to relieve pain.

Gangrene

Gangrene is defined as the death or rotting of tissue in a part of the body resulting from insufficient blood circulation in the affected tissues. Gangrene may be caused by embolism, arterial thrombosis, diabetes, Raynaud's disease, ergot poisoning, trauma, chemical destruction of tissue and extremes of temperature. The patient with occlusive arterial disease develops gangrenous areas by the occlusion of the vessels and an infarction of the tissue they fail to supply. Vasculitis may be an early sign of impending gangrene. Absence of pulsations and circulation to the part are symptoms of gangrene. The part is cool to touch; function, color and sensory perception are lost. The etiology of gangrene is based on a complete obliteration of arterial supply to the affected parts. Samuels (1962) recognized the presence of mycotic infection as an exciting factor in gangrene. Gangrene may be either dry or moist.

Dry gangrene is the loss of nourishment to a part followed by mummification. The affected limb becomes dry, indurated, black, shriveled and parchment-like. Dry gangrene has little tendency to spread and is only mildly painful. Arterial occlusion results in a well-defined line of demarcation separat-

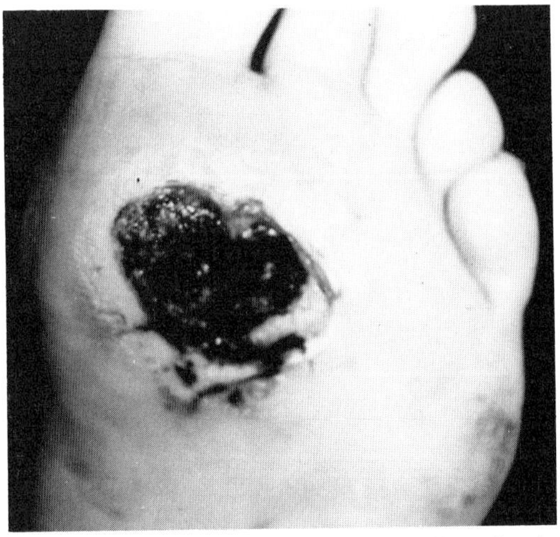

Fig. 8.17. Infective gangrenous diabetic ulcer.

ing the healthy from the pathologic tissues. The distal end of a toe in ainhum may undergo necrosis and gangrene in the advanced stages.

Treatment. Exercise is therapeutic and vasospasm should be controlled with drugs such as sublingual nitroglycerine prescribed by the internist. A clean, dry site should be maintained to allow mummification and a line of demarcation to develop. The patient should avoid use of tobacco. Reflex vasodilatation should be provided. Gravity aids blood flow.

When all soft tissues have become mummified and adjacent viable tissue appears well-vascularized pursue the following course. Anesthesia may not be necessary if mummification is present. Nerve block anesthesia with Xylocaine 1% plain may have to be used. Care must be taken not to embarrass viable circulation. Sterile preparation includes draping of the part. With scissors, cut through necrotic tissue at the line of demarcation and remove the gangrenous part. Care must be taken not to cut viable tissue. Rarely is anesthesia necessary. Dry dressing using antibiotic powder of choice is helpful. Heat in any form should not be used.

Support of local treatment by meticulous systemic treatment by a qualified medical doctor is mandatory. Sympathectomy is indicated. Amputation at site of adequate circulation proximal to necrotic tissue may embarrass circulation and allow for spread of gangrene.

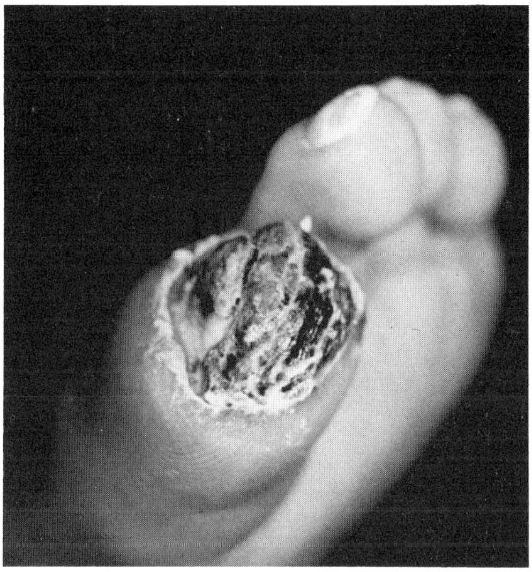

Fig. 8.18. Dry gangrene distal end of hallux.

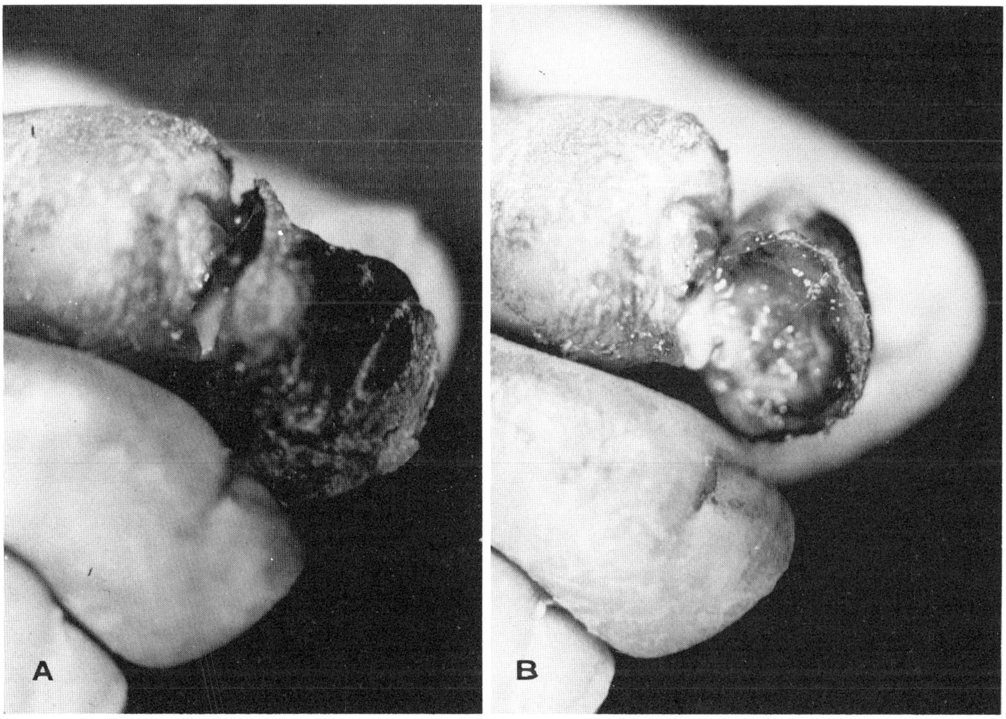

Fig. 8.19. *A*, dry gangrene showing line of demarcation. *B*, distal end of toe attached only by flexor tendon.

Foley (1958) recommended walking as a treatment for gangrene of the feet and legs. He states that "one of the greatest stimuli to the development of collateral blood flow in the legs is walking."

Samuels (1957) and Downie and O'Connor (1957) advise the use of conservative treatment before mutilating amputation of an infected foot. Incision and drainage followed by a topical broad-spectrum antibiotic often relieves the tissue of embarrassment allowing collateral circulation to take over. Systemic antibiotics cannot reach the infected tissue if circulation is diminished.

Blau (1960) described a conservative treatment in 64 cases of vascular insufficiency and gangrenous ulceration. Treatment consists of debridement, non-irritating foot soaks, Panthoderm with 0.5% neomycin, and oral nylidrin HCl, a peripheral vascular dilator. The patient was encouraged to be ambulatory to aid in vasodilitation. I have used modifications of this treatment with moderate success.

Dubois and Arterberry (1962) described five cases of gangrene due to systemic lupus erythematosis which they treated with fair success using large doses of steroids. Lassen *et al.* (1968) cited five cases of gangrene that were improved by increasing blood pressure about 15 mm. of mercury. This was accomplished by using fluorocortisone or deoxycorticosterone to induce moderate hypertension.

Jones *et al.* (1970), in a review of exposure to cold, recommended rapid thawing of the frozen extremity, bed rest, nourishing diet, antibiotics and antitetanus if infection occurred. Apparent gangrene may only involve superficial layers of skin. Delays of 60 to 90 days in amputation is desirable.

Rakow (1972) notes that osteopathy secondary to peripheral neuropathy must not be construed as osteomyelitis and impending gangrene. Incision and drainage may embarrass the circulation.

Wet gangrene is a necrosis of tissue followed by destruction due to excessive moisture; decomposition occurs through the action of putrefactive bacteria. Gases accumulate in the tissues and the line of demarcation is ill-defined. The extremely painful part is purple and swollen. Wet gangrene may be due to venous thrombosis and bullous lesions may be evident early. Diabetics commonly develop this type of moist gangrene when widespread infection exists.

Treatment. This type of necrosis spreads rapidly and is not easily controlled. Consultation must be sought with an internist or vascular surgeon. Bacterial sensitivity tests and early use of systemic and local antibiotics of choice may control the fulminating character of this disorder. Use of peripheral vascular dilators may be helpful. Sympathectomy is indicated.

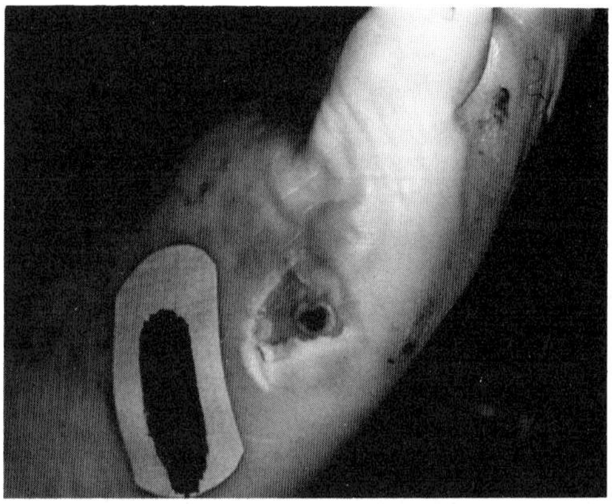

Fig. 8.20. Infective gangrenous ulcer.

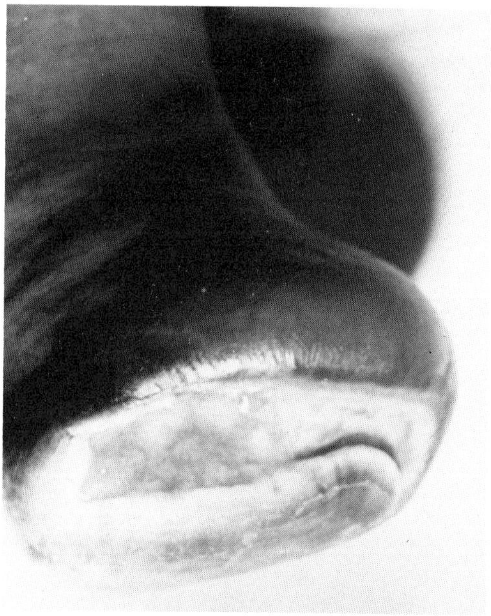

Fig. 8.21. Transmetatarsal amputation with healing by third intention.

Amputation at a site of viable and well-vascularized tissue proximal to all necrotized parts may be the treatment of choice. Amputation should await the results of sympathectomy, thrombectomies, by-pass and arterial grafts. Amputation becomes necessary if persistent and unbearable pain develops, when infection cannot be controlled by antibiotics and septicemia is imminent or if destruction of tissue makes skin healing and skin grafting impossible.

Levine (1971) proposed a treatment regimen for control of infection in gangrene. It consists of the following measures. Bandages soaked in Povidone-Iodine solution (Betadine solution containing 10% Povidone-Iodine) are applied to the affected area. An overlay of plastic film is applied to make an occlusive dressing which is changed twice daily for up to 6 weeks. This is followed by treatment with Betadine ointment containing 10% Povidone-Iodine (1% available iodine) twice daily.

9

Skin Structure and Diagnostic Skin Tests

Many years of podiatric practice have shown the importance of alterations in color, texture and physiology of the skin in evaluating foot health. When the foot is examined with the patient in a recumbent position, the general color and texture of the skin are observed. The significance of marked specific color changes and texture of the skin is described in earlier chapters. These changes especially those of rubor, cyanosis and pallor, in addition to the presence or absence of hair, evaluation of texture and deformity of the foot and toenails are vital clues to a patients' foot problems.

Skin Structure and Composition

The skin is made up of the epidermis and dermis. The outermost layer of the skin is the stratum corneum, developed from a cornification process of the viable epidermal cells. The deeper layer of the stratum corneum is highly specialized and is capable of serving as a "barrier" to absorption of substances through the skin. This layer is called the "barrier area."

The granular layer beneath the stratum corneum is a cellular layer containing basophilic granules. Below the granular layer is the cellular epidermis consisting of the stratum malpighian and the palisading layer stratum germinativum.

The dermal-epidermal juncture is where the epidermal cells meet the connective tissue beneath. The dermis (corium) is that section of the skin lying between the subcutaneous fat and the epidermis. This layer of the skin contains blood vessels, nerves and such specialized epithelial tissues as sweat glands and ducts and hair follicles and their sebaceous glands.

The surface film on the epidermis is the product of the metabolic functions of the skin and interferes with absorption of noxious agents, serves as an antiseptic, lubricates the corneous layer while it maintains adequate moisture and buffers acid and alkali.

Stoughton (1959) notes that the chemical content of the surface film differs on different parts of the body. Some of the contents of the surface film have been analyzed as derived from the following: sweat glands, lactic acid, amino acids, urea, uric acid and ammonia; sebaceous glands (not found on the soles of feet), triglycerides, free fatty acids and wax alcohols, cornification process, sterols, amino acids, pentoses, phospholipids and complex polypeptides.

Sano *et al.* (1965), in a study of pathologic keratinization, evaluated glycogen, pentose, hexosamine and β-glucuronidase in normal and pathologic keratinization. In noninflammatory keratoses these substances were present in normal amounts, but, in the scales of psoriasis, erythrodermia and eczemas, abnormally high amounts were present. It is concluded that abnormal products of metabolism may be excreted from the epidermis as a scale.

Keratin is a fibrous protein in the

horny layer of the skin and is probably derived from cytoplasmic filaments in the granular layer. It is interesting to note that while fungus infections commonly occur on the soles of the feet, free fatty acids—which are highly fungistatic—are not normally found on the soles.

The horny layer of skin on the soles of the feet is thickest where external trauma is greatest. The stratum corneum increases in thickness with trauma. The outer layers peel off as new cells are formed continuously to maintain the thickness. It is not clearly understood what binds these loose, non-nucleated cells together. It may very well be this "binding" process that contributes to the development of corns and calluses.

The nerve supply of the skin is both sensory and motor. The sensory provides for perception of touch, temperature and pain. The involuntary sympathetic motor nerves control the sweat glands, arterioles and smooth muscle of the skin.

Skin Cultures

Interpretation of clinical findings by the use of skin tests and sophisticated diagnostic equipment is essential to early diagnosis and treatment. Magnification of the lesions seen on the extremities is available by a high-power magnifying lens or by smears, sections and cultures of lesions examined grossly and under the microscope. The presence of a specific type of bacteria can be ascertained by careful macroscopic and microscopic examinations of cultures and smears.

One of the common uses of the microscope in podiatry is to examine in a few minutes a scale or fluid from a suspicious vesicle, scale or scraping in looking for the presence of mycelia in mycotic skin disorders.

The technique for this examination is to cleanse the skin with 70% alcohol. The infected material is obtained from the spreading margins of the skin lesion or from the roofs of vesicles and placed on a clean slide. Potassium hydroxide in a 10% strength is applied by dropper to dissolve the specimen. The use of ink in combination with KOH may allow for better visualization of the mounted specimen. After several minutes of microscopic examination, networks of threads and filaments in chains and interspersed spores or clumps of spores appear if the smear is positive. One must be trained in differentiating mycelial threads from cotton fibers, wool fibers, hair or feathers. Mycelial threads are usually thin, light green and refractile.

In *Epidermophyton* invasions, the mycelia may be numerous. In *Trichophyton rubrum* infections there are few threads. In *Candida (Monilia) albicans* infections, one may see budding cells in the specimen.

Test tube cultures are made by implanting the tissue or scraping into a medium previously selected for growth of the suspected organism. The medium must be free of impurities and incubated at 37°C. for 2 days to rule out contamination before using. Beef extract broth is a frequently used liquid medium. Beef extract, agar and gelatin are used in the solid medium. Sabouraud's slants are widely used in raising colonies of fungi. Conrad (1961), in a series of experiments to produce a more luxuriant growth, found that potato broth and carrot broth in combination with vitamin B complex gave best results.

Growth Reactions in Culture Media. The following changes are seen and may be interpreted in the colony growth of fungi.

Trichophyton gypseum. On culture media, the surface of the colony is white to cream color and may have a powdery or fluffy surface. The substrate pigment changes from red to brown in old colonies. In new colonies there is very little pigment.

Trichophyton rubrum. On culture media, the fluffy surface of the colony may be white to rose or purple. The substrate pigment is red or purple.

Epidermophyton floccosum. On culture, the colony is green to buff color. The surface is velvety or felt-like. There are usually many irregular folds in the surface; at times there are small, white fluffy areas present on the colony.

Candida (Monilia) albicans. On culture media the colony appears as a cream colored, moist, yeast-like growth.

Methods for diagnosis of fungus disease include the direct examination, where pus, exudate, scrapings, scales and hair may be examined microscopically after careful but simple preparation of a slide.

Examination by magnification is the use of a magnifying lens on certain small lesions in ascertaining the type of lesions being dealt with. The magnifying glass is an aid in differentiating gross lesions that are small in size and difficult to see with the naked eye. Very often petechial hemorrhages, uncommonly shaped skin lesions and other characteristic skin changes may be noted on examination by magnification under good light, preferably daylight.

The culture method discussed above shows characteristic colonies and identification of the species.

Filtered ultraviolet radiation creates a fluorescence of the fungi in the infected tissues. Wood's black light is used for this purpose. Normal skin appears as a weak blue color under Wood's light. The presence of fungus shows up as a greenish yellow and in erythrasma a pink fluorescence is noted.

Cutaneous Tests

Tests for Hypersensitivity

Patch Test. The patch test is used primarily to demonstrate the etiologic basis for contact dermatitis, allergies or dermatitis venenata. The United States Public Health Service (1964) has defined a *primary cutaneous irritant* as "an agent which will cause dermatitis by direct action on the normal skin at the site of contact, if it is permitted to act in sufficient intensity or quantity for a sufficient length of time." The Public Health Service refers to a *cutaneous sensitizer* as an agent which does not necessarily cause demonstrable cutaneous changes on first contact but may effect such specific changes in the skin after 5 to 7 days or more; further contact on the skin of other parts of the body will cause dermatitis.

A small portion of the suspected sensitizer material is applied to normal skin and covered with impermeable material, such as plastic wrap and sealed to the skin by adhesive plaster. The test is varied in accordance with the materials being tested. When a liquid sensitizer is being used for the test, a piece of gauze ¼-in. square is saturated with the solution and covered by cellophane. One must make sure that the adhesive binding on the patch is not setting up a reaction which may interfere with the real test.

Powders are placed on a small gauze patch which has previously been dampened to hold the powder better. Solids are dissolved in a suitable solvent and the saturated solution remaining is used for the patch. Ointments are tested in the same manner as liquids. In all tests the examiner must determine the extent of the sensitivity and a careful evaluation is made of the skin changes that result.

Interpretation. The reaction to the patch tests is graded as 1+, erythema under the patch; 2+, erythema and edema; 3+, erythema, edema, papules and few vesicles; 4+, erythema, edema, many vesicles and sometimes ulcerations. Reactions to different concentrations of the same material may differ in the same individual. Reactions should be checked after 48 hr and for delayed action at least 5 to 7 days after the patch has been removed.

Contact dermatitis is rarely seen on the soles of the feet. Allergic dermatitis occurs where the keratin is thinnest.

In a shoe, the backing, tongue, inner sole and lining may be the cause for sensitivity but rarely is the outer leather the cause; often the tanning chemicals, shoe dyes and adhesive materials are at fault. Patch tests of sock and sock lining are indicated in suspicious foot dermatitis.

Tuberculin patch tests can be used by the podiatrist in a commercially prepared form when a foot lesion suggests tuberculous infection.

Scratch Test. After selecting a suitable place which is free of hair—such as the forearm, upper arm or back, it is cleansed with alcohol and dried. Two or three series of very superficial scratches about 1/8 in. in length and 1 in. apart are made with no bleeding. One drop of 0.1% NaOH is placed beside each scratch. The proteins of suspected materials in powder form are carefully combined with the NaOH and rubbed into the scratch using plain NaOH as a control. A positive reaction shows up in about 30 min. if the protein used is the offender. The reaction is shown by a wheal and surrounding erythema larger than that in the control.

Intradermal Test. Here about 0.05 ml. of an extract diluted 0.001 mg. of protein to 1 ml. is injected intradermally. Care must be taken to inject the protein into the epidermis and not under the skin.

Trichophyton Test. An antigen prepared commercially from fungi grown from mycotic skin infections is injected intradermally. About 0.05 ml. of the standard preparation is used either by injection or by a patch test. The positive intradermal test presents an erythematous area from 1 to 3.5 cm. in diameter within 45 hr. The patch test results in a papulovesicular dermatitis in from 4 days to 2 weeks. The value of this test is questionable.

Sensitivity Tests

Podiatrists must at all times have sterile swabs and transport media available. When an ulceration or infection does not respond readily to conventional treatment it is necessary to ascertain quickly the type of antibiotic that is most suitable in combatting the offending organism. Under proper incubation in the laboratory and with testing the colony growth for sensitivity to different antibiotic agents, the podiatrist prescribes the medication that serves best as a bacteriostatic or bacteriocidal agent.

10

Helomas

The uncomplicated heloma durum can be described as thickness of the skin composed of desquamated, impacted, crenated, distorted and keratinized dead cells of the epidermis localized at a site of great pressure and friction. The lesion is found most commonly about the toes and can occur wherever great pressure and friction are present. The color may vary from a white to gray-yellow, brown or red. The texture may vary from a dry, horny mass to a waxy, hyaline appearance.

Helomas may be caused by a variety of extrinsic factors. The more common etiologic factors are shoe pressure from ill-fitting footgear and irritations from irregularities in the shoes or hose. Intrinsic problems, such as bony prominences, enlarged bursae or faulty foot function and structure, may cause corns. Altered foot physiology due to occupational stress, deformity and pathology of the skin and underlying structures create friction and pressure producing helomas.

Gamble and Yale (1966) noted several types of bone involvements as being etiologic. They described irregularly-shaped toe bones, roughened bone margins, exostoses and malalignments. Toes are often entirely in varus or parts assume a varus postion.

Bonavilla (1968) supported the concept of inflammation rather than degeneration of cells where heloma dura occur. He demonstrated by histologic study the presence of a thickened layer of cornified epithelium. Polymorphonuclear leukocytes invade the thickened epithelium. The dermis demonstrates an increase in capillary vessels, arterioles and collagen fibers. Bonavilla also concluded that the pain and chronicity of a heloma durum is probably due to perineural scarring of the nerve filaments in the skin.

I have recognized a rotation of the proximal phalanx on its long axis with a prominent condyle serving as the source of intrinsic irritation and corn formation on the fifth toe. I hypothesize that corns and calluses are the result of multiple minimal trauma sufficiently severe to disturb the mechanism that releases the horny layer cells from each other. Thus, instead of desquamation, there is an over-activity of the binding process resulting in a laying down of one cell upon the other that causes the development of a hard, horny mass.

Penneys *et al.* (1970) noted that cell proliferation is not limited to the basal layers but also occurs in the more superficial cells. Mitotic division in the stratum germinativum is stimulated by removing a few of the many layers of the stratum corneum (Pinkus, 1951). McCarthy and Habowsky (1972) studied the structure of the heloma durum and presented electromicroscopic evidence of their findings.

Pathogenesis. Repeated trauma may result in dilitation of capillaries and redness of the skin. If the trauma occurs over a long period of time, the subcutaneous tissue reacts to create an adventitious bursa to cushion the underlying bone. The irritation may go on to

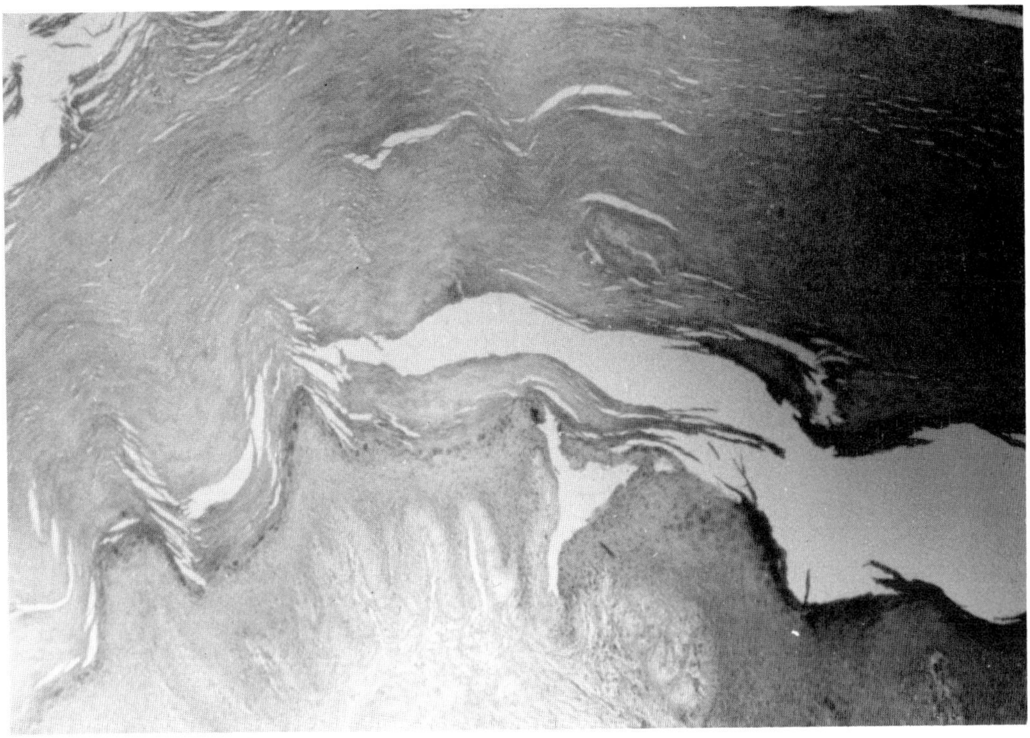

Fig. 10.1. Low-power magnification of heloma durum. Note the typical thickening of the epidermis consistent with hyperkeratosis. Courtesy of J. F. Yale.

the development of a bullous lesion. In most instances, the trauma is so subtle that the superficial epidermal cells pack down as a thickened mass. Repeated trauma disturbs the binding functions of the exfoliating stratum corneum which results in a localized thickening of the skin painful to digital pressure. The surrounding skin shows evidence of inflammation and the subcutaneous tissue is edematous. Complicating bursitis, traumatic arthritis, lipping, osteophytes, exostosis, sinus tract formation and ulcerations may require treatment for relief and cure of the heloma. On microscopic examination of 76 toes from cadavers, Freed (1969) noted the following sequence of events: 1) inflammation of soft tissues about the bone, 2) enlargement of cortical bone by homoplastic bone formation, 3) swelling of the skin and corn formation.

Pathology. A broad conical of hard hornified mass of thickened stratum corneum is noted. It may be white, yellow, red or brown in color. A heloma may be dry or waxy in appearance. It appears over a bony prominence or at a site of pressure from ill-fitting footgear or malaligned toes. The lesion may be compressed so that its superficial surface is even with the skin surface or it may be elevated with a broad base and peaked top. Digital pressure from side to side is not as painful as direct compression into the underlying inflamed skin, bursa and bone. Helomas may occur at the distal ends of the toes, usually the second, third and fourth toes and on the dorsum of all the lesser toes and over their proximal and distal interphalangeal joints. The fifth toe is commonly affected. Misuse of commercial corn remedies may produce a heloma overlaid with white, macerated, and necrotic tissue.

Heloma dura located at the distal ends of the second, third and fourth toes often pose a major problem. This type of lesion is commonly found in elderly

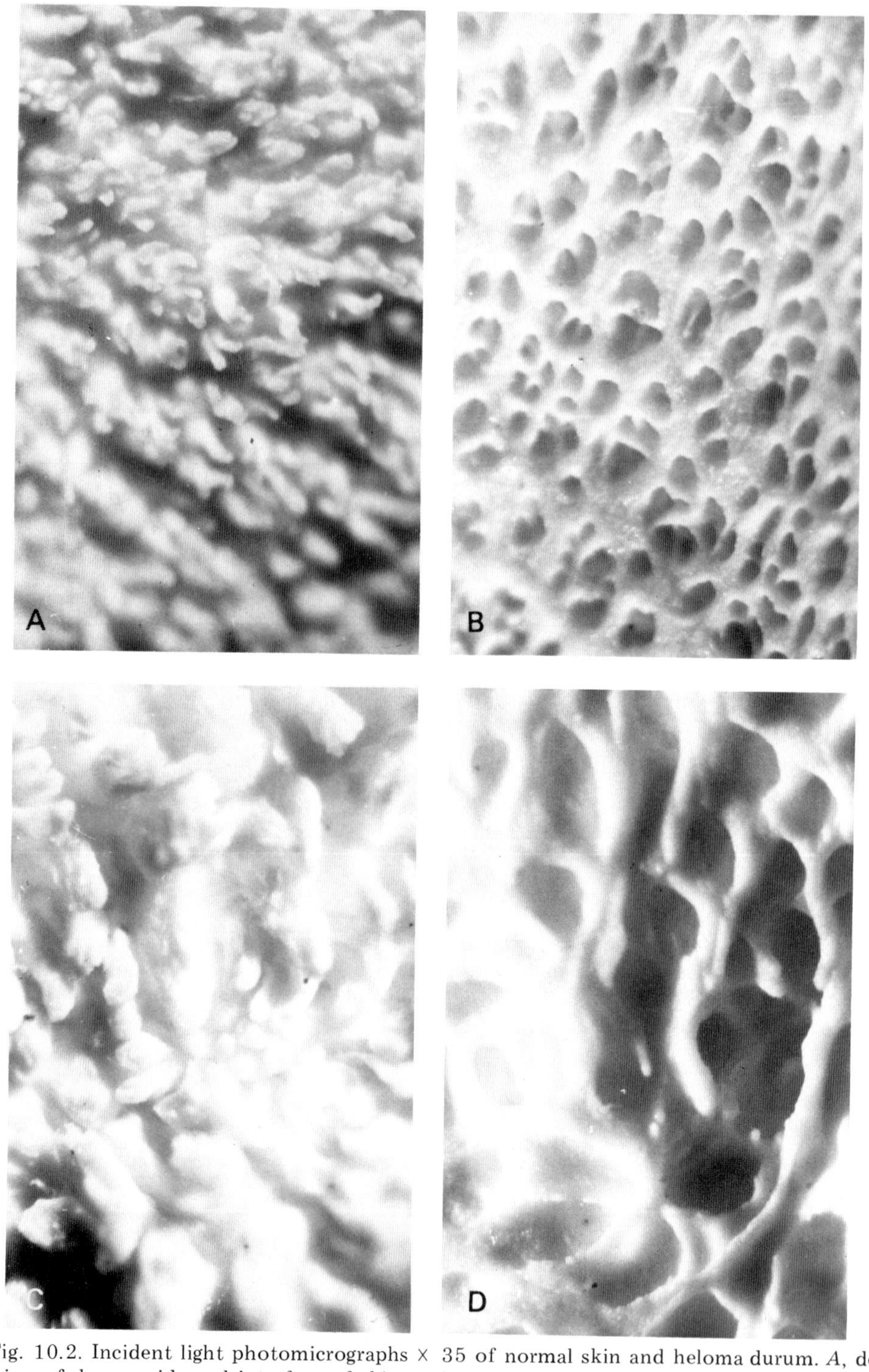

Fig. 10.2. Incident light photomicrographs × 35 of normal skin and heloma durum. *A*, dermal portion of dermoepidermal interface of skin excised from the interphalangeal region of a normal fifth digit. Dermal papillae show a uniformity of height and are spaced with regularity. *B*, epidermal portion of dermoepidermal interface of skin excised from the interphalangeal region of a normal fifth digit. Rete ridges are interconnected in an orderly fashion and are structurally discrete. *C*, dermal portion of dermoepidermal interface of surgically excised heloma durum of the fifth digit. The dermal papillae are hypertrophied with foot-like projections on the superior aspect seemingly from a coalescence of several papillae. Papillae orient in several directions. *D*, epidermal portion of dermoepidermal interface of surgically excised heloma durum of the fifth digit. Rete ridges are considerably wider and irregular making a bizarre pattern for receiving the grossly altered dermal papillae. Courtesy of D. J. McCarthy and J. E. J. Habowsky, J. A. P. A., *62:* 305, 1972.

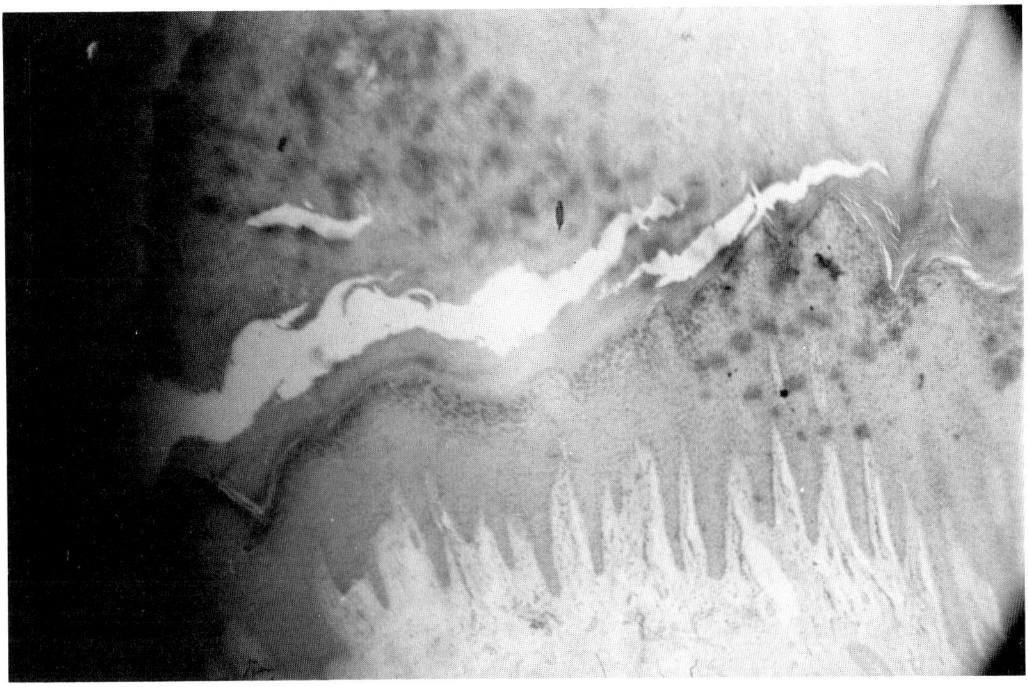

Fig. 10.3. Low-power, cross-section, plantar heloma. Numerous changes including markedly elongated dermal papillae in the area of the nucleus. Courtesy of A. T. Sharpe, Department of Pathology, Pennsylvania College of Podiatric Medicine.

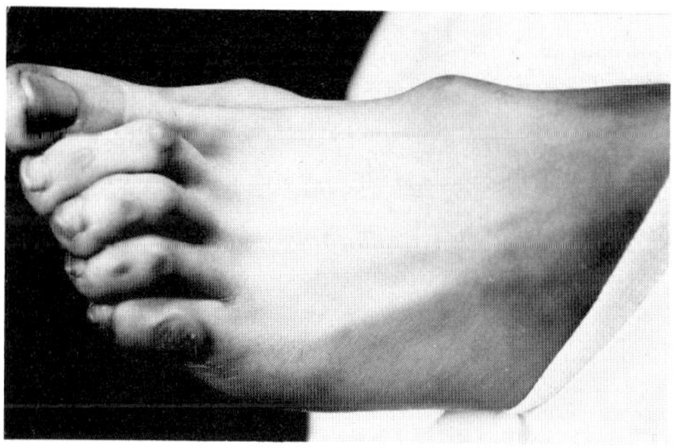

Fig. 10.4. Hypertrophied first metatarsocuneiform joint with keratotic mass overlying prominence.

patients with degenerative disease involving the interphalangeal joints. The flexion deformity is generally accompanied by a dorsal prominence, contraction of both the skin and flexor musculature on their plantar surface and a broadened distal end of the toe. Intermittent trauma to the distal end of the digit creates a painful heloma or tyloma. The toenail is often hypertrophied by trauma and the toe takes on the typical appearance of a modified or well-advanced hammertoe. The lesion at this site may break down with multiple minimal irritation and eventually ulcerate. This is especially true in patients with diabetes or peripheral vascular problems since fragility of the capillaries predisposes to ulceration.

The patient may become a "heel walker" in an attempt to relieve pressure. Adaptation becomes a sub-

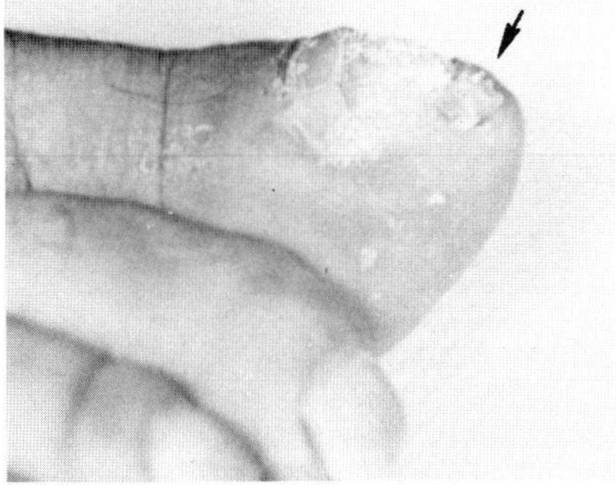

Fig. 10.5. Subungual heloma uncovered following removal of hypertrophied plate and debridement of nail bed.

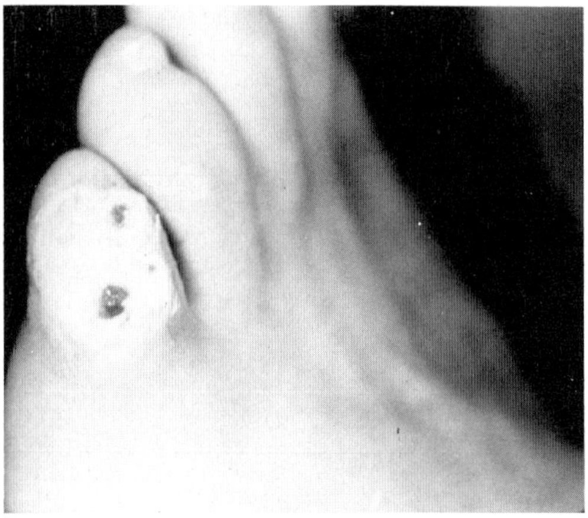

Fig. 10.6. Salicylic acid burn due to commercial "corn cure."

conscious command. With continuing pain, the stress and irritation must be removed early to avoid complications. This is accomplished palliatively or surgically depending on the patient and the attendant risk. Treatment must embody an active or passive adaptation for the pathology.

Treatment. Treatment of these painful helomas depends on their etiology and on their size, consistency, number and location, and on the patient's age and health.

The heloma durum, wherever its location and regardless of other circumstances, must be treated judiciously by a podiatrist. A hyperkeratotic skin mass by its very pathologic state is capable of causing further difficulty. Treatment is simple and is accomplished by softening the hyperkeratosis with a keratolytic, analgesic, antiseptic solution before reduction.

The corn may be excised by sharp dissection using a sharp scalpel, a small sharp chisel or sharp skin forceps. A line of demarcation is noted between the dead horny mass and the healthy pink underlying skin. Removal of the keratotic mass is often accomplished by use of sandpaper disks, diamond or steel burrs. In the more painful lesions a complete toe block or field block anesthesia is used to relieve pain. I use lidocaine, Carbocaine or procaine 1% solution plain. A 1:200,000 epinephrine solution can be used in combination with the anesthetic where the circulation is good; however, the constriction causes slower absorption and often increases postoperative pain.

Once this treatment has been accomplished, the site of reduction is properly shielded and an ointment dressing is applied. A crest pad may be used. Sansone (1970) described the very successful shielding of excrescences of all types and on all locations by parallel strips of adhesive felt. These are placed behind and in front of the lesion or in parallel fashion to each side.

Etiology and Pathology in Further Treatment. After reduction of the hyperkeratotic heloma, it is the responsibility of the operator to evaluate the etiology, the degree of damage to the skin, the extent of inflammation of a bursa that commonly forms beneath the corn, the presence of a toe deformity and the size of bone enlargements on the underlying phalanges. Very often the phalanges are rotated on their longitudinal axis. Radiographs are taken to ascertain the extent of the underlying pathology.

Deffinger (1962) describes neuromas occurring on the digital nerves to the toes as being the primary cause of severe pain in a heloma.

At this point in treatment, the podiatrist plans the desirable treatment for the particular pathology. The patient is usually relieved by the skillful excision, reduction and shielding of the lesion, but complete eradication of the heloma must be sought. Treatment may require consideration of the degree of faulty func-

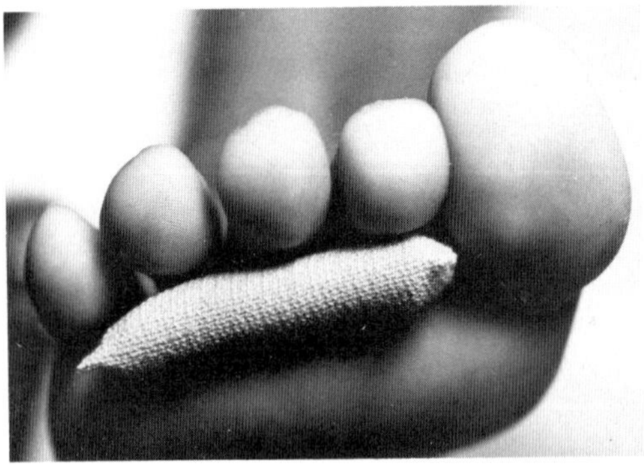

Fig. 10.7. Crest pad. This pad can be dipped in latex after it has been worn and shaped for 5 days. It may also be covered with silicone paste, closed in plastic to keep from adhering to hose and completed with subsequent coatings of silicone.

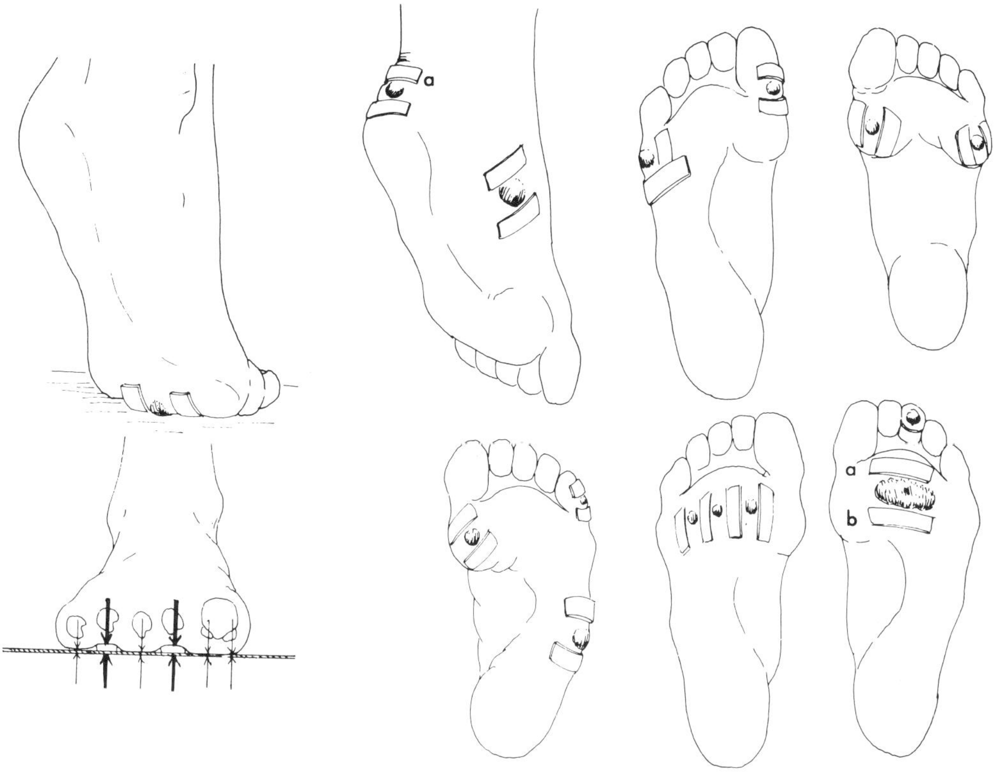

Fig. 10.8. Parallel pads and strip pontoons as described by Sansone. Courtesy of R. Sansone.

tioning of the foot, which must be corrected. Ill-fitting footgear must also be replaced according to the podiatrist's instructions or prescription. If a complicating circulatory or diabetic problem exists, further treatment is conservative. This may include periodic examination and reduction of the excrescense and instruction of the patient as to basic rules for foot care. The patient and his family are taught to recognize incipient problems and are advised to refrain from use of home remedies and "bathroom surgery." The uncomplicated heloma in a patient with arteriosclerosis, diabetes, or other peripheral vascular disorder may be protected by permanent removable shields and pads that are constructed to plaster impressions or made over the affected toe. These are made of liquid latex, liquid plastic, silicone, foam, sponge rubber, felt, self-adherent bandages and a variety of other materials.

Construction of Permanent Shields. Sivitz (1957) describes the construction of crests and shields from acrylic plastic resin (Vernon Resin No. 61956).

M. Polokoff (1958) describes a latex shield made with tubular gauze directly on the affected toe. Many variants are constructed based on Polokoff's original techniques.

The following method is a typical approach to permanent shielding of the painful excrescense not amenable to surgery.

A 4-in. length of No. 1 tube gauze is slit about 2 in. at one end. The toe is coated with rubber cement and the tube end of the gauze is slipped over the toe and cemented down. An aperture pad or a suitable shield shape designed by the podiatrist is placed around the excrescence for protection. The shield and tube gauze on the toe is covered with rubber cement. The split end is given a half-twist, worked back over the pad covered toe and adhered on the dorsum of the foot behind the toe.

The entire shield is then coated with liquid latex and covered with thin plastic sheeting to protect the hose. The shield is kept on the toe

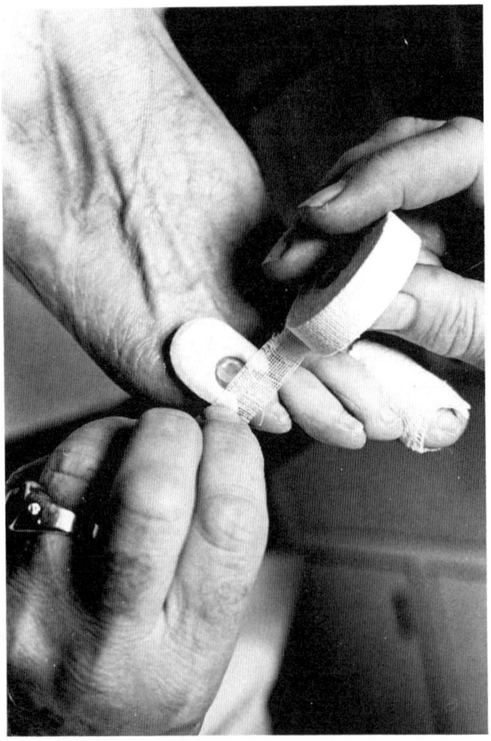

Fig. 10.9. Heloma shield.

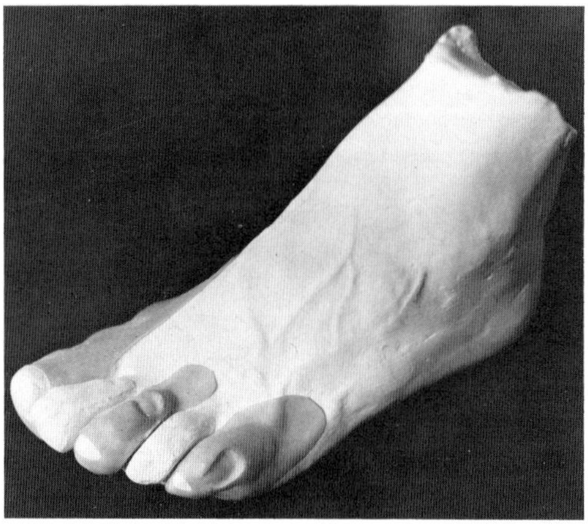

Fig. 10.10. Latex prosthesis. In diabetics, arteriosclerotics or in people unable to tolerate surgical correction, the use of latex prostheses constructed to plaster casts is advisable. Impressions are taken of individual toes and sent to the laboratory for construction of prosthesis. Courtesy of Liquid Rubber Appliance Laboratory.

for about 4 days. When the patient returns, the shield is trimmed, coated once again and dried with a hot air blower or a spray of equal parts acetic acid and alcohol to speed up curing of the latex. The podiatrist may wish to use silicone gel or other plastic substances in lieu of liquid latex.

Ulcer and Sinus Tract Formation. If the subhelomal tissue presents an ulceration or sinus tract, it is imperative that the operator stimulate repair with suitable medication and physical measures. The sinus tract may be cauterized with silver nitrate from 5% to 50% to stimulate or destroy the fibrous tract. If an infection is present, incision and drainage may be necessary. Total excision of the sinus tract may be the desirable approach if the tract is calcified and intractable. Wet dressings of aluminum subacetate, physiologic saline or dilute boric acid solutions may be necessary to facilitate drainage. Hexylresorcinol as a wet dressing is best used for only short periods of time. If an ulceration exists, follow the principles outlined for ulcerations. If an infection is present, bacterial sensitivity tests are performed to ascertain the antibiotic of choice.

Subheloma Bursitis. Very often an adventitious bursa develops in the subcutaneous tissue beneath the heloma. If acutely inflamed, the toe is swollen in circumscribed fashion around the perimeter of the keratotic mass. It may be red, indurated or fluctuant, and exquisitely painful to touch. If the lesion is chronic, a radiograph may disclose a calcareous degeneration of the bursa and often a secondary osteomyelitis.

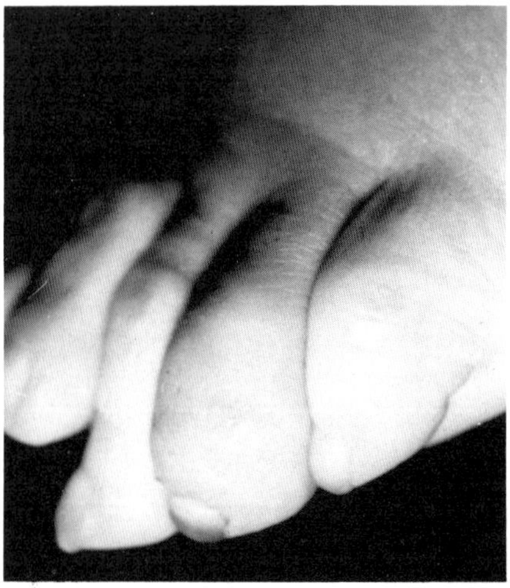

Fig. 10.11. Swollen fourth toe, osteomyelitis, sinus tract.

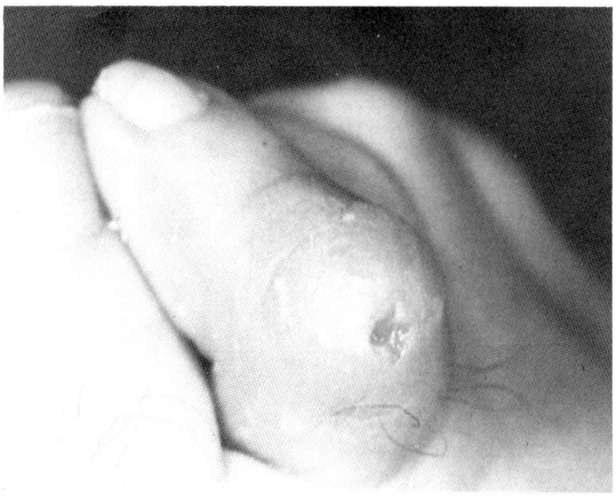

Fig. 10.12. Hammertoe. Sinus tract beneath heloma durum.

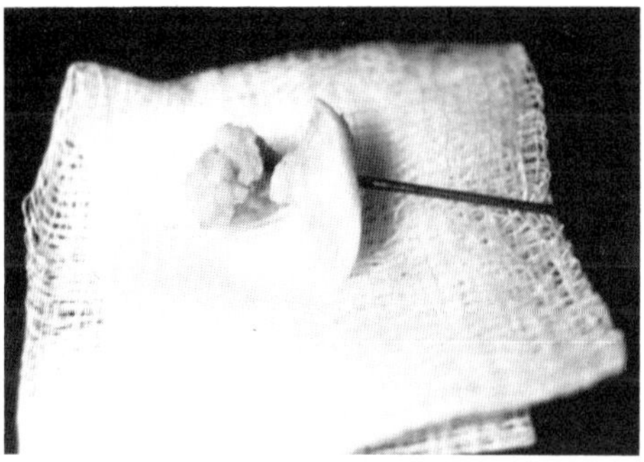

Fig. 10.13. Gross specimen, sinus tract, osteomyelitis.

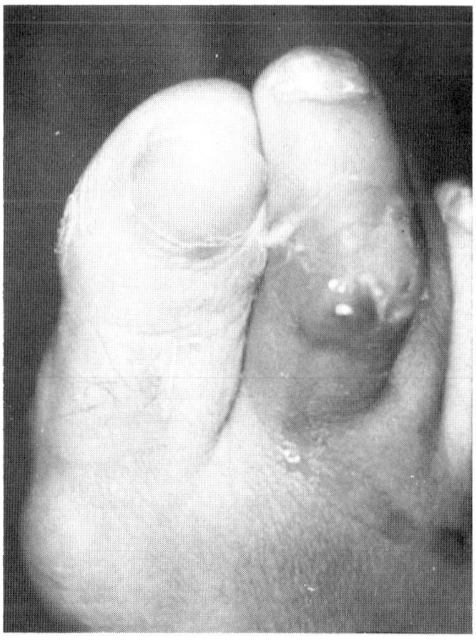

Fig. 10.14. Infection, cellulitis, swelling, discoloration, draining sinus tract, second toe. Pain with impending gangrene.

Treatment of the bursitis may be necessary to relieve pain. This is accomplished by meticulously aseptic use of field block anesthesia and infiltration of lidocaine 1% plain into the bursal tissue. If calcific deposits are present, they must be broken up by needling. This consists of multiple subcutaneous punctures of the calcified bursa following the initial injection. This is followed by aspiration of the intrabursal fluid using an 18 to 20 gauge 1-in. needle.

With the aspirating needle within the bursa, the barrel of the syringe is replaced by one containing 0.3 to 0.5 ml. of a corticosteriod anti-inflammatory solution which is injected into and around the bursal sac. Results have been gratifying where betamethosone (Celestone), triamcinolone (Aristocort) (Kenalog) and methylprednisolone (Medrol) have been used. Chymotrypsin, 0.2 ml. to 0.6 ml. (Chymdase tabs; Chymoral 100) may be used instead of a corticosteroid. Streiker (1961) was impressed by the results of chymotrypsin injections in treating helomas and related disorders. A suitable protective dressing is applied to relieve pressure. Physical therapeutic measures consisting of saline soaks, heat or cold, infrared rays, short wave and ultrasound may be used for fast relief of pain. Oral analgesics or combinations of analgesics and narcotics such as APC and codeine up to 1% or Tylenol with codeine potentiated by promethazine are indicated where the pain is severe.

On occasion, the treatment of choice is

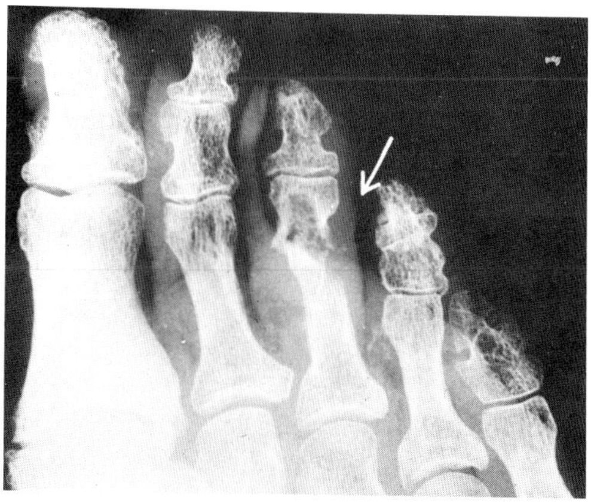

Fig. 10.15. Heloma durum, proximal interphalangeal joint. Osteomyelitis secondary to infected sinus tract. From F. O. Gamble and I. Yale, *Clinical Foot Roentgenology*, The Williams & Wilkins Company, 1966.

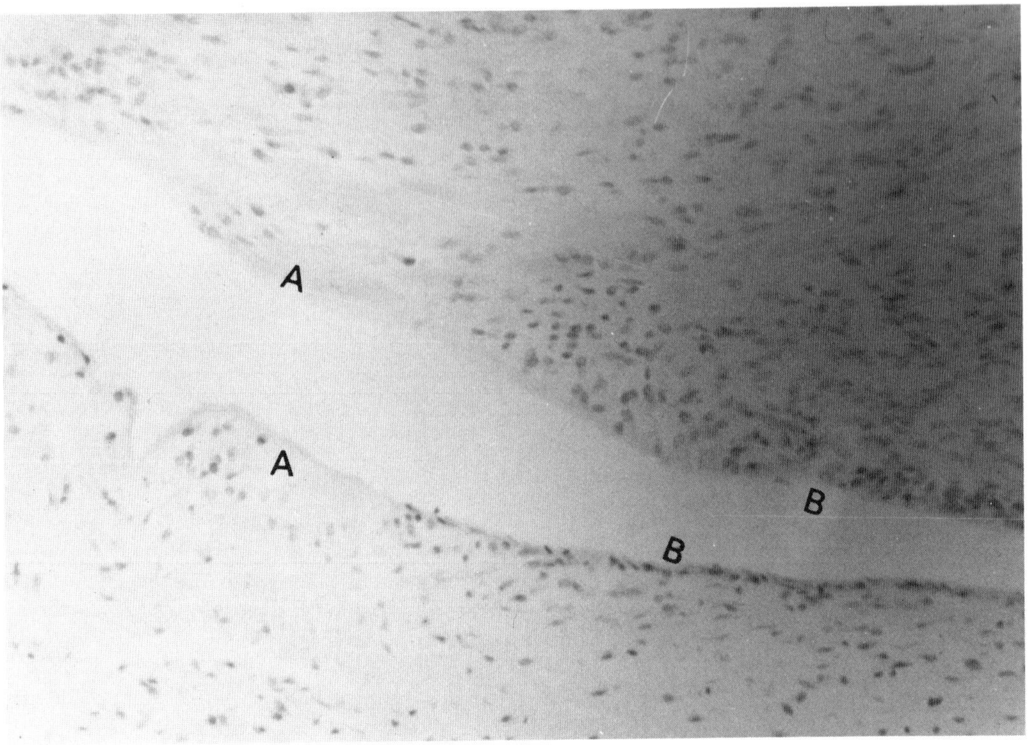

Fig. 10.16. Bursal lining: *A*, epithelium has degenerated consistent with late change; *B*, note epithelial cells lining bursa. Courtesy of J. F. Yale.

surgical excision of the chronic bursa or calcific deposits. This may be accomplished by semi-elliptical incisions around the heloma to remove an elliptical section of tissue to expose the bursa. The bursa is grasped by Allis forceps and sharply and bluntly dissected out by Sistrunk scissors. If a prominence of bone, either thickened cortex, an exostosis, or osteochondroma, is present, the overgrowth is removed by bone forceps and rasping. Closure is completed by suturing with 4-0 cotton, silk or nylon.

Palliative treatment for hard corns on the dorsum of the interphalangeal joints of the lesser toes includes reduction of the excrescence and adequate protection and use of a corrective force to realign the deformity. Reduction is accomplished in the usual manner. Pain is relieved by injections of local anesthesia and corticosteriods. Shielding includes the use of a variety of materials, including felt, moleskin, foam, adhesive and latex.

Splinting the toe or using adhesive strapping to bring a flexed toe into better forefoot relationship is often necessary to facilitate relief. Construction of a crest pad to realign the toes is helpful. Shoes with extra depth will relieve pressure from dorsiflexed toes by providing an additional ¼ in. in the toe region when properly corrected. The ¼-in. insole is removed and the forepart removed or ground to a feather edge. Acker (1964) did some early research on subcutaneous implantation of a soft tissue substitute (medical Silastic) for the relief of helomas. To date, the treatment has not been sufficiently perfected to be considered effective.

There are many approaches for this condition, including surgical correction of de-

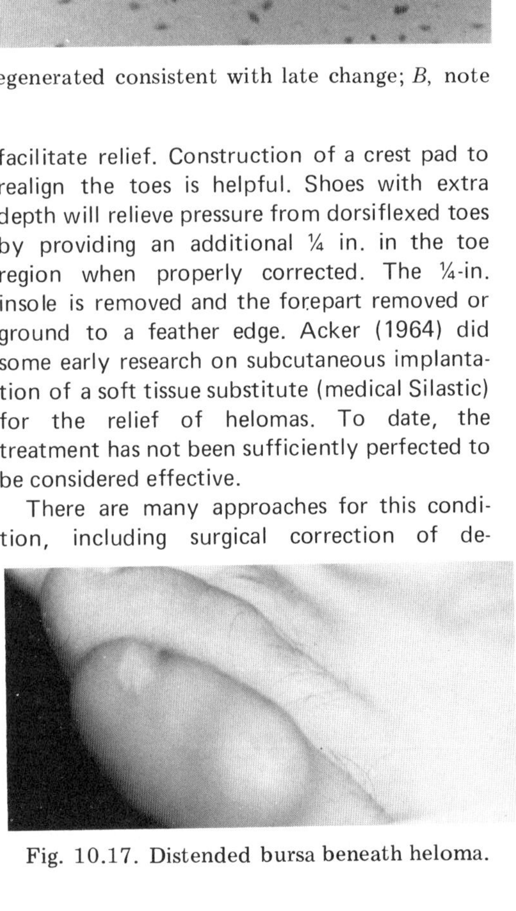

Fig. 10.17. Distended bursa beneath heloma.

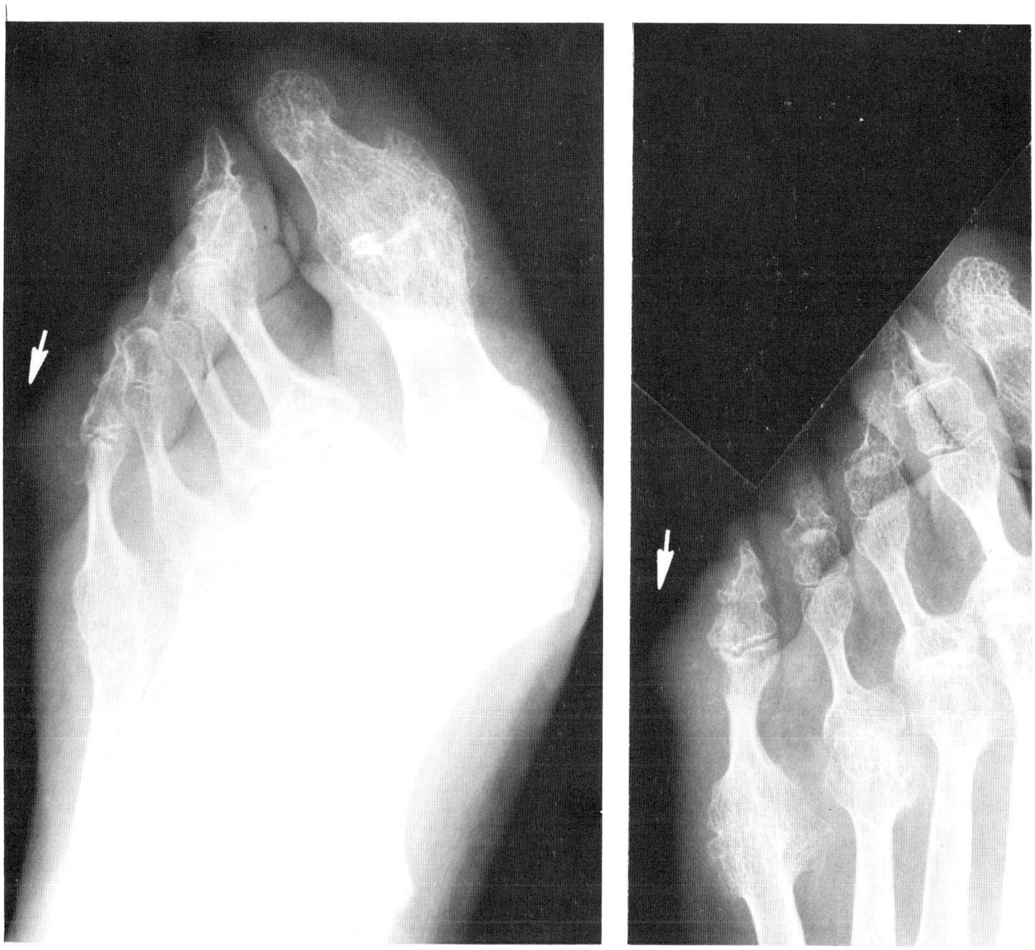

Fig. 10.18. Heloma, secondary complication. Infected bursa—rheumatoid arthritis. Sinus tract enters infected area of destruction at the head of proximal phalanx.

formities and the injection of local anesthesia, sclerosing agents, dispersion media, corticosteriods and vitamin A for the relief of pain or alteration of the subhelomal pathology. The techniques are described below.

In a painful heloma with an underlying bursitis or capsulitis without bone pathology or infection, the use of a local anesthetic by infiltration or field block is often helpful. The hyperemia created by the local inflammatory reaction to stress is often relieved by alterations in the local tissue chemistry following use of local anesthesia. Injection is best made by using a tuberculin syringe and 25- to 26-gauge 1-in. needle. The solution I prefer is lidocaine 1% with 1:100,000 epinephrine. Epinephrine must be used with care especially when circulatory inadequacies are present. However, the use of epinephrine to constrict the markedly distended capillaries is essential to the relief of symptoms. The amount of anesthesia is kept at a minimum. About 0.5 ml. of anesthetic per lesion is adequate.

Kaplan and Kashuk (1971) report no serious complications either systemically or locally in over 65,000 digital surgical procedures where epinephrine in proper concentration was used with the anesthetic for vasoconstriction. Steinberg and Block (1971) report the successful use of lidocaine with epinephrine in over 200,000 injections with proper selection of the patient and good injection technique.

The injection is directed from the proximal side of the lesion, infiltrating behind, beneath and to outer sides of the heloma and its underlying bursitis. The injection has the

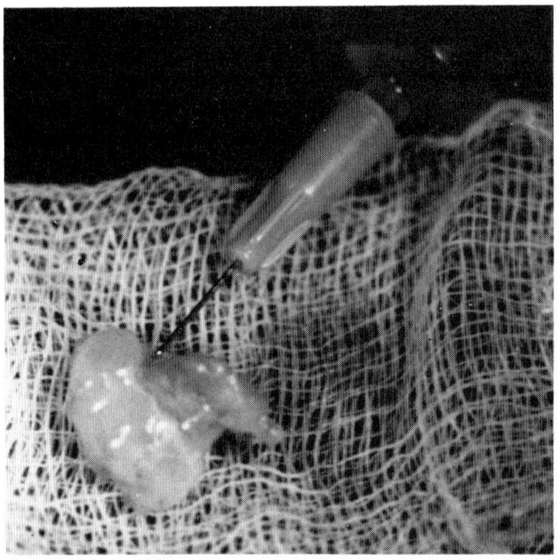

Fig. 10.19. Distended bursa beneath heloma durum. Gross specimen.

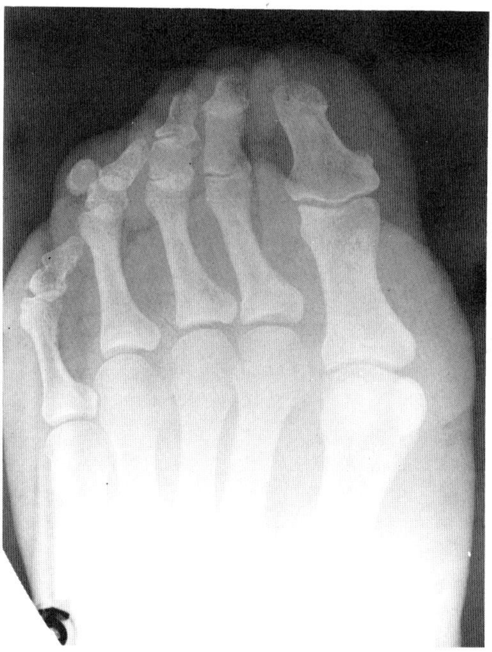

Fig. 10.20. Osteochondroma fourth toe. Heloma durum occurs over deformity.

immediate effect of relieving pain. Gross appearance is one of blanching of the area injected as the distended capillaries constrict. Subsequent observation reveals a decrease in swelling and inflammation. Bursae are usually reduced in size.

Austin (1950) demonstrated fibrous adhesions between the chronic heloma and the underlying fascial or capsular tissue. He recommended the infiltration of local anesthesia by pooling beneath the heloma. This, in effect, results in a mechanical stretching and tearing of the fibrous adhesions beneath the excrescence. Austin also suggested incising the fibrous adhesions. To get the same effect, Jacobs (1960) treated 107 cases by suction using specially prepared applicators attached to a 1/6 horsepower aspirator-suction machine. He notes that "severing adhesions will very likely go on to result in more adhesions. Repeated administration of negative pressure at regular intervals should mobilize the adhesion so that the surface tissue will not be bound down, but will be freely movable." The reflex hyperemia produces an alteration in tissue fluid chemistry and relief from pain.

Sclerosing agents must be used with great care. I find little use for this technique in the treatment of helomas. Hyaluronidase (Alidase) in 250-unit vials acts as a dispersing media when used with other drugs. When injected under a heloma in combination with a local anesthetic, we can expect better and more complete infiltration of the degenerated subhelomal tissue. The use of corticosteriods in intradermal, intrabursal and intracapillary injections as recommended by Locke (1956; 1958) and by Ashur *et al*. (1961) has been found useful as an anti-inflammant in acutely sensitive

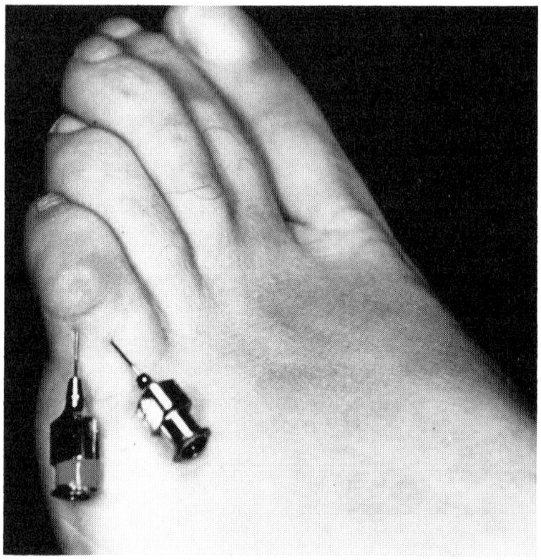

Fig. 10.21. Position of needle for injection of the anesthetic followed by an injection of a corticosteroid with banded needle. Courtesy of R. K. Locke.

non-infected helomas. Locke (1958) notes that the "newest water soluble corticosteroids have proven of special value in soft tissue injections." Cameron (1966) reported the use of aqueous suspension of betamethasone disodium phosphate by injection, claiming 10 to 15 times greater anti-inflammatory effect than prednisolone produced. The average dose is 0.2 to 0.4 ml. If the excrescence is complicated by a calcareous deposit beneath the heloma, it is often possible to break up the calcium deposit through needling. Needling can be described as the multiple injections of a local anesthetic under the excrescence into the calcareous deposit. The deposit is broken up and aspiration may be productive.

Multiple punctures without withdrawing the needle from its original site of insertion are made into the calcium deposit to break up the mass into small fragments. A wide-bore 18-gauge needle is used for this purpose and an attempt is made alternately to inject and aspirate the anesthetic with the purpose of trying to remove some of the flaky or paste-like calcareous deposit. When the deposit is in an early paste-like state, this treatment is adequate for relief of pain and removal of the deposit. Where the calcareous deposit is extensive or old, it is advisable to resect the mass *in toto*.

Levy (1958) studied the efficacy and safety of the corticosteroids injected for the treatment of clavi and callosities. One group treated with injectable steriods was compared with the results of a control group. Levy states that, "in the control group, 58.6% of the sites were successes. This is compared to 42% of the sites which were successes in the steroid treated group. Forty-two percent of the sites treated with corticosteroid solutions developed the following side effects: Ulcers 12%, severe pain 16%, subdermal atrophy 14%. There were no side effects in the control group injected with the vehicle alone."

The oral use of vitamin A, 50,000 to 100,000 units daily, has been prescribed by many as an anti-hyperkeratotic agent and it has been effective in decreasing the extensive hyperkeratosis in many helomas. The injection of Steinberg's solution, Keramin, has been used successfully in decreasing the keratinization in inflamed helomas. Silverman *et al*. (1958) cited patients who were successfully treated with injections of a high-potency, aqueous solution of synthetic vitamin A palmitate containing 50,000 U.S.P. units/ml. The heloma is anesthetized by infiltration with an anesthetic of choice. This is followed by the injection of Keramin solution intradermally under the heloma. The direction of the 25-gauge needle is practically on a horizontal plane. I prefer a field block or complete toe block prior to injections of vitamin A. This is followed by infiltration of the vitamin solution from the periphery of the lesion intradermally using from 0.1 to 0.3 ml. according to the size of the heloma. The needle is held in its puncture for 2 min. before removing it quickly to avoid loss of the injected fluid. Injections are repeated if necessary for 2 to 6 successive weeks.

Surgical treatment depends to a great degree upon the presence or absence of pathology as visualized on the radiograph. If the distal interphalangeal joint is involved, removal of the middle phalanx is in order. This middle phalangectomy has been used with success by many podiatrists. In this technique, the resection of the middle phalanx enables the podiatrist to bring about a normal alignment when the middle phalanx is disarticulated and removed. The flexion deformity and pressure on the distal end of the toe are corrected.

Another surgical technique, the condylectomy or arthroplasty is performed by removing the head of the proximal phalanx. A longitudinal or transverse semi-elliptical incision is the usual surgical approach to the bone. When the heloma occurs on the plantar surface, it may be excised in a similar fashion.

McCain illustrates a technique where the flexor digitorum brevis is severed at its attachments, split and, following removal of the proximal phalangeal head, the tendon is carried upward, overlapping and attaching to the neck of the proximal phalanx. This results in the proximal phalanx being brought down to a more horizontal plane.

Polokoff (1962) describes his technique of raspostectomy in removing exostoses that develop beneath excrescences. Following toe block anesthesia, he makes a small incision in the skin adjacent to the lesion and passes a narrow chisel through the skin opening to the pathology. The exostosis is chiseled down, a file of the necessary size is inserted through the same wound and the exostosis is rasped smooth. The grit and coarseness of the files and

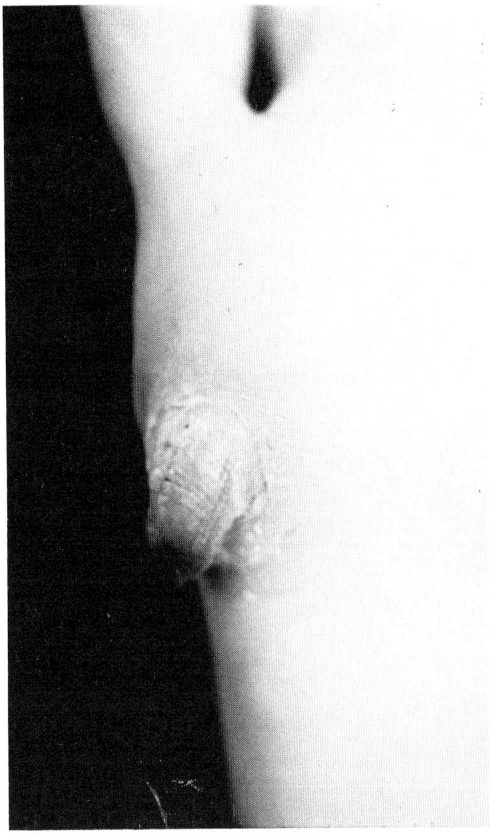

Fig. 10.22. Heloma on the head of fifth metatarsal. Treatment is radical excision and suturing. Plantar condylectomy based on x-ray findings. Construction of balanced accommodative appliance. Skin graft may be indicated.

rasp depend on the size of the bony prominence. Polokoff (1962) states that results have been favorable in 600 raspostectomies of lesser toes and 20 subunqual exostoses. Osteotripsy is the new terminology for this technique. This mini-surgery has been popularized by Probber, Perrone and a growing group of their disciples. Hymes has also demonstrated the value of rasp techniques in podiatry. Power equipment has been developed for definitive mini-surgery.

Selecting the proper treatment for the individual pathology is mandatory. There is no special technique or best procedure for eradicating helomas. Levin (1958) briefly lists acceptable procedures as follows: condylectomy, midphalangectomy, partial midphalangectomy, complete removal head of proximal phalanx, smoothing of the base of the middle phalanx, and a variety of combinations of the above.

Treatment of helomas on the dorsum of the toes depends on the location, pathology and operative technique. Austin (1950) suggested placing a scalpel under the heloma in such a manner as to cut the subheloma fibrous strands. This is done under local anesthesia using a puncture wound at the periphery of the corn and then inserting the blade.

In the event of contraction of the extensor tendons creating stress on the dorsum of the toe or toes, it is practical to do a tenectomy or tenotomy to bring the toe down to a proper relationship. Very often this is accompanied by a "Z" plasty of the skin in order to correct the contraction of the skin. Infiltration of anesthesia is effected with a 1% solution of lidocaine or procaine hydrochloride. The site selected is about 1/16 in. to one side of the extensor tendon over the metatarsophalangeal joint. The incision is only long enough through the skin and superficial fascia to expose the extensor tendon. A ¼-in. incision using a No. 15 blade is usually adequate and least traumatizing. The exposed tendon is grasped by Allis

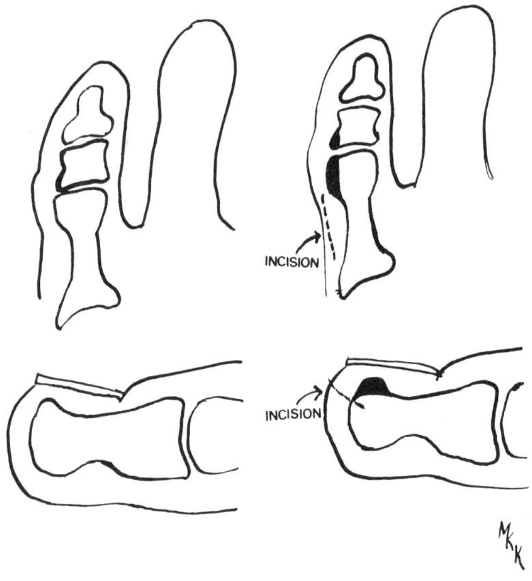

Fig. 10.23. Osteotripsy for removal of enlarged condyles at the articular margins of phalanges has proven successful. Note the entrance site for the condyles and also a subungual exostosis. Technique after Polokoff.

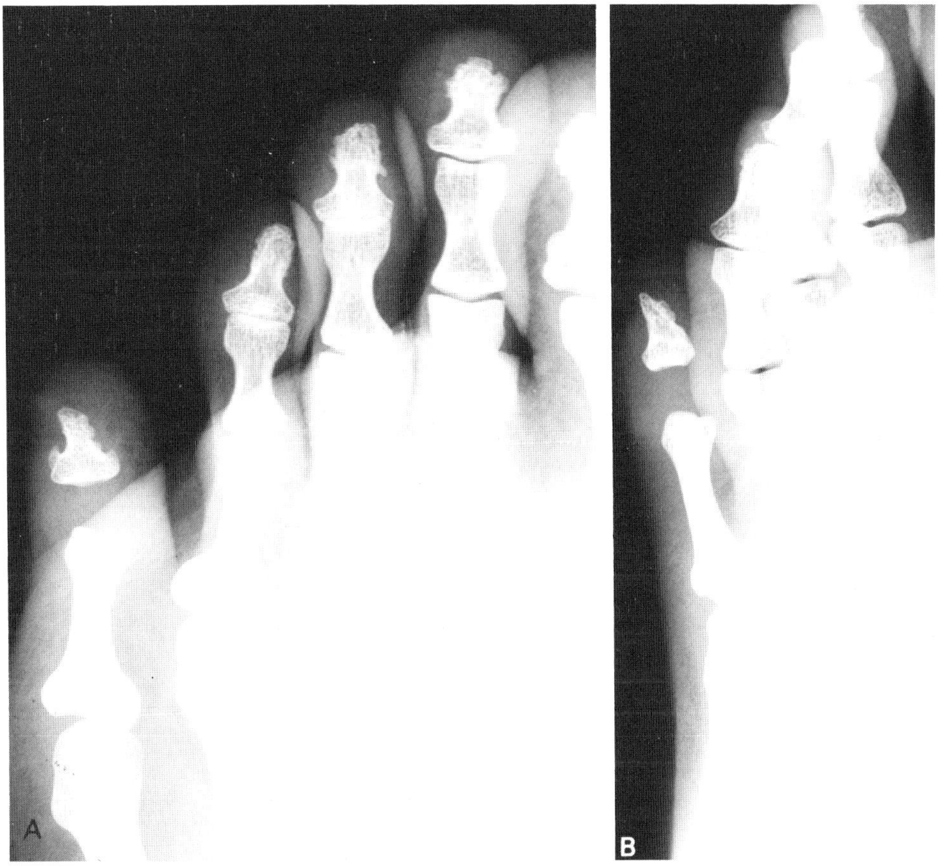

Fig. 10.24. Correction of chronic heloma durum, middle phalangectomy fifth toe. *A*, dorsoplantar view, *B*, lateral view.

forceps and pulled up into the surgical wound. An incision is made at the distal margin of the forceps through the tendon. The toe is thus released. A second incision on the proximal side of the Allis forceps allows for removal of about 0.5 cm. of the extensor tendon.

I do not believe that the so-called punch tenotomy is a good or even adequate technique. The blind plunge of a narrow scalpel blade through the skin and tendon can prove to be dangerous.

In the technique described above, the skin incision is to one side of the tendon, thereby diminishing the possibility of scar tissue developing over the incised tendon. The incision is small enough to close by sterile Steri-Strips, butterfly suture, or a single interrupted dermal silk suture.

It may be necessary to do a "Z" skin plasty with the tenectomy for best results. This is accomplished through infiltration, field block or nerve block anesthesia. A longitudinal incision about 1 in. long is made to one side of the tendon and is deepened to include the superficial fascia exposing the tendon; the tendon is grasped by Allis forceps and is incised. A small section is removed as stated above. The dorsal capsule is incised. Subcutaneous closure is accomplished by interrupted 5-0 plain gut sutures. The skin is closed with 3-0 dermal silk. However, the ends of the longitudinal incision are allowed to remain open. The toe is flexed to a maximum, indicating the extent of the tendon correction. The amount of skin contraction is noted and skin plasty is accomplished to allow further release. A transverse incision about ¼ in. to ½ in. is made through the skin only at right angles and laterally from the distal incision. A second transverse incision as above is made medially to join the proximal end of the long incision. Now when the toe is flexed, the transverse skin incisions open wide removing the previous restriction. No sutures are used; repair is by second intention while the toe is kept flexed or splinted in a correct position until complete repair takes place. The completed incision looks like a "Z" with the center sutured and the ends healing by second and third intention.

Another approach to the surgical cure of helomas is the removal of the subheloma bursa. The technique is used in the uncomplicated heloma without bone pathology. This is an operative procedure which can be instituted together with the tenectomy. The heloma is excised by the elliptical incision around the excrescence and deeply around the underlying bursa. The skin margins are sutured using 3-0 dermal silk. Repair is rapid and results are good. Still another technique is the use of a semi-elliptical incision around the heloma. The underlying bursa is exposed and dissected out. Any underlying exostosis is removed by rongeur and/or bone rasp. The incision is closed, a dry Telfa dressing is applied and the usual postoperative care is followed. More radical procedures for correction of dorsal heloma are the same ones used for the correction of hammertoes.

The approach for condylectomy may be either the longitudinal, elliptical, semi-elliptical or transverse incisions. These may be a single incision or take in an elliptical section overlying the affected tissue. The longitudinal incision over a hypertrophied, markedly flexed joint is made on the dorsum of the toe medially or laterally to the hyperplasia. It extends ¼ to ½

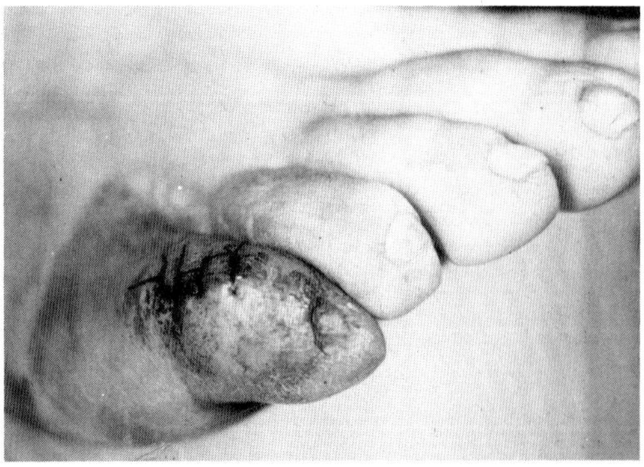

Fig. 10.25. Heloma durum—exostosis. Longitudinal incision fifth toe for exposure of deformity.

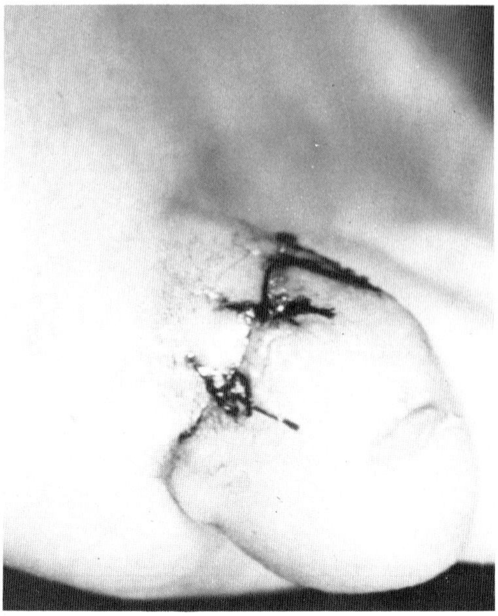

Fig. 10.26. Correction of heloma durum; transverse incision. Excision of the heloma, arthroplasty of the head of the proximal phalanx.

in. behind or in front of the joint and exposes the extensor tendons over the neck and head of the proximal phalanx and the base and shaft of the middle phalanx.

The transverse elliptical incisions are made directly in front of the highest point in the hypertrophied joint and in front of and behind the heloma. The incision is confined to the dorsum of the toe and care is taken not to incise the digital vessels on either side of the toe.

If a chronic heloma and/or bursa are to be resected, an elliptical incision is made around the lesion as previously described and a section of tissue is removed. This may be either longitudinal or transverse. The dorsal aponeurosis is thus exposed. Here a transverse incision is made through the flat fibrotendinous tissue and the joint capsule. It is wise to make this incision anterior to the prominence of the joint since experience has shown that the lipping at the joint margin obscures the joint space. Such an incision facilitates easy division of the articular ligaments. Also, one must keep the scalpel close to the bone to avoid damage to the circulatory supply. Transverse incisions are then made through the lateral collateral ligaments on either side of the joint resulting in an immediate release of the articulations. The head of the proximal phalanx is delivered up through the surgical wound. The capsule is retracted and the neck is exposed. The head and neck are excised by bone rongeur, forceps or saw. The margins are rasped smooth and corners are rounded. Care must be taken to remove all bone fragments and debris from the wound. Flushing with physiologic saline is advisable. A trial co-aptation is made and if there is a restriction to correction or to motion, more bone should be removed. Locke and Strauss (1964) recommend local instillation of corticosteroids in minimal dosage for reduction of postoperative pain and edema.

I use interrupted sutures exclusively in uncomplicated digital surgery. A single, deep vertical mattress suture may be used for closure of the joint. If the incisions have been transverse, the capsule may be picked up with a vertical mattress or interrupted deep suture. Further closure is based on one's appreciation of the need. Sutures are actual splints for the toe and skillful closure facilitates maintenance of position and early uneventful repair.

A middle phalangectomy is accomplished as above. Incisions are the same. However, the dissection of the middle phalanx must be close to the bone to avoid the digital vessels. A good technique makes for minimal trauma and rapid repair. Our experiences have shown that a middle phalangectomy is less traumatizing than resection of the head of the proximal phalanx. Thus, when faced with a choice of surgical technique for correction of hammertoe, removal of the middle phalanx is advised. This is especially desirable if the middle phalanx is short.

Kaplan (1964) corrected overlapping toes by detaching the extensor digitorum tendon from its attachment to the proximal and middle phalanx. The head of the proximal phalanx is resected, a capsulotomy at the metatarsophalangeal joint is performed and the extensor tendon is sutured to the proximal third of the proximal phalanx. The skin is closed and an elliptical section of tissue is removed on the plantar surface of the toe at the crease in the web. The toe is then sutured down into position.

Proximal phalangectomy can be used to correct a hammertoe with a dislocation dorsally at the metatarsophalangeal joint. I do not believe this surgery should be used—except on special occasions—in hammertoes involving the interphalangeal joint. The approach to proximal phalangectomy may be a dorsal or lateral plantar longitudinal incision. The dorsal approach is as described for hammertoe except that the incision is extended back over the metatarsophalangeal joint. The proximal phalanx is sharply dissected out and, if damaged, the tendon tissue is repaired with 5-0 plain gut. The skin is closed in the usual manner.

The lateral plantar approach is made by an incision along the side of the shaft of the proximal phalanx. The phalanx is dissected out from the lateral approach.

Whatever the approach or technique, the foot surgeon must evaluate the need for either severing or lengthening the flexor digitorum longus tendon. A "Z" plasty on the plantar skin may also be necessary to obtain correction.

Fusion or arthrodesis is accomplished by removing the head of the proximal phalanx and the base of the middle. Thus, the two opposing bleeding surfaces are free of cartilage and are opposed. I find that the use of a Kirshner wire is unnecessary for these small joints. Splinting of the part following suturing usually suffices to bring about arthrodesis. The use of bone cement may also serve to obtain fusion.

Medication. Preoperative medication must provide mild sedation and rest for the anxious patient. Glutethimide (Doriden), 0.5 g., the night before surgery and 0.5 to 1.0 g. 1 hr. before anesthesia may help relieve a patient's anxiety. Short-acting barbiturates are helpful preoperatively. Pentobarbital (Nembutal) in 30-, 50- and 100-mg. capsules or by injection and secobarbital (Seconal), 50- and 100-mg. capsules, provide the desired effects.

In foot surgery that is traumatizing, administration of anti-inflammatory enzymes 24 hr. before surgery and after surgery helps reduce pain and swelling. Chymoral tablets, 100 mg. b. i. d.; Papase, Orenzyme, Elase, and other natural enzymes are absorbed readily when taken 1 hr. before mealtime.

Postoperative daytime sedation may be provided by Doriden 0.125 to 0.25 mg. t. i. d. after meals. Other nonbarbiturates for postoperative rest are ethinomate (Valmid), 0.5 mg.; methaqualone (Quaalude), 150 and 300 mg.; ethchloroynol (Placidyl) in 100-, 200- and 500-mg.

capsules; and methaqualone HCl (Parest), 200 mg.

Analgesics essential for relief of pain are described in detail elsewhere in this text.

Keratotic Implants

Often after surgery on the foot or the nails, fine, deep-seated, horny plugs of cornified tissue develop at the site of suture markings. Faulty technique in suturing skin may result in a few dermal cells being carried deeply into the subcutaneous tissue where they commence growing. A dull hypodermic or suture needle or poor apposition of the skin may create this problem. Radical nail surgery with removal of the nail lip may result in subsequent epithelial implants when technique is faulty. In the subcutaneous tissue the displaced cells grow and proliferate producing an irritating sharp implant. The presence of a low-grade inflammation which is aggravated by pressure and friction is noted early at the previous site of surgery or at the suture markings. Dry skin is an etiologic factor.

These implants differ from the ordinary heloma in that they grow from within outward to the external surface. When removed they usually measure 0.75 to 1 cm. in length and rarely exceed 2 mm. in diameter. Usually, they are straight and long but often will curve with the outline of subcutaneous structures such as bone.

I have found that frictionizing the affected skin area with a sanding burr separates the implant from the surrounding tissue and allows for easy removal by scalpel or tissue forceps.

Field block or infiltrating anesthesia followed by sharp curettage or sharp excision is often a successful procedure. Local intradermal injections of aqueous solutions of vitamin A, 50,000 U.S.P. units, have proven helpful. Subcutaneous injections of an acetylated corticosteroid may relieve discomfort.

Electrodessication, fulgeration or coagulation followed by sharp curettage of the necrotic tissue may destroy the lesion. Good judgment must be exercised where a lesion is over a bony prominence or prominent weight-bearing area.

Shielding and padding the painful lesion are indicated. The use of foot appliances to accommodate the pathology is necessary where there is a loss of adipose tissue.

Treatment of keratotic implants may include treatment for extremely dry skin. A vitamin deficiency should be corrected by prescribing emollients such as oils, lanolin and Acid Mantle-based vitamin A creams. This is fortified by daily oral use of 50,000 units of high potency vitamin A capsules. Foot baths in moisturizing agent-reinforced solutions are generally helpful. A variety of bath oils and over-the-counter or prescribed products for dry skin may be used.

It is necessary to remove chronic keratotic plugs. They may be burned out with strong keratolytics and acids capable of creating a liquefaction necrosis. Monochloroacetic acid, bichloroacetic acid, fuming nitric acid, salicylic acid in highly concentrated 20 to 70% strengths, and compounds of vesicants such as cantharides may be used.

It is occasionally necessary to apply 20 to 40% salicylic acid to the lesion in a plaster. The patient returns in 5 days, the foot is soaked in warm water and the implant may lift out with the plaster. Several treatments may be indicated and sharp section or curettage may be necessary to complete the treatment. Occasionally the keratotic implant has a large inclusion cyst attached to its base.

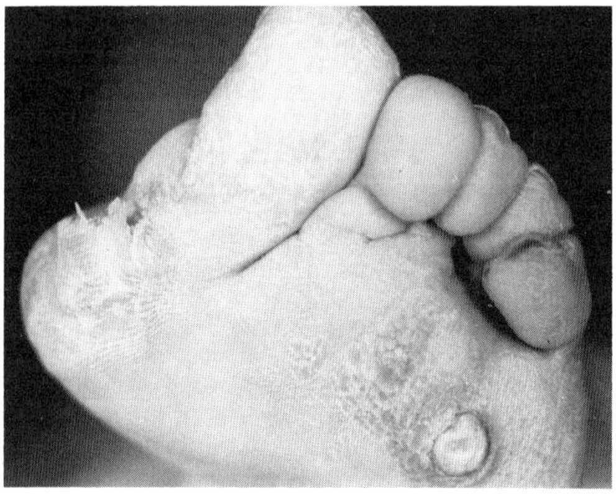

Fig. 10.27. Keratotic implant—tyloma, dry skin at base of rotated hallux. Deep keratoma of the fourth metatarsal. Anidrosis—arteriosclerosis.

Miliary Helomas

Miliary helomas consist of multiple localized spotty areas of hyperkeratosis measuring about 1 to 3 mm. in diameter. They are found alone or in tylomas, helomas or tissues that are markedly anhydrotic. They occur on the plantar surface of the balls and heels of the feet but are capable of developing on any site. Occasionally miliary helomas are located over a hallux joint, in heloma or tyloma on the dorsum and distal ends of the toes.

Pathogenesis. Lesions are noted singly or multiply over weight-bearing areas within tylomas and helomas. The skin is dry and presents a marked scaling and hyperkeratosis over areas that are not necessarily subjected to trauma. Miliary helomas are pearly-white to yellow, pinpoint to pinhead in size. They are multiple, deeply imbedded hyperkeratotic lesions in the feet and often on the palms at sites of friction and pressure. Mibelli lesions according to Wheeless (1969) become hyperkeratotic and slowly enlarge to a diameter of 1 to 2 cm. coalescing to form larger plaques. They may become verruca-like and itch and break down at the heel causing deep fissures. Mullins (1956) noted resolution of this lesion following 3 to 5 injections of vitamin A (Steinberg's Solution) by dispersion beneath the lesion. Hall (1958) anesthetized and injected the solution from the dorsum to the plantar depositing the medication subjacent to the lesion. Locke (1956) advised the injection of corticosteroids beneath this recalcitrant lesion. Results appeared promising at that time. To date, they have proven helpful in eradicating the lesion or relieving pain for longer periods of time following treatment. I prefer to anesthetize the lesion by field block and inject a corticosteroid sublesionally. About 0.2 to 0.3 ml. of solution is the average dosage required for relief of pain.

Injection techniques are of no value in the presence of an inclusion cyst.

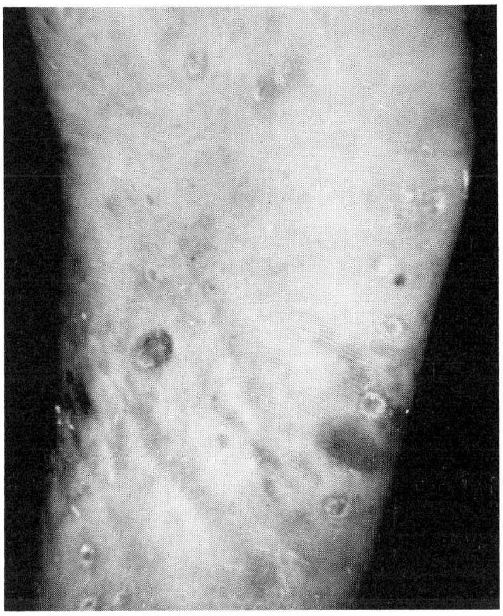

Fig. 10.28. Diffuse miliary helomas.

Etiology. It is believed that loose threads in hose or irregularity in insoles may contribute to this lesion. Evidence of this type of keratosis has been observed in patients suffering from avitaminosis A.

Trice (1955) noted complete resolution of miliary helomas in patients undergoing treatment for fungus infections. In further studies, he cited cures of this condition using undecylenic acid compounds and other forms of antimycotic treatment. He tabulated results in the treatment of 25 cases, 23 exhibiting microscopic evidence of fungus conditions and 21 with clinical evidence of the disease. All 25 responded to treatment.

Treatment. To treat miliary helomas, the tissue is softened with a keratolytic solution. Each lesion is enucleated by scalpel or sharp tissue forceps using sharp section, sharp curettage or sharply pointed tissue forceps. Antimycotic treatment as prescribed by Trice (1955) may be used. Kleiman (1958) applied a 10% silver nitrate ointment with good results. Sharp curettage under local anesthesia may cure the lesions.

Heloma Neurofibrosum

Heloma neurofibrosum is the common name of lesions which pathologically resemble verrucae but in clinical appearance look like a heloma with ill-defined hyperkeratotic margins and a central core of fibrous, verrucoid tissue. This is an excruciatingly painful lesion with a throbbing, burning and stabbing pain found in an area of extreme friction and pressure or at a site of direct trauma. The underlying heloma takes on a yellowish-gray to white appearance with vascular elements that appear to be a superficial plexus of nerves following along the course of the capillary plexus in the skin.

Pathogenesis. These lesions have a rather irregular outline and an appearance of hyperkeratosis that differs from the usual heloma. It is both superficial and deep with hypertrophy of the capillary layer and extreme fibrosis of the deeper layers of the skin. This neurofibrous lesion may be related to warty masses and it may also be secondary to tylomas that have hemorrhaged or been irritated from injudicious cutting or extremes of trauma. These are very often seen in a patient with endocrine disorders and are often characterized by their mosaic appearance and fibrous characteristics. They may occur at points of great friction and pressure such as the dorsum of the fifth toe, medial aspect of the hallux joint, lateral aspect of the fifth metatarsophalangeal joint and the plantar of the first and fifth metatarsal head. On surgical resection of these lesions where the heloma was localized, compact and conical, I have noted that an underlying bursa and frequently an inclusion cyst were present in the deeper layers of the skin. Resection of these tissues cures the condition.

Treatment. There are several approaches to removal of a heloma neurofibrosum. One method involves reduction of the overlying callus to expose the painful lesion. This is followed by the application of concentrated silver nitrate and 40% salicylic acid plaster slightly larger than the mass. The patient returns in 3 to 5 days and the necrotic tissue is removed by sharp section. Treatment is repeated until the entire verrucoid lesion is cleared of pathologic tissue. However, other escharotics may also be used to destroy the pathologic tissue. Sixty percent (60%) salicylic acid in a suitable base, pyrogallic acid and many vesicants such as cantharides, Dry Ice and monochloroacetic acid have been used. Liquefaction necrosis often occurs.

It has been my experience that if the lesion is excruciatingly painful under careful treatment that a subcutaneous inclusion cyst may be found in the center of the lesion. Its superficial, sharply demarcated, white fibrous element is deceiving. A local anesthetic and deep probing often uncovers an inclusion cyst beneath the corium.

Another approach to treating heloma neurofibrosum consists of local anesthesia by nerve block or field block followed by sharp excision by sharp section or curettage of the pathologic tissue. The wound is cauterized by electrodesiccation and a dry dressing applied.

I have excised these lesions by removing an elliptical section of tissue including an underlying inclusion cyst, chronic bursa or fibrolipomatous mass. The wound requires suturing in most cases but sometimes may be allowed to granulate in by third intention. Gelfoam controls bleeding.

Permanent results may require supportive therapy such as balance inlays or appliances for relieving pressure on the affected part.

Heloma Vascularis

Heloma vascularis is like heloma durum but the hyperkeratotic tissue becomes hemorrhagic. The extravasations which stand out as orange, red to yellow linear discolorations are separated by a callus and covered with dry or moist hyperkeratotic tissue.

The pathogenesis of heloma vascularis is similar to that of heloma durum with this exception: the presence of vascular elements within the heloma may be secondary to severe pressure and friction or injudicious cutting of the heloma. On occasion, the splitting of the superficial capillaries beneath the heloma may be secondary to systemic disorders which create fragility of the capillaries. These may be classified as metabolic, endocrine or circulatory disturbances of the extremities. The presence of vascular elements may also be the result of previous infection with resultant hypertrophy of the papillary layer of the skin.

The pain in this lesion differs from a typical heloma durum in severity. The pain may be excruciating and sometimes throbbing and burning in nature. The common site for the development of these lesions is at points of great pressure such as the dorsum of the fifth toe, the plantar surface of the first and fifth metatarsal heads, the distal ends of the lesser toes, or the plantar surface of the interphalangeal joint of the hallux. These lesions may be compact, conical, vascular, hyperkeratotic masses. They are characterized by the presence of capillary loops and a coagulum beneath and within the hyperkeratotic mass. The surrounding tissues may be mildly red due to inflammatory changes. A sinus tract may be found along the course of one of the capillary loops.

Gross Pathology. The presence of a heloma durum with underlying capillary loops that appear thickened together with a hemorrhagic coagulum within the hyperkeratotic mass is typical of heloma vascularis.

Treatment. The reduction of the hyperkeratotic tissue without creating hemorrhage often relieves pain in these lesions. The metabolism of the localized tissue must be decreased, the hypertrophied capillaries should be destroyed or decreased in size and the underlying systemic problems must be treated to alleviate capillary fragility. Subhelomal ulceration may be present. Shielding and padding of the part is used to relieve continuing trauma. The construction of appliances designed to remove pressure from the part is also indicated. Large doses of vitamin C and systemic medications for reducing capillary fragility is helpful. In the acute phases of this lesion, adequate protection and use of 25 to 50% silver nitrate stick or solution decreases the size of the hypertrophied capillary layer of the skin. If the patient is a good surgical risk, it is often advisable to perform corrective surgery as in a heloma durum. Surgery must include complete dissection of the pathologic tissue.

Occasionally, painful helomas or tylomas become infected and the patient develops cellulitis, lymphadenopathy, lymphangitis, ulceration or even gangrene. Antibiotic therapy is given when infection is present. Treatment of local infections may be by warm saline soaks or with sodium hypochlorite soaks (Chlorazene) as a wet dressing. Enzymatic debridement using an antibiotic-enzyme combination is useful.

Systemic antibiotics are prescribed as dictated by bacterial sensitivity and extension of the infection, cellulitis and evidence of systemic symptoms. Penicillin, tetracycline, erythromycin or cephalexin monohydrate (Keflex) are often useful systemically where needed to combat sensitive bacteria.

Topical antibiotics such as Bacitracin, neomycin, gentamicin sulfate (Garamycin) and corticosteroids may be necessary. Nitrofurazone as Furacin may be used as a pad, powder, solution, cream, soluble dressing or stretch gauze roll. Nitrofurazone is available with hydrocortisone or as a cream.

Locke (1942) recommended shoe sponging as an aid in removing pressure from plantar lesions. The technique consists of applying an indelible marking on the sole of the foot at the site of the painful lesion and having the patient step into the shoe to locate the site on the insole that falls beneath the lesion. When this area is located, the site of weight transfer is ground out of the insole into the shoe filler by a drill. A piece of sponge is cemented into the ground-out section of the insole enabling the patient to walk in comfort. The ground-out insole area should be larger than the lesion to provide for movement during gait.

Soft Corns

A heloma molle is essentially a heloma that has absorbed a considerable amount of skin moisture which produces a slight edema and increased dermal pressure. The skin may have a dull redness which progresses to acute irritation and the development of a bullous lesion that may eventually dry and become atrophied and develop a mild hyperkeratosis.

Continued pressure results in an additional moist, hyperkeratotic mass deeloping over the primary site of irritation. In the presence of moisture, pressure may create a heloma molle, usually on the interdigital abutting surfaces of the toes. The lesion may be white, gray or yellow and spongy in texture. It may be localized and circumscribed over a bony enlargement, usually the head of the proximal phalanx of the fifth or at the base and the head of the proximal phalanx of the fourth toe. On occasion, diffuse type of excrescence may develop within the web itself secondary to friction in that area. Secondary infections are common with cellulitis and development of ulcerations and sinus tracts. A heloma molle may develop between any of the toes, especially where excessive perspiration has been permitted. Cellulitis, lymphangitis and inquinal lymphadenopathy are not uncommon with infection of the soft tissues and osteomyelitis.

Palliative Treatment. The affected tissue may be resected by the judicious use of a scalpel and a tissue forceps. Many podiatrists use a special instrument called a soft corn spoon which is quite effective in the resection of this spongy hyperkeratosis. Following reduction of the hyperkeratotic tissue, the hyperidrotic underlying skin may be dried thoroughly by the use of a 5 to 10% silver nitrate solution. This solution also decreases the metabolism of the skin. Protecting the opposing toe surfaces by inserting lamb's wool or foam rubber or similar substance may be quite effective in relieving irritation. Where an ulceration or sinus infection exists beneath the excrescence, it is wise to use an antibiotic to control infection. Wet dressings of an astringent such as potassium permanganate or aluminum subacetate solution should also be used in such cases.

Corrective Treatments. The physical treatment of a heloma molle may necessitate the shielding and padding of the excrescence and the underlying enlargement of bone. It may require the use of an anti-inflammant to decrease the inflammatory changes within a bursa common over the bony enlargement under the corn itself. Very often the elevation of the fourth metatarsal has a tendency to alter

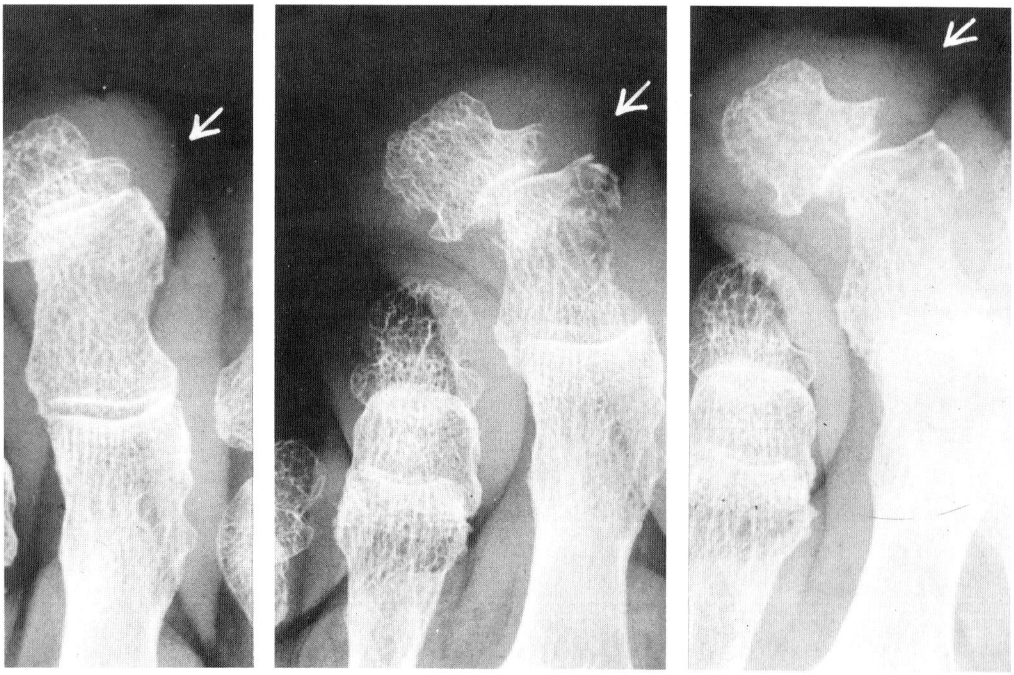

Fig. 10.29. Infected soft corn, sinus tract, and osteomyelitis distal interphalangeal joint. As destruction increases, the joint becomes dislocated. From F. O. Gamble and I. Yale, *Clinical Foot Roentgenology*, Baltimore: The Williams & Wilkins Company, 1966.

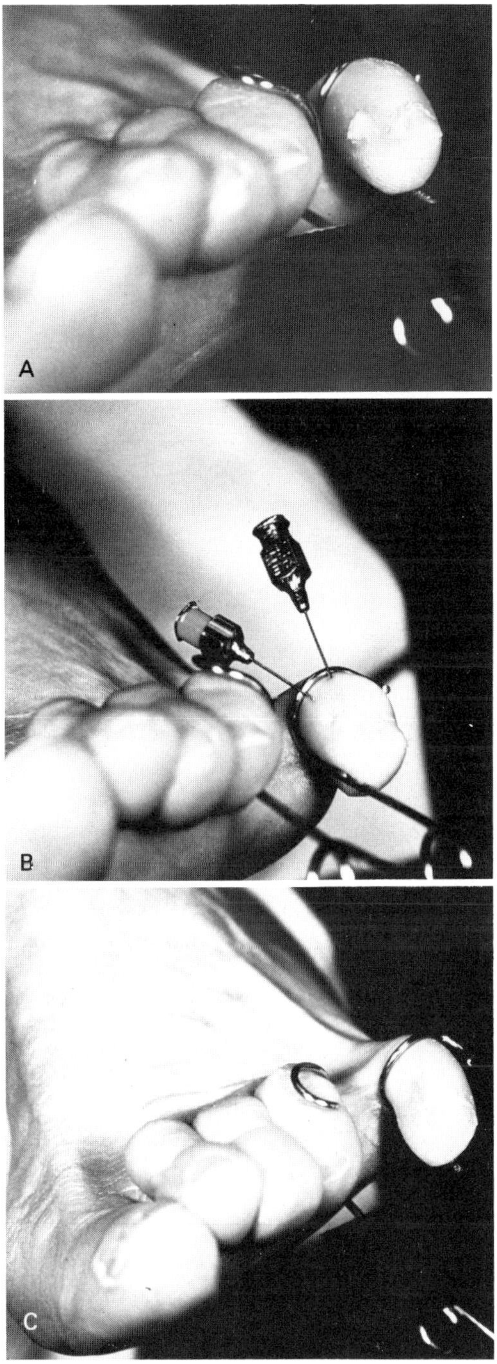

Fig. 10.30. Treatment of soft corn. *A*, lesion; *B*, anesthesia and injection of corticosteroid; *C*, regression of lesion. Courtesy of R. K. Locke.

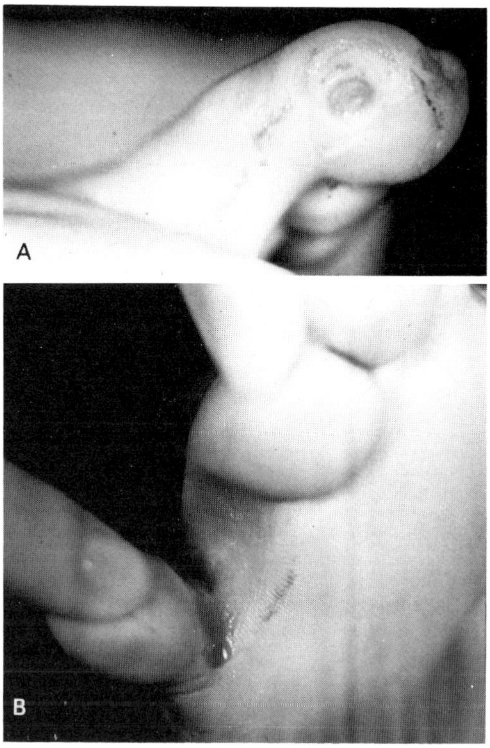

Fig. 10.31. Ulceration secondary to multiple minimal trauma in diabetic patient with soft corns (*A*). *B*, Infected fourth interdigital space. Staphylococcus cellulitis secondary to infected soft corn.

the relationship of the fourth and fifth toes eliminating some of the abnormal pressure that exists. Certainly the removal of irritating forces such as ill-fitting footgear including stretch hose is indicated.

Surgical Treatment. Many of the surgical techniques used for removing a heloma durum are indicated in the treatment of a complicated heloma molle. However, where an exostosis exists, an incision should be made over an area that is not easily irritated or aggravated by friction or pressure from adjacent toes. Occasionally, resection of the base of the proximal phalanx of the fourth toe is indicated. Resection of the head of the proximal phalanx of the fourth toe is often necessary where there is hypertrophy of the head or an exostosis. Resection of the proximal interphalangeal joint of the fifth toe for the permanent removal of a heloma durum is equally effective for removal of some soft corns. A surgical syndactyly of the abutting toes is useful in some intractable cases.

Mini-surgical excision by raspectomy or osteotripsy has proven successful in some cases.

11

Tylomas, Verrucae and Related Entities

Tylomas

A callus is a broad-based hyperkeratotic mass commonly found at the ball of the foot at a site of friction, irritation and pressure. It occurs often over a bony enlargement or at a site of abnormal weight distribution. Symptoms include burning, tenderness or a throbbing ache.

The common site for a callus may be at the perimeter of the heel, at the medial aspect of the heel, at the talar head or a prominent tuberosity of the navicular, the dorsal surface of the first metatarsal-cuneiform joint, the medial aspect of the hallux joint over a hallux abducto valgus, the plantar medial aspect of first metatarso phalangeal joint, the medial and plantar aspect of the great toe, the plantar surfaces of each of the metatarsal heads, especially under the first, second and fifth heads, lateral aspect of the fifth metatarsal head and occasionally at a prominent base of the fifth metatarsal. The yellowish-gray lesion is flat, often raised and spread over a wide area.

Pathogenesis. At first a hyperemia is present followed by a thickening of the skin. Later a packing down of the superficial layers of the skin is noted as desquamation takes place and creates a broad hyperkeratotic mass. Unlike the discrete margins of helomas, the margins of tylomas are not clearly defined. Surgical reduction may reveal an adventitious bursa; sometimes a sinus or suppurating ulceration is found beneath the thickened callus tissue. An intractable plantar keratosis is often a complication of a simple tyloma.

Microscopic examination shows hyperemia with increased epithelial cell formation, cornification, with dehydration of the localized tissue and atrophy of the sudoriferous glands.

X-ray examination of the foot may disclose a biomechanical problem resulting in abnormal stress on the affected parts. There may also be present an exostosis or calcareous deposit on the bone or within the soft tissues beneath the affected part.

Palliative treatment of painful tylomas is generally used concomitantly with measures to correct the etiologic basis for the development of the lesion since the callus is the objective reaction to the stress of friction, pressure and irritation caused by faulty weight distribution and deforming pathology.

The following procedures are used in palliative treatment of tylomas. Absorbent cotton is placed over the thickened excrescence and a suitable liquid antiseptic keratolytic agent is applied to the cotton and allowed to remain for at least 3 min. The agent used may be an aqueous solution of 2 to 5% phenol, a solution of tincture of green soap in warm water, a softening and wetting agent, moisturizing solutions, hydrogen peroxide, or one of the numerous commerical products compounded for this purpose. The ideal solution is one that has the properties of being keratolytic, antiseptic, germicidal, analgesic and relatively nonsensitizing.

After the initial contact with the softened

calloused tissue, the moist cotton is removed and a suitable instrument is used to reduce and excise the callus. Some podiatrists use chisel blades; others prefer a scalpel. Electrically-powered burrs and disks may be used. I prefer a No. 20 scalpel blade for reducing most callosities.

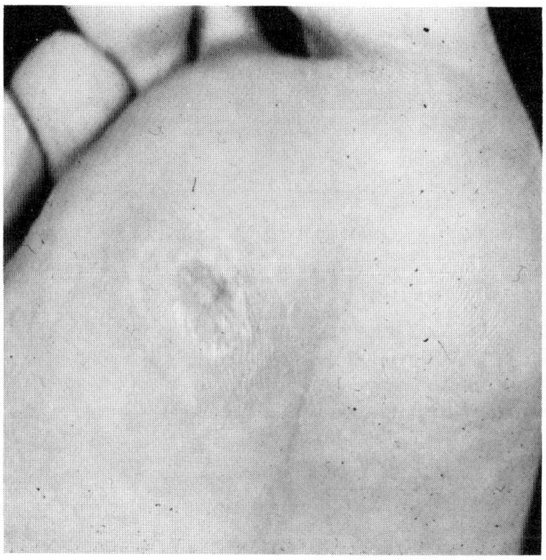

Fig. 11.1. Typical tyloma.

Surgical Treatment. Two surgical techniques are commonly used to reduce calluses. Total excision of the tyloma in one section requires an initial incision at a line of demarcation at the periphery. This loosens and separates the pathologic mass from the underlying healthy skin. The loosened margin is grasped with forceps, hemostat, or thumb forceps held with the left hand and gently retracted. As the callus is retracted, the blade of the scalpel or chisel in the right hand follows the line of cleavage between the pathologic hyperkeratosis and the pink, healthy underlying skin. As the scalpel advances, the tyloma is gently pulled up and away until the entire mass is removed. This technique is only suitable for thick calluses and deep-seated helomas.

The second method is universally used by podiatrists and consists of removing the softened callus by scalpel or chisel in small slices. The skill of the foot specialist is demonstrated when he knows how deep to cut and how close to reduce the hyperkeratosis in

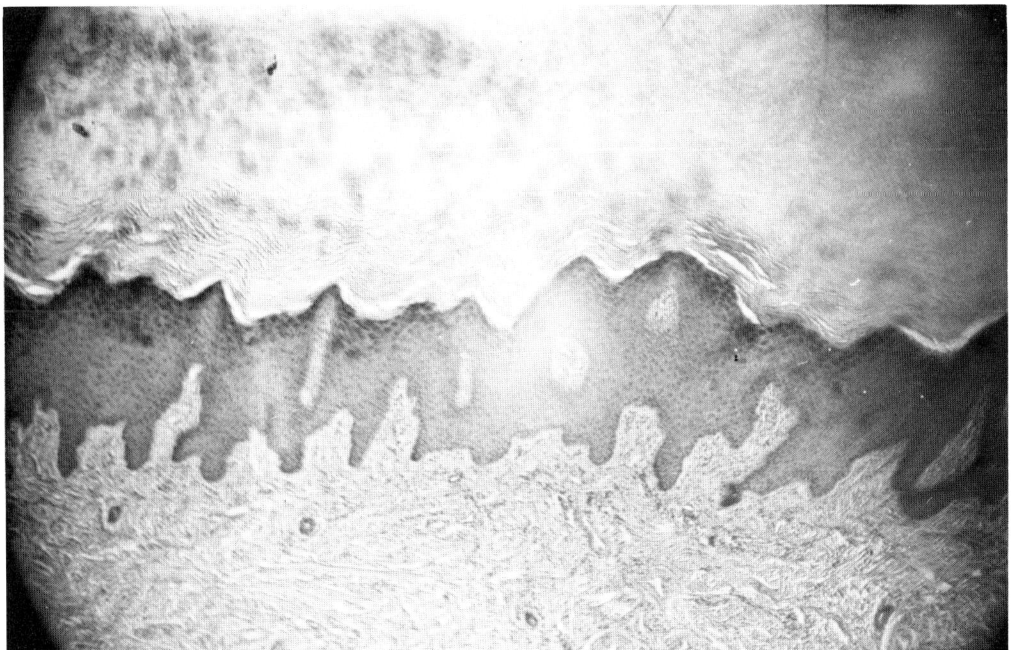

Fig. 11.2. Low-power cross-section, plantar tyloma. Note: thickened corneum (hyperplasia); exaggerated and hyperchromatic stratum granulosum (dysplasia); engorgement, edema, cloudy swelling of dermis. Courtesy A. T. Sharpe, Department of Pathology, Pennsylvania College of Podiatric Medicine.

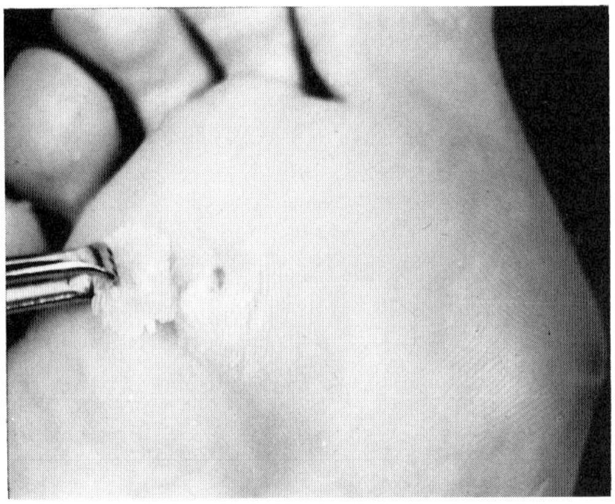

Fig. 11.3. Intractable plantar keratosis—total excision of hyperkeratoses. Must be differentiated from verrucae.

order to obtain relief of symptoms. The technique requires the sensitivity of a violinist to feel the different textures of the underlying tissues through the operative instrument. Proper wrist motion, finger dexterity and sensory perception are developed only after years of practice.

Other methods for reducing heavy keratoses are the use of such keratolytic agents as salicylic acid in 10 to 30% solutions or creams. Twenty to 40% salicylic acid plaster is often applied to a callus for 3 to 5 days. This is followed by hot soaks and removal of the white necrotic tissue by sharp scalpel.

Some foot specialists use a podiatric drill with a diamond or steel burr and a variety of fine and coarse sandpaper disks to reduce the painful lesion dependent on skin texture.

Balkin (1966), in a preliminary report, discussed use of liquid silicone injections of fatty acids beneath the plantar keratosis. This technique induces local anesthesia by field block or posterior tibial nerve block. An 18-gauge needle is used to remove the liquid silicone from its vial. Using a 25-gauge 1-in. needle, 0.5 to 1.0 ml. of the silicone preparation is deposited beneath the lesion from a proximal insertion of the needle. This minimizes migration of the solution since the tendency in walking is to force the fluid forward. This treatment with refinements may prove to be most effective in the resolution of plantar keratosis.

Regardless of the treatment used to remove the tyloma for palliative relief, the etiology must be understood. The etiologic basis for tyloma development is stress over the affected part beyond physiologic limits. This stress is primarily initiated by disease, deformity, injury and biomechanical dysfunction.

It is not the purpose of this text to delve deeply into the realm of foot biomechanics. Yet it is imperative that we discuss the broad factors leading to production of the callus.

Faulty weight distribution acts as a *stressor* and, therefore, must be corrected. Obviously, this stressor creates other problems in the tissues immediately subjacent to the tyloma. For example, we must be concerned with inflammation of the true skin, verrucoid lesions in the dermis not of viral origin but related to pressure, subcutaneous bursae, calcifications, tenosynovitis, fascitis, neuromas, inclusion cysts, ganglia, giant cell tumors, capsulitis, fibrositis, degenerative changes in the affected joint secondary to trauma, spurs, exostoses, osteophytes, and lippings. These lesions often occur beneath calluses and must be relieved and corrected.

Let us review the stressors in broad fashion. Ill-fitting footgear may force the toes back or limit function at the metatarsophalangeal joints. This creates faulty function of the forefoot. High-heeled shoes often throw undue stress on one or more metatarsal heads or on the bases of the phalanges and cause calluses to develop. Soft, flexible soles fail to protect the malfunctioning foot and allow for abnormal stress. Elasticized stockings may force toes back causing friction at the ball of the foot. Narrow shoes often cause the medial and lateral borders of the foot to bear weight on seams where the upper and the insole of the shoe come together. It is necessary to recognize here that imbalanced feet, foot deformities, toe deformities, paralysis, shortages, traumatic disturbances, functional and structural weaknesses, and developmental and acquired disorders may act as stressors. The reaction to this stress may manifest itself in the objective finding of tylomas and their sequelae. Adaptation to the stressor may be demonstrated by a conscious or subconscious effort to offset the pathology. Alterations in gait to remove pressure and friction from the callus, using foot and leg musculature incorrectly, and acquiring sedentary habits are but a few of the adaptations to the reaction of stress.

Treatment of the Marginal Heel Callus. Shoes with a well-constructed heel seat, firm rubber heel and a fit that allows for a broad distribution of body weight often relieve pressure from the marginal heel callus. A plastic heel cup may be necessary to reinforce the lateral spreading of the soft tissue in the heel. A pendulous abdomen and lordosis of the spine in obese individuals throws the center of gravity backward on the heels and this must be corrected. Loss of weight is indicated. A full foot orthotic or appliance worn in the shoe, constructed for the foot to a cast or by a variety of molding methods may be necessary to control weight distribution.

Calluses at the medial plantar aspect of the heel are generally the result of rotation of the calcaneus in foot disorders involving pronation with a positive Helbing's sign. Correction of the foot disorder to restore physiologic functions is necessary to keep an excised callus from reoccurring. Thomas heels and extended counters are helpful in controlling ankle valgus.

Tylomas overlying prominent talar heads require maintenance of the integrity of the midtarsal and subtalar joints. This requires adequate footgear, corrective orthotic thrusts, and, in old, uncorrectable subluxations, accommodative foot balancers to remove pressure.

Spence and Shields (1968) describe a closed cellular Neoprene insole which will absorb 1 cm. of fore, aft and lateral shear with 25 degrees of rotary shear. The insoles and material which they are made from are commercially available for professional use. An inlay depth shoe with a ¼-in. Neoprene insole covering the metatarsal heads is helpful.

Felt pads may be designed to relieve weight-bearing stress on painful tylomas. Sansone (1970) presented a system of parallel strip padding with adhesive felt of various widths, lengths and thicknesses—3/16-in., 1/16-in., 1/8-in. This technique is used following the reduction of calluses to protect the area from friction, irritation and pressure. With time and persistent effort, the excrescence should undergo resolution. According to Sansone, these pads act as pontoon stabilizers, disbursing and diffusing the weight stresses. They induce flowing action over tissues of various densities. The pontoon strip pads act as a buttress and encourage the flow of weight to follow the line of least resistance.

The parallel pads assist weight distribution and exert a little pressure upon the structures of the foot. Because of their minimal bulk, accommodation is relatively simple. They detour weight from the areas of pain to the

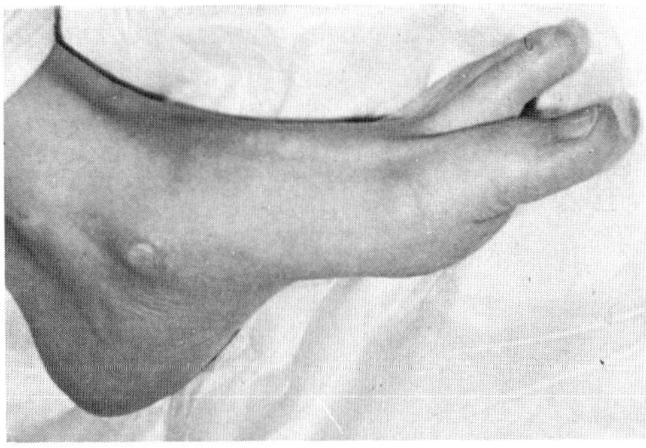

Fig. 11.4. Os tibiale externum. Note callus on prominence.

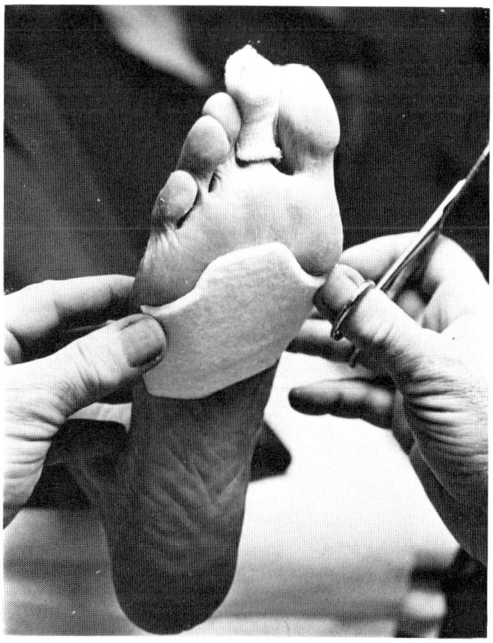

Fig. 11.5. Typical pad for relief of calluses under first, second and fifth metatarsals. May also be useful for sesamoiditis.

pontoons. They are intended to accept the additional stress and remove it from the area of insult (see Fig. 10.8).

Callus formation on the dorsum of the foot over the first metatarsocuneiform joint may be due to an accessory ossicle, exostosis or simple hypertrophy of bone. Wearing low-cut shoes may help. However, these problems usually occur in a structurally disabled foot that requires a firm, highly laced 5 to 6 eyelet tie. It may be necessary to either remove the metal eyelets overlying the bony prominence or to lace the shoe in a manner to avoid the calloused area.

Correction can be provided by surgically excising the extra ossicle or bony prominence along with correction of the faulty foot function. This procedure may also be necessary at a prominent tuberosity of the navicular or where an os tibiale externum is present at the medial aspect of the arch. Full foot radiographs are essential for study. Occasionally accessory ossicles create pressure and callosities.

Where tylomas develop over a bunion joint, accommodation by bunion-last shoes may eliminate the callus. A bunion shield is helpful in relieving pressure from the part. Surgical correction is necessary if the joint is markedly enlarged and deformed as in hallux abducto valgus.

Callus at the medial plantar aspect of the first metatarsophalangeal joint is generally secondary to pronation and ankle valgus which must be corrected.

Tylomas at the plantar and plantar medial aspect of the hallux at the interphalangeal joint result from the part acting as a fulcrum due to a limitation of function of the hallux or an equinus deformity of the first metatarsal. A hallux limitus or rigidus does not dorsiflex and results in the hallux taking the brunt in the "take-off phase" of walking.

Tylomas on Rim of Heel and Under Metatarsal Heads. Abnormally high arches usually cause the weight of the body to be borne on the heel and ball of the foot in stance. This often results in callus formation around the rim of the heel and under the first and fifth metatarsal heads, especially beneath the sesamoids. This may result in the formation of an intractable keratosis.

After palliative reduction, the callus is relieved by constructing a foot appliance to allow for the arch of the foot to bear some weight, thus distributing the weight broadly across the foot. Often the appliance provides for cutouts under the first and fifth metatarsal heads to take pressure off the calloused parts. A rigid orthotic device may be used to correct the usual forefoot varus.

Polokoff (1967) described a removable shield for lesions around the fifth metatarsal. He refers to it as "MH5" and again in a simple approach he fashions a suitable pad from 1/8-in. Polokoff felt measuring 2 x 3 in. An off-center oval is cut out of the pad so the base of the fifth toe is encircled by a soft felt and the callus on the plantar surface of the metatarsal head is suitably protected. The pad is trimmed and beveled to conform to the shape of the metatarsal head. A 1/2-in. elastic adhesive is placed around the base of the toe and encircles the foot with the adhesive side up. Rubber cement is placed on the skin and the

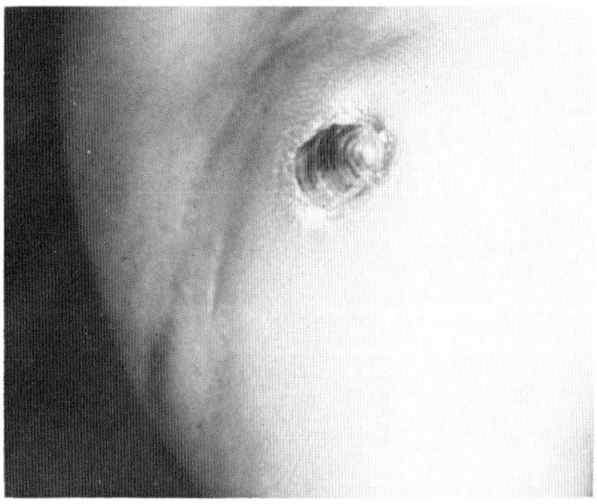

Fig. 11.6. Intractable plantar keratosis.

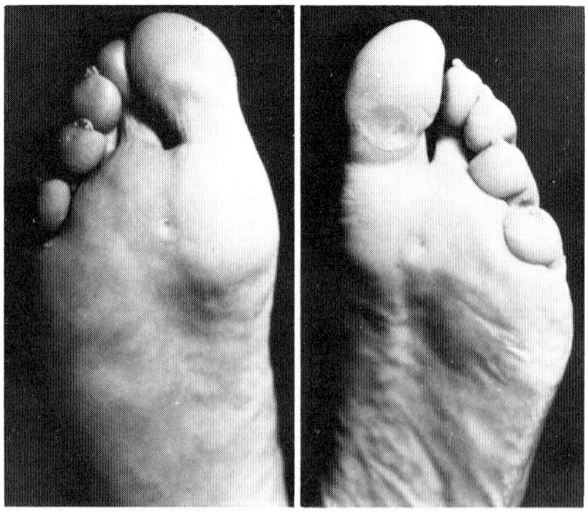

Fig. 11.7. Intractable plantar keratosis.

pad. The pad is then slipped over the fifth toe and adhered. A second strip of elastic tape covers the first enveloping the pad. Excess material is trimmed and the entire pad and encircling strap is coated with latex. The pad may be built up and covered with plastic solutions to complete the protection.

Where the metatarsal parabola is disturbed, and in the presence of erratic metatarsal length patterns, tylomas will develop on those metatarsal heads receiving the greatest stress. Where hypermobility of the first or fifth metatarsal segments exist, tylomas form on the central metatarsophalangeal joints. Thus, wherever possible, the foot deformities and abnormal structural and functional states must be corrected or accommodated to remove pressure and stress that cause the painful objective symptom of callus. Improved foot mechanics may be augmented by shoe therapy, shielding, padding, wedging and metatarsal build-ups.

Mixtures of rubber butter (liquid latex and cork or wood dust) spatulated into a shoe or on a Celastic insole are often used to create dynamic molds. Dynamic molds can be constructed for plantar tylomas and placed in shoes much like an insole. They are usually a rubberized or vinyl material capable of being compressed and shaped by the weight-bearing foot.

Roven (1958) describes a latex forefoot device made to a plaster impression cast in dental stone. The particular appliance was constructed to remove pressure from a painful bursa overlying the hallux, dissipated pressure from a painful plantar neurofibrosum and compensated by bi-plane pads for the imbalance of the forefoot.

Surgical Resection of the Metatarsal Head. Surgical correction techniques consisting of resection of the metatarsal head for intractable callus has demonstrated excellent results in many cases. T. Amberry described a technique used in 1200 resections with fine results. French surgeons have been using variations of this technique for many years. Plantar condylectomy described by DuVries has met with varied success. Henenfeld and Walkes (1960) describe a modification of DuVries' plantar condylectomy which involves removal of the base of the proximal phalanx as well as the plantar condyle.

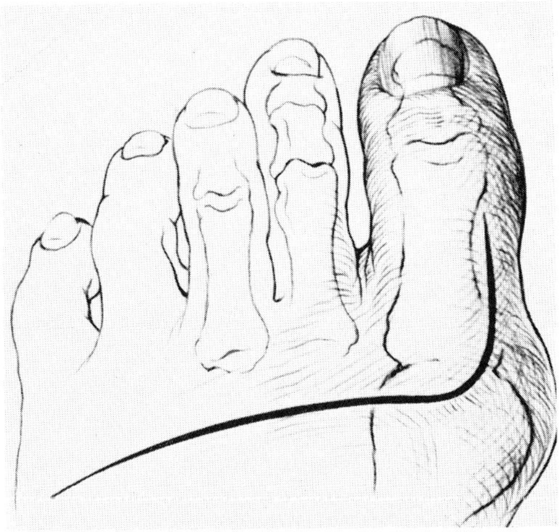

Fig. 11.8. Incision used for resection of metatarsal heads for relief of multiple intractable plantar keratoses. Courtesy of Hall International, Inc.

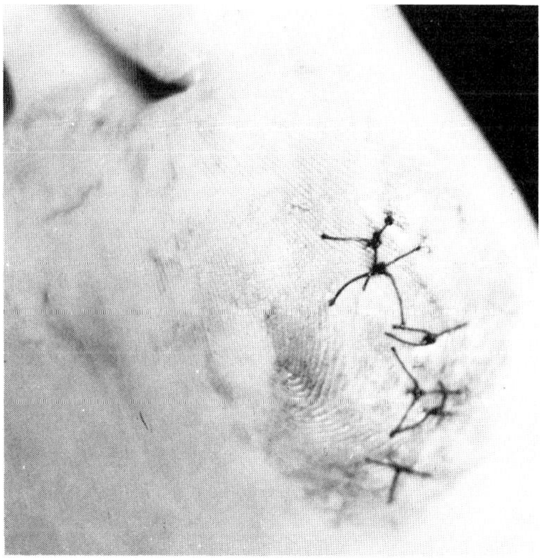

Fig. 11.9. Excision intractable plantar keratosis, first metatarsal head. Note the line of incision follows the normal skin markings.

I have noted the presence of an adventitious bursa under chronic, deep-seated tylomas. The excrescence is resected by semi-elliptical incisions around the mass to include the subcutaneous tissue. Invariably a bursa is found beneath the excrescence. The entire mass is excised by sharp and blunt dissection and sutured.

Excision of Plantar Tylomas. Although surgery on the plantar surface has generally been discouraged, I feel that excision of plantar

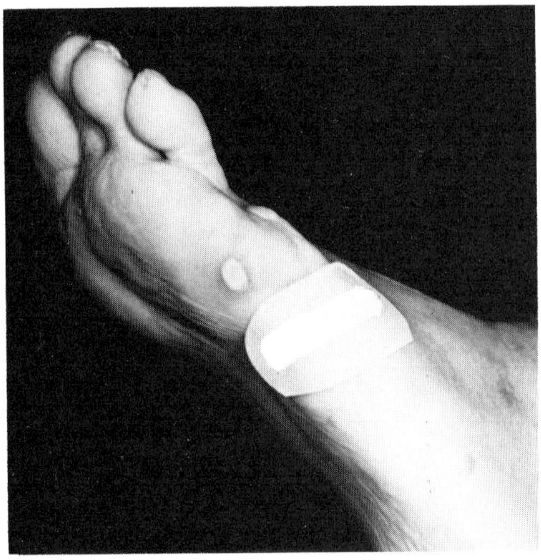

Fig. 11.10. Reactive chronic keratosis—amputated fifth toe followed by localized reactive keratosis head of fifth metatarsal which acts as a fulcrum in gait. Note grayish-white scar tissue in base with irregular border. Gunshot wound and keloid resulting in deformity requiring dynamic mold.

lesions can be a useful procedure when it is attempted only following careful evaluation of previous treatment results and in those cases where pain remains acute and which have proven resistant to palliative treatment.

Henenfeld and Walkes (1959) recommended excision of the proximal phalanx where subluxations of the metatarsophalangeal joints exist. They note marked improvement in the pathology on the plantar surface of a metatarsal head where a callus exists, correction of a hammertoe and elimination of a dorsal excrescence as well as reduction of the subluxation. I have used this technique successfully to relieve forefoot keratosis.

In nucleated plantar tylomas, Bronston (1967) recommended a soft tissue approach in selected cases. Using a 2% lidocaine solution mixed with Decadron in a 10:1 ratio, he induced anesthesia from the dorsum over the involved metatarsophalangeal joint and continued to infiltrate the plantar site of the nucleated tyloma. A snap tenotomy is accomplished on the extensor tendon dorsally through a 1/4-in. linear incision. A second incision on the plantar surface distal to the lesion is used as an approach for adhesiotomy between the tyloma and its underlying attachments. The incisions are closed with a single suture and a length of tube gauze applied to the toe and bound down. The end of the tube gauze is carried under the foot and adhered to the ball of the foot with the toe in flexion.

Personal discussions with R. K. Locke indicate that promising results may be obtained in intractable plantar keratoses by inducing a surgical fracture of the affected metatarsal at the surgical neck. Repair generally results in a slight elevation of the head of the metatarsal following immobilization. Osteotomy performed at the base of a metatarsal is also effective if proper postoperative care is given.

Porokeratosis Plantaris Discreta

Steinberg and Taub (1969-1970) described porokeratosis plantaris discreta as an obstruction by pressure of the terminal portion of the plantar sweat pore with the formation of a lamellated horny plug commonly occurring in the age group 22 to 55. Their exhaustive studies in 649 consecutive biopsies indicate that the lesion penetrates about 1.5 cm. in depth. Pressure so great as to obstruct a sweat gland is thought to be the exciting etiologic factor. The investigators concluded that this pathologic

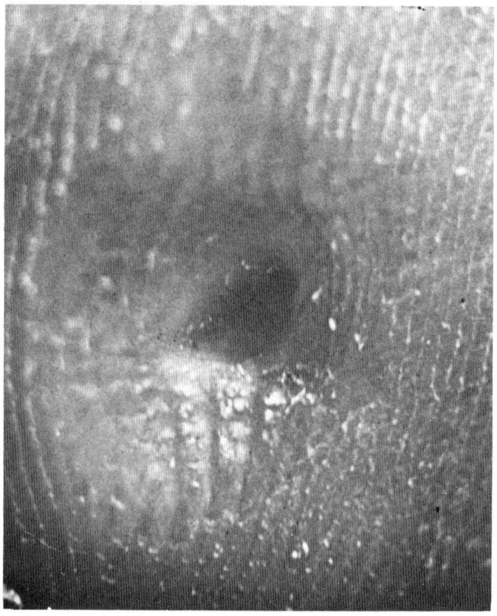

Fig. 11.11. Nucleated plantar tyloma.

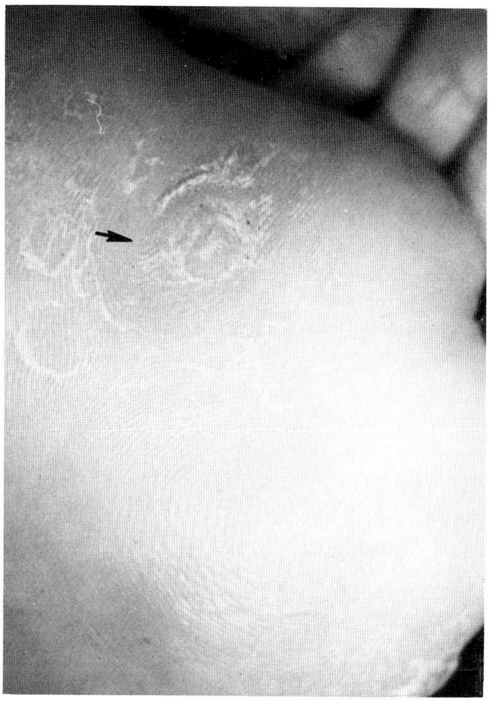

Fig. 11.12. Porokeratosis plantaris discreta.

entity was characterized by a "hyperkeratosis of the epidermal sweat duct with the formation of a cornoid lamella, absence of stratum granulosum and acanthosis of the epidermis and dilitation of the sweat apparatus in the corresponding deep dermis."

Eccrine Poroma

Eccrine poromas appears as painless, nonpigmented, superficial, partially flattened lesions with intertwined bundles of small cells with dark-staining nuclei from the epidermis down into the corium. No keratinization nor melanin has been seen in the reported cases. Only 2 of the 10 cases reported occurred in males. Kipping (1962) reported a case of eccrine poroma in which the lesion occurred on the sole of the foot and was believed to originate from the "intraepidermal sweat duct unit."

Okun and Ansell (1963) note that eccrine poroma is a benign slow-growing tumor composed of poral-epithelium occurring generally in patients over the age of 40. It resembles a granuloma pyogenicum, amelanotic melanoma, scar tissue with telangiectasia and dermatofibroma. The lesions are solitary with a sessile or pedunculated base.

Tanenbaum (1965) reported the first five cases of poroma on the glabrous surfaces of the foot and toes. They may appear on the soles, palms and digits. They enlarge slowly, are soft, gray or red, and by their appearance and location suggest a benign neoplasm. Gibbs (1969) describes the lesion as being a smooth-surfaced and pedunculated mass which is usually located interdigitally.

Treatment. Treatment of choice is complete surgical extirpation by wide excision with a field block anesthesia or infiltration of 1% lidocaine HCl, 1:100,000 epinephrine solution.

Curette is placed at the line of cleavage and pressed deeply into the lesion with a sweeping type of motion. The hard mass with its characteristic pearly base is removed *en masse*. Steinberg and Taub (1969) recommended that extirpation extend subcutaneously to include 1/16 in. of normal tissue. A dry compression bandage is applied and repair is usually uneventful. If bleeding persists, the cavity is packed with surgical sterile coagulating gelatin foams, powders or cellular coagulants. Gelfoam an absorbable gelatin and SURGICEL an oxidized cellulose have proven useful in podiatric procedures.

Verrucae

Verrucae are benign, highly vascular epithelial neoplasms occurring singly or multiply and are characterized by excruciating pain on weightbearing, especially when arising after a period of rest. They may be classified according to anatomic location such as verruca digiti, metatarsi, plantaris, calcanei, etc., or according to their characteristic texture, as moist (humida) or dry (verruca arida). When warty lesions are moistened with alcohol or glycerine, their topography is sufficient to differentiate them from helomas or tylomas.

The etiology of these lesions is obscure with many theories having been

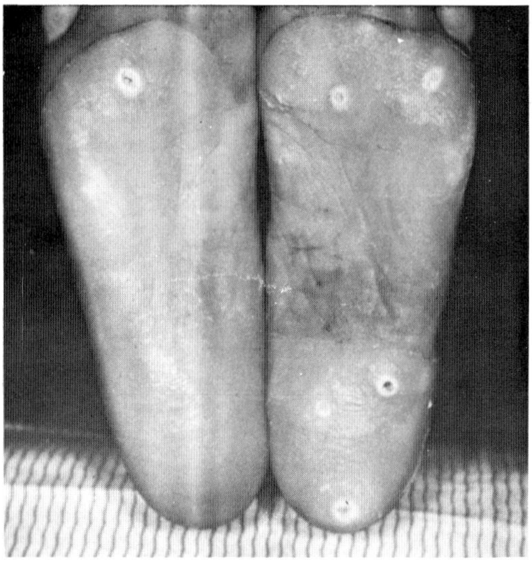

Fig. 11.13. Multiple plantar warts following initial treatment with chemotherapy.

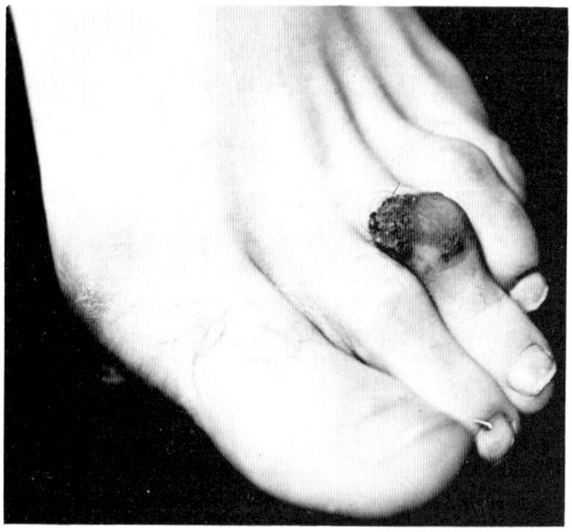

Fig. 11.14. Verruca dorsum third toe—digiti flexus.

proposed as possible etiologic factors. Recent study has shown the cause to be a filterable infectious agent, a virus. Irritation by stone bruises, shell cuts, improper weight distribution and ill-fitting shoes are believed to be contributing causes. Psychologists point to the possibility of a psychosomatic factor being etiologic as these growths are often cured by psychotherapy. Other investigators feel that the endocrines and metabolic disorders in children of adolescent age are etiologic.

It is significant to note that these warts are most commonly found in adolescents, in young married women and in individuals with "stone-wall" worries. Several cases in pregnant women disappeared without treatment after delivery. Conversely, in many other cases, growths have appeared after delivery of a baby. Generally, the patient comes into the podiatrist's office after many weeks or months of neglect with a history of having had a single small growth the size of a pinhead which has since enlarged. Often the enlargement proves to be a coalescing of two or more growths with many satellite tumors about the periphery. These growths may vary from the size of 1 mm. to as much as 1.5 cm.

Under electron microscopic study, plantar warts present unusual cytologic variations such as virus-like particles, intranuclear inclusion bodies and growth characteristics. Clinical appearance and reactions to treatment may vary with cellular characteristics. It is conceivable that antibodies may develop in the presence of infectious agents. Verrucae in other parts are known to stimulate anti-viral or other immunologic reactions.

Warts are believed to be ectotropic affecting only skin and mucous mem-

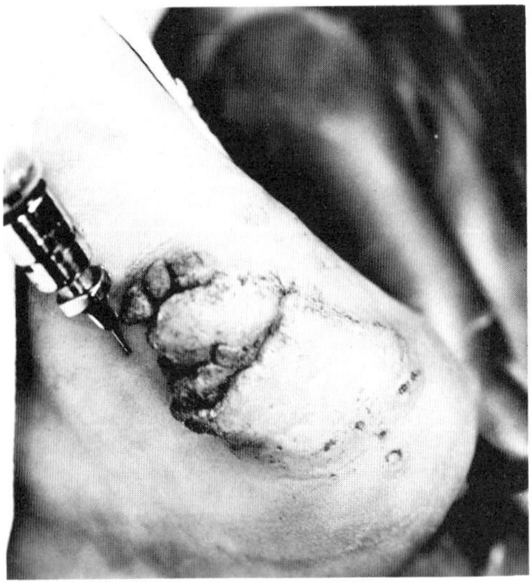

Fig. 11.15. Verruca vulgaris and keloid posterior heel. Courtesy of D. Mowbray.

branes, and invade only cells of epithelial origin. Papillary acanthosis and hyperkeratosis is characteristic with elongated rete ridges and papillary processes that appear to come together at the base in cone-like fashion. Microscopic examination also reveals a thick stratum corneum, enlarged cells and many mitotic figures. There is much controversy about the appearance of the nucleus, cytoplasmic and intranuclear processes. Lyell and Miles (1951) noted that the whole verruca was not uniformly affected. The central part appears to be more involved with less pathology at the periphery. Mendelson and Kligman (1961) demonstrated the isolation of wart virus in tissue culture. The ultrafiltrate of the infected tissue culture injected with human skin can cause a wart to develop.

Where virus-like particles are found, it is also noted that the lower layers of the stratum corneum are nucleated directly above the verruca. The parakeratosis is characteristic of only those warts that present cytologic changes (viral-particles and intranuclear inclusion bodies). Apparently the viral-particles interfere with the normal development of epidermal cells from the basal cells to keratinization. Walter *et al.* (1965) did fluorescent microscopy studies confirming the presence of wart virus antigenic material in the nuclei of the upper prickle layer, the granular layer, and the nuclear residues of the keratin layer.

The individual lesions are usually clearly circumscribed, papillary masses, characterized by a corrugated and somewhat spongy surface of fibrous tissue intermingled with hypertrophic papillae. The lesions may be clear, wax-like, or translucent in character. Plantar verrucae are surrounded and covered by a keratotic tissue. Verrucae involving the periungual and subungual tissues require special treatment to avoid permanent damage to the nail.

The mosaic verruca is a patchy lesion with an irregular border and dry, granular, friable, horny top. The surface appears rough and hemorrhages readily on reduction.

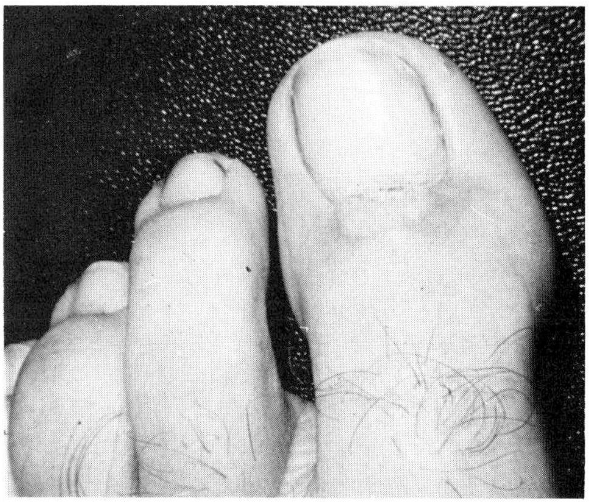

Fig. 11.16. Verruca, posterior nail fold. Courtesy of J. F. Yale.

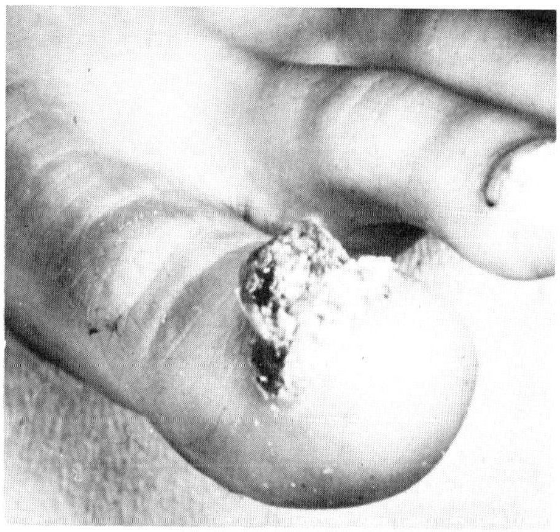

Fig. 11.17. Verruca in nail bed.

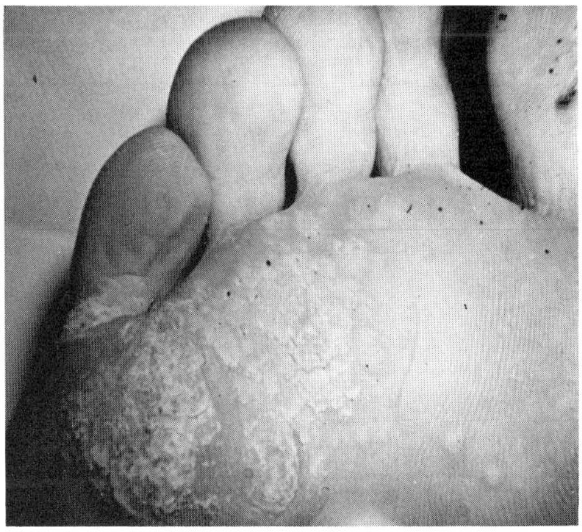

Fig. 11.18. Multiple mosaic verrucae, ball of foot.

Treatment. Verrucae are treated successfully by many techniques. Specific treatment for the etiologic viral infection has not yet been developed. Removal of warts may be achieved through excision or destruction or a combination of both methods.

Treatment depends on the patient's general health and the number of warts and their location, type and size. Treatment may range from chemotherapeutic techniques (a variety of acids and strong salts) to treatment with carbon dioxide snow, surgical excision, sharp curettage, electrodesiccation, fulgeration, coagulation, electrosection, negative galvanism (electrolysis), injection techniques, oral vitamin A therapy, psychotherapy and ultrasound therapy.

The most popular treatment and one that has proven effective in the majority of cases is chemotherapy. Many chemicals including monochloroacetic, bichloroacetic, fuming nitric, pyrogallic and salicylic acids; cantharidin, vitamin A, and silver nitrate and a variety of sclerosing agents are used alone or in combination.

Surgical excision of verrucae is practical when a single lesion exists or if multiple lesions are widely separated. Excision of lesions over bony prominences or on weight-bearing areas of the foot must be properly evaluated to eliminate scar formation.

Liquid nitrogen or liquid oxygen applied to a plantar wart causes instantaneous freezing. This is painless but pain commences with thawing and is increased for several hours. A bullous lesion develops and the patient returns in 1 week for excision of necrotic tissue. The wound is dressed daily and may take 3 to 4 weeks to heal. This treatment is especially effective for mosaic warts.

The presence of scar tissue following surgery may well plague the patient throughout his life. Chemosurgical approaches handled judiciously rarely cause scar formation.

Chemosurgical Technique. A circular cut-out—an adhesive plaster—slightly larger than the wart is placed over the lesion to cover the healthy tissue and expose the wart. An applicator or capillary tube (Woolf, 1959) is dipped into the agent of choice and applied to the wart. The hole in the adhesive is filled with 60 to 70% salicylic acid ointment or suitable commercial compounds and a protective 1/8- or 1/4-in. U-shaped felt pad is applied to the part to relieve weightbearing. The entire dressing is covered and the patient is cautioned to keep the part dry.

After 3 to 5 days, the wart appears slightly raised, white, soft and spongy and often has undergone a partial necrosis. A liquefaction necrosis may not occur until several applications of the above treatment have been completed. Debridement usually discloses an ulceration.

Repair of the ulceration caused by the acid is usually rapid and if a severe destructive reaction takes place with cellulitis and severe pain, it can be relieved by hot saline soaks.

Churnly (1961) advised against destruction of plantar warts and advised shielding in "anticipation of spontaneous remission."

In 180 cases of mosaic verruca, Lieberman (1960) reported good results in 165 cases. A half cup of sea salt to a quart of warm water as a foot soak daily for 15 min, and vitamin A, 50,000 units twice daily. The average cure took place in 2 to 10 weeks. The lesions were seen weekly and cauterized with silver nitrate.

Levey (1958) recommended the use of topical applications of 3% formaldehyde with

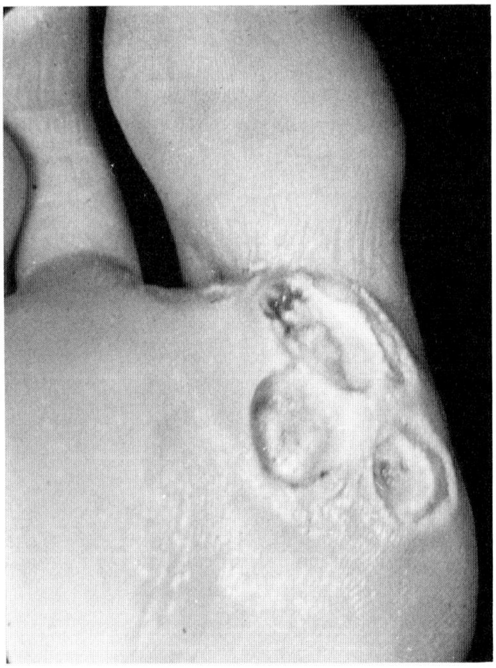

Fig. 11.19. Chemosurgical removal of three plantar warts. Note crater-like destruction and removal of necrotic masses.

oral vitamin A capsules as a regimen for selected cases of plantar warts.

Lerner (1959) claims a 91% rate of success using a method of excision and curettage and believes that reoccurrences are the result of faulty technique. The technique consists of a posterior tibial nerve block or direct infiltration of a local anesthetic of choice. A No. 11 or 15 scalpel blade is used to incise around the perimeter of the wart. This incision is deepened to include the entire mass. An iris scissors is used to excise the mass and trim the wound. A mastoid curette of desired size is used to remove verrucous elements. A compression (Gelfoam) dressing is applied.

Bornstein (1963) in describing the procedure by Lerner (1959) noted that he had a 43% decrease in healing time when oral chymotrypsin was prescribed, (e.g., 2 tablets Chymoral q. i. d. 2 days preoperatively and 4 to 6 days postoperatively.

Antahades (1963) used refrigeration anesthesia in the surgical excision of plantar verruca of non-mosaic type. He applied Dry Ice to organize, solidify and anesthetize the wart and assure hemostasis. With a sharp curette, the lesion was immediately excised while hard and anesthetized. Three or four sterile gauze pads were applied with pressure for hemostasis. Postoperative pain is negligible and repair is rapid.

Suppan and Besterman (1963) described a similar approach to the treatment of verrucae using curettage and chemocautery. This essentially consists of field block or infiltration anesthesia, followed by sharp curettage of the wart. The base is then cauterized for from 3 to 5 min. with a cotton swab and 88% phenol solution.

Buske (1963) cited bismuth Cevitamate as his method of choice for injection into the verrucous mass. He cautions the operator to use no more than 0.5 to 1.0 minims on the toes but demonstrates the effective use of 1.0 to 3.0 minims on other parts of the foot. The 27-gauge needle is injected from the periphery directly into the base of the lesion. Resistance is felt if the medication is being properly placed. Smernoff (1969) used successfully a combination of bismuth Cevitamate and 1% Sotradecol mixed with an anesthetic and administered by Panjet. This is followed by a 60% salicylic acid ointment in a lanolin base.

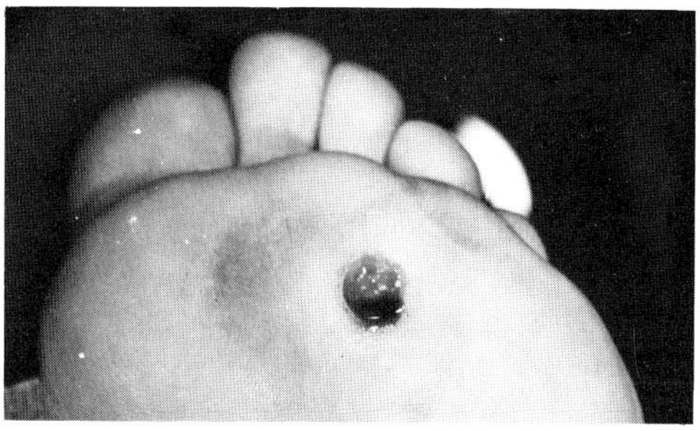

Fig. 11.20. Verruca plantaris. One week postoperative excision *in toto* of plantar wart, packed with Gelfoam. Ulceration repairs by third intention.

The area is debrided and eventually undergoes a liquefaction necrosis. In chronic cases, bismuth sodium triglycollamate (Bristrimate), an oral systemic bismuth therapy was prescribed 2 tablets, t. i. d. (adult). This dosage appears to stimulate and reinforce other treatments being used in the treatment of warts. (A dark discoloration of the gums is one of the contraindications to the use of bismuth.)

Grady (1962) used a high-speed drill with a steel burr to grind out plantar verruca while the patient was anesthetized by infiltration of an anesthetic with epiniphrine. Results in 20 patients were remarkably good with a single failure attributed to the presence of diabetes.

Dry Ice Technique. In this procedure, the cartridge of carbon dioxide gas is released into a suitably-sized plastic applicator as Dry Ice or carbon dioxide snow. The applicator, slightly larger than the wart, is held firmly over and surrounding the wart for 2 to 4 min. until the wart is white, hard and frozen. Applying a warm, moist, gauze sponge allows for a rapid thaw and less discomfort. The part is covered by an adhesive protective dressing.

In about 7 to 10 days the patient returns for treatment. Typically the area appears as a bullous lesion which is removed and drained. The remaining ulceration repairs slowly and the results are good. This destructive measure has limited application as it is most effective only on the soft, non-weight-bearing parts of the foot.

Kingland (1962) discussed the treatment of 86 patients using cryotherapy. Sixteen warts were destroyed in one treatment, 24 in two treatments, 16 in three treatments, 22 in four treatments, 5 in six treatments and 1 in seven treatments. Goldman and Stillman (1963) recommended Dry Ice followed by electrodesiccation as a painless treatment for warts.

Electrosurgery. The technique of electrosurgery is preceded by local anesthesia. The part is anesthetized with 1% lidocaine, or other suitable injectable anesthetic. 1:100,000 epinephrine is desirable for hemostasis. A needle electrode on a short wave machine or other electrodesiccating and coagulating equipment is applied intermittently to the lesion by use of a foot pedal. The current emitted may be electrodesiccating or one that fulgerates or coagulates the tissue.

The operator starts at the periphery of the lesion working inward, and in one sitting he destroys the verruca by inserting the needle as it is sparked into the mass. The coagulum (necrosis) is either removed by sharp curettage or allowed to remain. If allowed to remain, the destroyed wart acts as an irritant to the underlying tissue. A liquefaction necrosis occurs and this can be evacuated in about 10 days. The remaining ulceration must be kept clean and treated as a third degree burn.

The technique of electrosection is handled the same way. I use a cutting loop electrode. The wire electrode can be carried about and underneath the verruca with a sweeping motion. The resulting ulcerative cavity must be treated as a third degree burn and ulceration.

Superficial lesions may be dried or desiccated. Others are coagulated or cooked. Some masses are fulgerated or charred.

Injection-Therapy. Injections of a local anesthetic directly into a verruca has been helpful. Needling of the lesion under local anesthesia has been described as successful. Smallpox vaccine has been used as another method but is not recommended because of the possibility of adverse reactions. Vitamin A taken orally 50,000 units b. i. d. for several weeks has been advocated by some.

Injection of vitamin A or injectable solutions of sclerosing or necrotizing agents intracapsularly has been used successfully in the treatment of warts. Following local anesthesia, 0.3 to 0.5 ml. of Steinberg's solution is injected intradermally. Cataldi (1959) and others confirmed Steinberg's results. Steinberg (1956) developed a technique using a solution of vitamin A palmitate, alpha tocopherol, sesame oil, polysorbate 80, and distilled water (Keramin).

Yale (1940) recommended the injection of a solution containing Nupercainal, benzyl alcohol, quinine hydrobromide and physiologic saline. Prolonged anesthesia was effective for use in the armed services, but positive results were not as good as other chemotherapeutic measures. However, Stern (1961) reported excellent results with the same formula, Quinocaine. Cramer (1958) did preliminary studies with good results injecting parenzyme in oil.

Radium or x-ray therapy should be reserved for the recalcitrant wart. The judicious use of ultrasoft x-ray therapy observing the usual precautions, dosage time, technique and good judgment must be observed.

A firm adherent fibrous connective tissue may develop at the site of radiation. Since radiation may be carcinogenic on the sole of the foot, I advise less hazardous methods of removal of this common disorder.

Summary Results of Other Techniques. Curettage alone under local anesthesia has been most effective when carried out properly. A scooping motion from the periphery is effective. Weinstock (1957) reports 87 cases with only 4 reoccurrences using this method.

Harris (1966) applied concentrated phenol to warts following electrodesiccation with marked relief of pain and good results.

Gilbert and Williams (1959) report an 18-month study on 100 patients with plantar warts treated with vitamin A (Keramin) injected into the lesion. Complete resolution occurred in 82% and relief of pain in 95%. If resolution did not occur in 3 to 4 treatments, injections were discontinued. Patients were able to return to work immediately.

Carpenter (1961) injected local anesthetics with 1:50,000 epinephrine intradermally with excellent results. The needle is directed into the base of the verruca remaining within the capsule. He believes the intradermal pressure creates a pressure necrosis that destroys the mass. Sixty-one percent of the total number of warts were eradicated with a single injection and 71% were rendered symptom-free. No more than three injections were administered in any of the cases.

Goodman (1960) recommends liquid nitrogen for treatment of warts. He describes the skin reaction as a fuming sensation for a few hours, followed by a blister formation in about 3 days. Bullae should be opened if pressure builds up but the smaller blisters will dry.

Crusts drop off in about 3 weeks. Applications of liquid nitrogen may be used at 3-week intervals.

Goldman and Palerma (1961) obtained necrosis in warts by applying a heavy, syrupy lotion prepared by mixing podophyllin 20%, trichloroacetic acid 25%, glycerin 25% and salicylic acid 30%.

Ormond (1962) recommends the purified active principle of cantharides in a collodion tincture vehicle, Cantharone, in the treatment of intractable lesions involving the germinal layer of the skin. An acantholytic agent destroys the germinal layer of the skin by a selective process. Cantharides are powerful vesicants which produce blisters. The wart is treated by direct application. The lesion is then covered with plastic tape. After 4 or 5 days, an aseptic bullous lesion develops. This is aspirated and should reveal a healthy base. At the first redressing the lesion looks like a blood blister; the second week a scab forms; about the third redressing, the scab comes off leaving clean, healthy-looking skin. The part is kept clean and a band-aid applied for protection at each visit. Scar tissue is minimal and healing is usually uneventful.

Locke and Zang (1969) found that the jet spray injection of sodium tetradecyl sulfate combined with mepivacaine intralesionally was "effective, efficient and a convenient method for verruca therapy" in 78.7% of the cases treated.

Block (1967) and Trapp (1967), in separate studies, used ultrasound in verruca plantaris with a fair degree of success. Trapp concludes that ultrasound is effective on single warts and closely-grouped multiple lesions. Mosaic warts are amenable to ultrasound but require longer treatments. Weekly treatments are desirable. Block states that the "anti-inflammatory, antiviral effect of ultra-sound has good therapeutic value in the management of plantar verrucae."

Falknor (1969) used direct physical trauma in the form of "needling" to bring about dissolution of plantar warts. Insertion of the same needle used for local anesthesia about 60 times directly into the center and at the periphery of the wart produced good results with a minimum of pain.

Keratoderma

Arsenical keratosis and keratoderma plantaris must be differentiated from

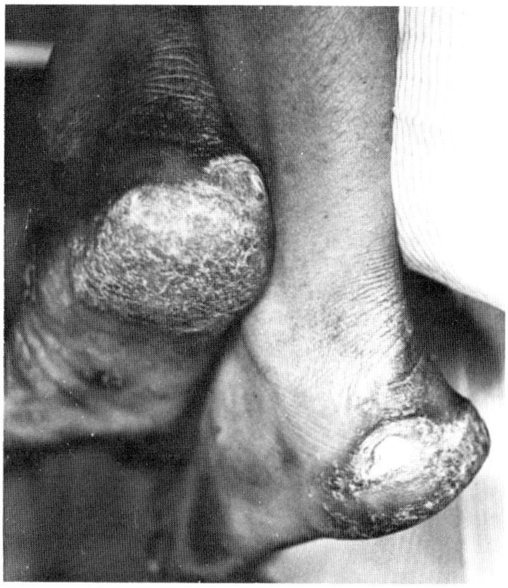

Fig. 11.21. Chronic reactive hyperkeratoses. Note callosities plantar and posterior of heel and heloma durum.

plantar warts. A history of long-term use of arsenicals helps establish the diagnosis of arsenical keratosis. Keratoderma plantaris usually has hereditary background. The lesions range from 1 to 3 mm. in size and may be larger. They affect the palms as well as the soles. These lesions manifest themselves as discrete hyperkeratotic papules. Their center is usually translucent. Friction and pressure seem to play a minor role.

Keratosis palmaris and plantaris is reported by Fred *et al.*, (1964), as being a heredo-familial trait transmitted as a Mendelian dominant. Keratoses of the soles may be of systemic or local origin. The systemic disorder may be caused by such inorganic drugs as arsenic and gold or an infectious systemic disease. The skin manifestations are usually generalized.

Superficial infections by *Tricophyton rubrum* may cause keratosis of the soles. Other keratoses may be idiopathic and present themselves as multiple, minute, punctate, hyperkeratotic skin lesions of unknown etiology.

Grayson (1965) reported a case of painful keratotic lesions on the hands and soles accompanied by papillomatous lesions of the buccal mucosa with opacities in the epithelium of the cornea. The combination is rare.

Treatment of keratoses varies with the etiology. Drug use is discontinued and systemic disorders are diagnosed and treated by an internist. Irritating chemicals are avoided and local treatment is institued. Many emollient creams containing vitamin A are helpful. Lanolin may help soften the hyperkeratosis. Reduction by scalpel, sandpaper or diamond burrs may relieve discomfort. Salicylic acid in supersaturated solutions combined with a 30 to 40% tincture of benzoin may serve as a keratolytic.

Heiss and Gross (1970) have described the successful clinical treatment of keratosis plantaris with topically applied vitamin A in 0.3% strength mixed in a base of petrolatum. Ammoniated mercury 10 to 20% may be helpful. Cocoa butter, mineral oil and a wide variety of emollients remove the scales. Exposure to sunlight has been recommended by some. Patients report relief of symptoms during warm weather.

Improvement of severe itching and scaling has been noted with the use of a betamethasone cream, Valisone as an occlusive dressing. Cordran tape may be applied, removed in 12 hr., and re-applied to remove scales and keratotic lesions and to relieve itching and other symptoms.

12

Disorders of the Sweat Glands and Mycotic Pathology

The two basic disorders involving the sweat glands are hyperidrosis, an abnormal increase in perspiration, and anidrosis, an abnormal decrease in perspiration. Both conditions are complicated by a variety of dermatologic lesions. The ability of the body to produce sweat and the ability of the sweat glands to deliver sweat are to be carefully considered in the treatment of these disorders.

Hyperidrosis is a functional disturbance of the sweat glands characterized by overactivity of the glands resulting in excessive perspiration. It is most commonly found in adolescents and in young adults. Extremely nervous individuals may perspire excessively when undergoing mental strain. Violent exercise produces an overactivity of sudoriferous glands in normal individuals. Unbalanced diets and such systemic disturbances as tuberculosis and anemia cause excessive perspiration. Salicylates and excessive ingestion of fluids may result in increased perspiration. Hyperthyroidism and hypoadrenalism cause excessive perspiration. Many individuals having hyperidrosis as a result of the stress of ill-fitting footgear, occupational stress or imbalanced feet are relieved of this condition when the underlying cause is removed.

Under physiologic conditions, sweating is associated with peripheral vasodilatation. Failure of normal evaporation of perspiration may result in symptoms of hyperidrosis. Certain conditions are generally accompanied by excessive perspiration and are complications secondary to physiologic or pathologic bodily alterations. An acid reaction of pH 4.5 to 6.0 results from organic substances being secreted which yield organic acids on hydrolysis.

Bromidrosis. Bromidrosis is characterized by excessive perspiration with a fetid odor caused by saprophytic bacteria. The normal flora on cutaneous surfaces are the micrococci diphtheroids and propionibacteria. Foot odor is caused by bacterial decomposition of skin secretions in the presence of moisture. The eccrine sweat combines with lipids and proteins resulting in a decomposition of the sweat followed by digestion of the debris by diphtheroids and micrococci. Combinations of antiperspirants and antibacterial agents retard multiplication of bacterial flora. Caprylic and lactic acids on the skin have antibacterial properties (Pillsbury, 1952). Rothman *et al.* (1947) feel that the organic acids on the skin have antifungal properties. Many times the odor is characteristic of certain dietary indiscretions with aromatic substances. The skin in some instances appears dry and even indurated when exposed to air allowing for evaporation of perspiration.

Chromidrosis. Chromidrosis is a rare condition characterized by a colored perspiration caused by abnormal con-

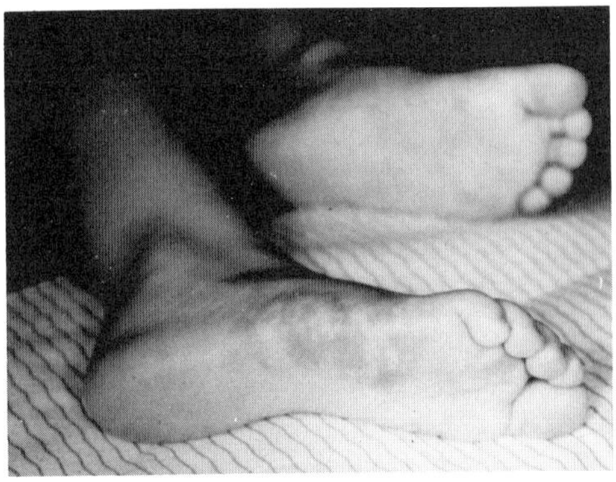

Fig. 12.1. Hyperidrosis. Note moist, white to mild red macerated skin on soles of feet.

stituents of sweat, bacterial action, chemicals in contact with the skin, synthetic materials in clothing and occupational stress.

Hematidrosis is a rare condition manifested by perspiration that is tinted by blood.

Hydrocystoma is a condition of elongation of the sweat glands or their ducts to form deep, noninflammatory papules resulting in tissue forming within the gland or duct that must be differentiated from verrucae.

Uridrosis is a condition of the sweat glands in which the excretion of urea in the sweat produces a urine-like smell in the perspiration.

Treatment. Treatment of the conditions of abnormal perspiration is aimed at normalizing the functions of the sweat glands and depends on the general physical status of the patient. It includes treatment of systemic disorders by an internist and correction of local physicochemical problems. Surgical excision of "plugged" sweat ducts may be necessary. When systemic disorders are not a factor the following procedures may be used.

A patient with abnormal perspiration should wear hose capable of absorbing perspiration and yet with a weave wide enough to allow for evaporation of insensible perspiration. Lightweight woolen hose or good quality absorbent cotten hose should be worn. Synthetic substances—such as nylon and Orlon—do not allow for adequate evaporation of excessive perspiration and may cause the skin to become soggy, irritated, macerated and painful.

Poorly constructed and ill-fitting footgear are a common cause of excessive perspiration. Shoes constructed of plastic or rubber compounds allow for continued accumulations of perspiration on the skin and subsequent maceration and discomfort. The following regimen has been used successfully to combat hyperidrosis and many of its complicating factors.

The patient should bathe the feet daily in lukewarm water and a tetramethylthiuram disulfide- or hexachlorophene-containing bacteriostatic product. The skin would be patted dry, not rubbed. A suitable astringent should be applied between toes and over areas exuding increased perspiration. A 15 to 25% aluminum chloride tincture with isopropyl alcohol may be helpful. Tannic acid, 5% in 70% ethyl alcohol in solution, is mildly astringent. A 0.25 to 0.5% Formalin solution (properly scented) may be swabbed daily over the perspiring feet and toes to decrease the excessive perspiration.

Hyperidrosis and bromidrosis may be helped by the addition of a dusting powder. Useful prescriptions for these conditions are aluminum chloride 3%, salicylic acid 3%, alum 10%, talcum powder 84% dusted on affected parts t. i. d.; and tannic acid powder, boric acid powder, zinc oxide, equal parts of each dusted on the feet 2 to 3 times daily. Such commercial powders as ZeaSORB medicated powder, BFI powder, Desenex, Efosorb, and Ammens foot powder are available.

Potassium permanganate soaks in 1:2000 solutions, t. i. d., for 20 min. help decrease the activity of sweat glands and the multiplication of odor-forming bacteria. Burrow's soaks 1:40 dilution is helpful.

In hydrocystoma, the firm papules are removed surgically. Care is exercised to remove the papule and its elongated sweat gland.

The use of sedatives and tranquilizers may be necessary in emotional and hypertensive patients. Effective drugs include chlordiazepoxide HCl, meprobamate (Equinil, Miltown, 200 to 400 mg. 3 to 4 times daily), phenobarbital, Benadryl. Phenaglycodol (Ultran) in 300-mg. pulvules and 200-mg. tablets may be helpful. Anticholinergic drugs such as Banthine (methantheline bromide) 50 to 100 mg. taken orally 3 to 4 times daily; probantheline bromide (Pro-Banthīne), 15 mg. and 7.5 mg.; and Pamine bromide (N-methylbromide of scopolamine), 2.5 mg. taken orally 4 times daily may be helpful.

In a preliminary study, David (1960) demonstrated the therapeutic potential of methenamine undecylenate for the treatment of hyperidrosis and bromidrosis. The controlled release of the active agents, formaldehyde and undecylenic acid, in effective but subtoxic concentrations provided relief of symptoms with very little skin irritation.

Anidrosis is a skin disorder characterized either by diminished function of the sudoriferous glands or mechanical obstruction of the sweat ducts and pores limiting the excretion of normal insensible perspiration and thereby causing dry skin. The skin is dry, scaly and sometimes parchment-like. The nails are dry, split and sometimes thickened. The nail grooves become calloused. Patients often complain of miliary helomas at sites of irritation such as the medial aspect of the first metatarsophalangeal joint, at seams of hose and at pressure points caused by abnormal weight distribution on the plantar surfaces. Heels crack and fissures develop as a secondary problem. Ulcerations may result. Plugging of sweat ducts may lead to the development of erythematous papules, vesicles and vesiculopustular lesions. Ichthyosis is a rare disease involving disfunction of the sweat glands.

The sebaceous secretion, sebum, accompanying normal perspiration, is lessened with a malfunctioning of the sweat glands. The subcutaneous adipose is often diminished and retention cysts may develop. Foot soaks avoiding excessive use of strong soap and hot salt water are mandatory. The disease may be aggravated or caused by diabetes, circulatory disturbances, a deficiency of vitamin A, hypothyroidism and con-

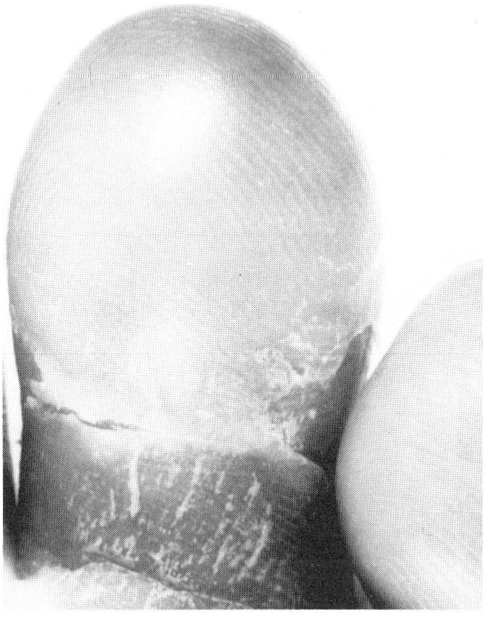

Fig. 12.2. Anidrosis. Fissure plantar surface toe—secondary to dry skin.

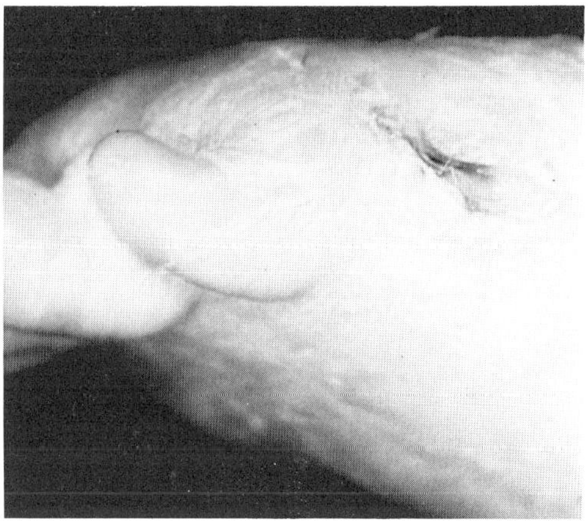

Fig. 12.3. Ulceration in anidrotic skin, fifth metatarsal head.

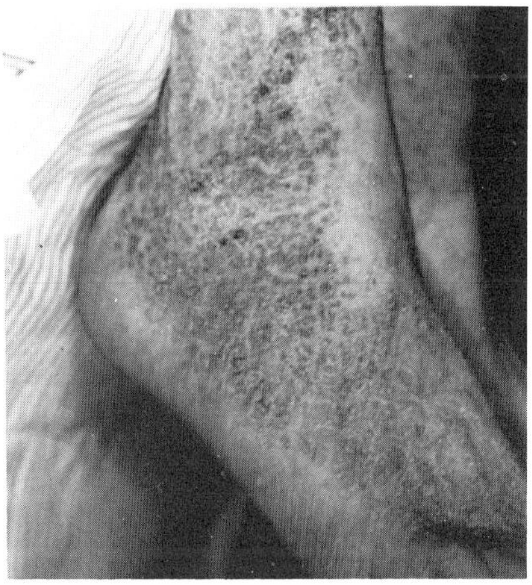

Fig. 12.4. Ichthyosis. Note dry thick scales and crusts. Usually systemic and present a variable degree all over the body.

genital absence of the sweat glands. Feldman (1958) states that "the cause of dry skin is due to a lack of water not a lack of oil or fat." Symptoms occur when the water content of stratum corneum falls below 10%.

Treatment. Excessive dryness of the skin must be treated both locally and systemically. The daily use of concentrated vitamin A in 50,000 to 100,000 U.S.P. units often improves the texture of the skin. The local use of emollient creams and moisturizing agents is suggested for maintenance of a healthy skin texture. Correction of systemic, metabolic and endocrine disturbances often improves skin texture. In advanced circulatory problems, a sympathectomy has proven to be effective in some instances. It is obvious that the skin must have proper application of moisturizing agents if the patient is to enjoy the comforts of supple skin.

A breakdown of skin into fissures and ulcerations may plague comfortable weightbearing and walking. Where fissures and ulcerations develop in anidrotic skin, it is advisable to use stimulating ointments or moisturizing agents. Fissuring of the skin is often relieved by application of tincture of benzoin compound. Use of heel cups or (Ignatoff, 1958) plaster of Paris heel casts give immediate relief and aid in repair of heel fissures.

Feldman (1958, 1959) recommends the use of a water-in-oil emulsion for dry skin consisting of 50% water in a hydrophilic ointment base, Polysorb. Patients were advised to apply Polysorb hydrate once or twice daily according to the severity of dry skin.

Prentice and Brezak (1958) recommend the use of hydrophilic water-in-oil emulsion in either whirlpool bath or as a foot soak before treatment. It may also be used in the form of a spray for its prolonged after-effect.

Boesenberg and Haas (1959) used capsules of 50,000 U.S.P. units of natural vitamin A in a water-soluble base twice daily for several weeks. Results were especially promising in the 48 cases treated. Hyperkeratotic lesions regressed in 71.4% of fissured heels, in 58.3% of yellow calvi and 53.8% of senile keratosis. Oral treatment was supplemented by inunction of a vitamin A cream.

Sturtz (1959) supports the use of oral vitamin A with hydro-dispersant emollients or lipoidal baths. He cautions against defatting the skin by using strong soap washings and recommends super-fatted soaps he calls "anti-dry soap."

Mulay and Urbach (1958) used proteolytic debridement in severe hyperkeratosis of the palms and soles. The soles of the feet were soaked for 30 min. in a 30% solution of commercial urea powder and water. The cutaneous horns and keratoses became white, translucent, slippery and soft. The hyperkeratoses were removed by scalpel until all thickened keratin was removed. This was repeated twice a day for 4 to 5 days. Rough spots were gently planed with a wire brush.

McFarlane (1962) discussed hyperkeratosis, ulceration and fissures around the heel. He noted that small fissures may be excised and sutured successfully but warned that underlying tissues of the heel cannot be mobilized successfully. Free grafts provide only a temporary cover; hyperkeratosis may occur between the graft and normal skin. The thickness between the graft and plantar skin differs and a keratin wall appears at the periphery. Prevention of this scar is accomplished by having the approximating edges of similar keratinized thickness. The fat and fascia must be about the same thickness and it is best accomplished by pedicle graft from plantar skin in an adjacent area.

Swanbeck (1968) found that high concentrations of urea allowed for an increase in the uptake of water by the horny layer of the skin. Seven patients with ichthyosis were treated with urea cream and 12 patients with atopic eczema were treated with combinations of urea cream and 1% hydrocortisone. Urea was found to be effective as a keratolytic agent and had the advantages of being nontoxic and nonallergenic.

Papa and Kligman (1966) state that in some cases return of sweating is affected by applying Scotch tape, and by pulling it off the stratum corneum is cleared from the porokeratotic duct.

In senile keratosis or actinic keratosis the use of a 5% fluorouracil (Efudex) creates an inflammatory reaction and exfoliation of skin. Treatment lasts for 2 weeks followed by a cessation of treatment to allow skin to clear.

Results have been excellent in those cases that had been treated by desiccation with only fair results.

Tinea Pedis. The diagnosis of skin lesions of the feet cannot be made on clinical findings alone. It is necessary to evaluate itching, peeling, vesiculopurulent areas on the feet by direct microscopic slides and culture studies. Too often the presence of the classical clinical signs of tinea pedis is not confirmed by microscopic examination of culture. The podiatrist must differentiate between tinea pedis and a variety of skin disorders ranging from chronic eczema, psoriasis, nummular dermatitis, dermatitis venenata, dermatitis medicamentosa and others. Steinberg (1956) noted a possible etiologic relationship between fungus infection of the human foot and rheumatoid arthritis through a complex antigen antibody effect.

Moisture, heat, dirt and alterations in pH on the surface of the feet create a media that is ideal for fungus growth. The normal range in pH of 4 to 6 is sufficiently acid to inhibit fungus growth. Kasdan (1970), in an interesting study of the environment and fungal morphology of *T. mentagrophytes*, was led into investigation of the enzyme systems of the granular and pleomorphic forms. His hypothesis that the pleomorph may well be the cause of chronic resistant cases of superficial mycotic infections is interesting, provocative and may well establish a treatment for permanent remission of symptoms.

Treatment. There are a number of approaches in managing mycotic infections. One of the first is for the patient to avoid synthetic hose which prevent evaporation of insensible perspiration and to wear lightweight wool or loosely knit cotton. Feet must be bathed frequently in a hexachlorophene preparation and dried thoroughly, especially between the toes. Exposing the feet to sunlight is helpful.

Other treatment depends on the type of fungus infection.

An acute eczematoid type of infection with blisters, crusts and scales either primary or secondary to an old tinea is treated with wet dressings of a dilute potassium permanganate solution about 1:12,000, aluminum subacetate solution or Burrow's solution in wet evaporating dressings to reduce inflammatory changes.

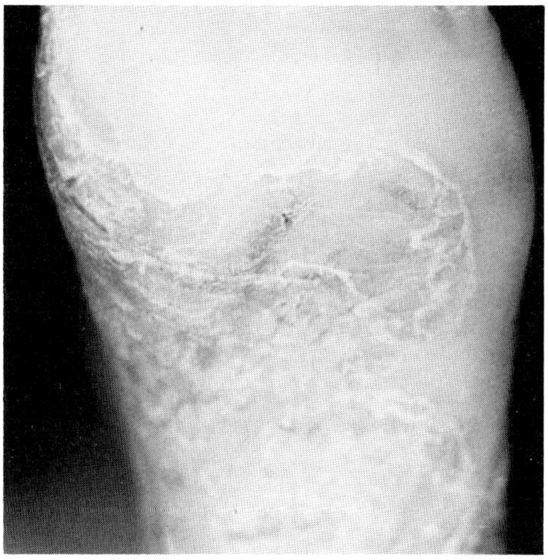

Fig. 12.5. Psoriasis. Note silvery white imbricated scales. Lesions also on elbows and knees.

Maskin *et al.* (1957), in a study of dermatophytosis from 1935 to 1954, point up the increase of *Trichophyton rubrum* as the cause of most dermatophytosis in this country.

Rothman *et al.* (1957) discuss tinea pedis as a source of infection in a family. A man with *T. rubrum* infection of the toes and heel placed his foot on the family toilet seat while treating his foot. His wife acquired a tinea circinata of the left buttock. Patients with tinea pedis must be warned of the contagious and autoinoculable characteristics of the infection.

Arancia *et al.* (1959) in discussing cutaneous moniliasis say that, "certain conditions of altered metabolism such as debilitation, obesity, diabetes mellitus, hyperhydrosis, and pregnancy predispose to cutaneous infection." They conclude that effectiveness in treatment of moniliasis of the feet was 50% better when nystatin was used in combination with other drugs. Relapses did occur and the addition of antibacterial agents to the nystatin shortened the course of therapy. Fluorohydrocortisone relieved erythema, burning and itching. Goldman and Unger (1959) found that when *Candida albicans* is the causitive organism the specific nystatin results in permanent control of the infection.

Hirschberg (1959) discussed a technique for destroying pathogenic microorganisms in footwear. The shoes and hose were placed in a non-hydrostatic polyethylene bag with a tablet containing trioxymethylene and hexahydrothymol (Zondex) as active ingredients. Hirshberg states that "95% of patients shoes tested before treatment contained spores of *M. albicans, T. gypseum,* aspergillus and *T. purpure.* After treatment with the fumigant for 24 to 48 hr., no evidence of the spores could be found on re-examination."

Walker (1959) evaluated 1 to 2% copper sulfate solution iontophoresis. He stressed the local effect, the low toxicity of the solution, its fungicidal properties and its deterrent effect on chronic recurrent eczema or "id" reaction. Patient's tolerance at an average of 10 milliamperes for 10 min. is considered desirable.

Goldberg (1959) showed that "clinically well feet seldom harbor pathogenic fungi and the shoes of these patients have little or no fungal elements."

Secondary reactions of cellulitis, lymphangitis and lymphadenopathy are treated with care to reduce sensitization from antibiotics. Systemic penicillin should not be used at this time for fear of sensitizing the patient. Wet dressings of sodium chloride as a warm physiologic saline or dilute potassium permanganate soaks are helpful. Aspirin, 2 tablets g. 4 h. with rest and elevation reduces fever. Neomycin sulfate is the antibiotic of choice. Griseofulvin is best used when the condition is subacute and in a quiescent state.

The chronic mycotic infection is manifest by dryness and scaling. Acute flare-ups can be avoided by reducing the scratch-itch syndrome. Unsaturated fatty acids such as undecylenic and proprionic acids in creams or ointments may be used effectively to reduce the infection. The feet are kept dry. Undecylenic and/or propionic acid powders used regularly between toes, shoes and hose inhibit the growth of fungi.

Oral griseofulvin may be prescribed for mycotic infections. Careful observation of the patient for sensitivities and blood dyscrasias is mandatory. Ultrafine griseofulvin, 500 mg., taken once daily seems to be effective. Lindenberg (1959) reported improvement in 25 of 28 cases studied under treatment with griseofulvin. Pruritis disappeared in 1 week. Minor headaches and occasional gastrointestinal disturbances were noted.

Gibbs (1970) simplifies the clinical varieties of tinea pedis as 1) a dry scaly interdigital type; 2) dry scaly plantar type; 3) vesicular type; dermatophytidic type. The dry scaly interdigital type presents erythrasma in the webs. It can be diagnosed by the reddish fluorescence of Wood's light even though cultures are negative.

The dry scaly plantar type of tinea pedis usually resulting in a moccasin-like diffuse scaling is pathognomonic of *T. rubrum* infection. Obviously, these lesions must be differentiated from primary irritant contact dermatitis. Unilateral vesiculation is probably of etiology other than fungus.

This may have to be differentiated from herpes zoster which is severely painful. Mycotic infections are rarely painful unless secondarily infected.

The "id" reaction on the hands secondary to mycotic foot infections have to be differentiated from dysidrosis and pustular psoriasis. Fungi are found in "id" lesions of the hands.

Apt (1967) notes that the clearing of a primary lesion results in disappearance of the "id" reaction. Since the "id" lesion is sterile of fungi it is not desirable to use antifungicides in treating it. Conant *et al.* (1963) recommend treating the "id" reaction with warm, wet saline or boric acid compresses, soothing lotions and creams.

The ringworm organism excretes an allergen to which the tissue is sensitized, or produces cytotoxic toxins affecting nonallergic skin. Apt hints that resistance or susceptibility may be genetically transmitted and that a high percentage of humans are naturally resistant to most dermatophytes.

Blask *et al.* (1959) described the typical response of tinea pedis to griseofulvin for relief of itching and burning in 2 to 6 days. Cultures and microscopic examination become negative in 2 to 6 weeks as vesicles and scales disappear completely. Topical keratolytic agents aid in eradicating fungi from the skin of the feet. Haas and Boesenberg (1960) reported cure or major improvement of 84% in the treatment of 30 patients with onychomycosis, dermatophytosis and patients with both diseases being treated concomitantly. Many patients had mixed culture responses such as *T. mentagrophytes* and *T. rubrum* or *C. albicans.*

Ashur and Farrar (1961) treated 104 patients with tinea pedis and 56 patients with onychomycosis using griseofulvin, 1000 mg. daily. The infecting organism was *T. mentographytes, T. rubrum* or *Epidermophyton floccosum.* Ninety-one patients with tinea pedis were cured and nine substantially improved. Of the patients with onychomycosis, 39 have been cured and 5 substantially improved. Tinea pedis was usually cured in 2 months and onychomycosis within 12 months. Clinical side effects were mild and transient and no pathologic changes were noted following regular examinations of blood and urine.

Ganley (1966) reported excellent results in treating 38 of 50 patients with mycotic infections with solutions of tolnaftate (1%). He notes disappointing results when pre-existing disease processes and associated illnesses exist. Results with this fungicidal agent in solution with a vehicle of butylated hydroxytoluene and polyethylene glycol have been good.

Stern and Fletcher (1966) in a study of 131 patients found that in their opinion Tinactin was the best treatment for acute and chronic tinea pedis. Tolnaftate is available in a solution, cream and powder for use b. i. d.

Carpenter (1966) in a 10-month controlled clinical study noted clearing of the clinical signs of infection using tolnaftate in solution on lesions between the toes and on the dorsum. He suggests that local treatment is best combined with systemic griseofulvin if controlled laboratory examination corroborate the diagnosis. His experience dictates that penetrability of tolnaftate is increased following the bath or foot soaks.

Ilowite (1967) concluded that, 1) dermatophytes cannot penetrate the stratum corneum unless irritation or maceration of the skin occurs, 2) disease ensues where tissue structure and function become deranged, 3) exposure to fungi plays a minor role in eliciting attacks of "athlete's foot."

Goldfarb *et al.* (1959-60) noted few undesirable reactions in a group of 137 patients treated with from 0.25 to 3.0 g of Griseofulvin per day. Therapy was discontinued when severe headache, persistent diarrhea or extreme fatigue occurred in rare cases. Despite relief of clinical symptoms, about one-third of the patients clinically cured continued to be mycologically positive.

Reiss and Kornblee (1963), in a 5-year study of tinea pedis treatment state that, "the average duration of treatment of patients was 8 weeks for those infected with *T. rubrum*; 6 weeks for those with *T. mentagrophytes*; 7 weeks for those with *E. floccosum*.

Estersohn (1966) noted in his study of 16 elderly patients with skin and nail mycotic infections that oral pulvule type ultrafine griseofulvin proved more effective, safer, and easier to administer than topical preparation.

Jones (1968) suggested that incision areas are often protected, dressed and medicated to prevent infection but create that very media for the over-growth of *Candida albicans.* The treatment of choice following positive identification of the sterile vesicular lesions around a postoperative site, is to remove occlusive dressings, use drying agents and medicate with drugs containing nystatin or amphoteracin B. Nystatin is provided in cream, ointment, powder, oral tablets and suspension form. Fungizone comes in a cream, lotion and ointment.

In treating mycotic infections, I recommend removal of all irritants, identification of the infecting organism and use of correct footgear. Local applications of tolnaftate in a cream solution and powder is effective as are undecylenic solutions, creams and powders. Systemic griseofulvin, 500 to 1000 mg. daily, may be a necessary adjunct if local treatment is ineffective.

13

Dermatologic Lesions and Ulcerations

Dermatologic Lesions

Madura Foot. Mycetoma pedis (Madura foot) usually occurs in young adults and is characterized by a painful enlargement of the forefoot which is pitted and presents multiple discharging sinus tracts. Regional lymph glands may be swollen and necrotic with a discharge containing fungi. Often the lesions are deep involving tendons, muscles and bone. The patient appears to have a markedly enlarged foot extending from an atrophic leg.

Treatment consists of incision and drainage of the sinus tracts followed by excision of the infected tissue. Skin grafts may be necessary. The drug of choice is Chlortetracycline 250 mg. q. 6 h. together with diamino-phenylsulfone 50 mg. daily for the first week, 100 to 250 mg. daily during the second week. Oyston (1961) described the lesions and the treatment in a study of 20 cases.

Pompholyx (Dyshidrosis). Multiple vesiculo-bullous lesions on the feet with intense pruritis in the presence of hyperidrosis may be pompholyx. Ingestion of sensitizing food may be etiologic. Pompholyx may develop in the presence of epidermophytosis and often is incited by allergic and toxic manifestations. It is usually resistant to treatment.

Haber and Wells (1959) described a subcorneal pustular dermatosis of the soles. The vesiculo-pustular lesions failed to respond to bed rest, local application of superficial x-ray therapy and a variety of internal and topical drugs.

There was no evidence of fungus infection on microscopic examination and cultures. Bacteriologic cultures were sterile. The bullae were filled with neutrophiles and the base appeared to undergo acantholysis. The great number of polymorphs under the stratum corneum produced a slight inflammatory reaction. The authors noted the similarity to the lesions described by Sneddon and Wilkinson (1956). No etiological explanation has been given for this subcorneal lesion.

Treatment of bullous lesions includes draining. Cultures are prepared. Undecylenic acid compounds are applied and the part is kept dry.

Atopic Dermatitis and Allergic Eczematous Contact Dermatitis. An eczematous eruption on the feet with a history of asthma, hay fever, urticaria or migrain headaches may be atopic dermatitis. Gibbs (1967) defines atopic dermatitis of the adult type as dermatitis appearing on the feet as a circumscribed scaly area, especially on the toes, or lichenified plaques around the ankles, dorsa of the feet and instep.

Contact dermatitis caused by shoes, hose, adhesive tape or other sensitizing materials or chemicals may primarily affect the dorsum of the foot, especially the skin overlying the hallux. It manifests itself as a scaling erythematous vesicular and bullous dermatosis which spreads to the dorsum of the adjacent toes. Secondary inflammatory reactions may develop from the itch-scratch syndrome. These include infections ac-

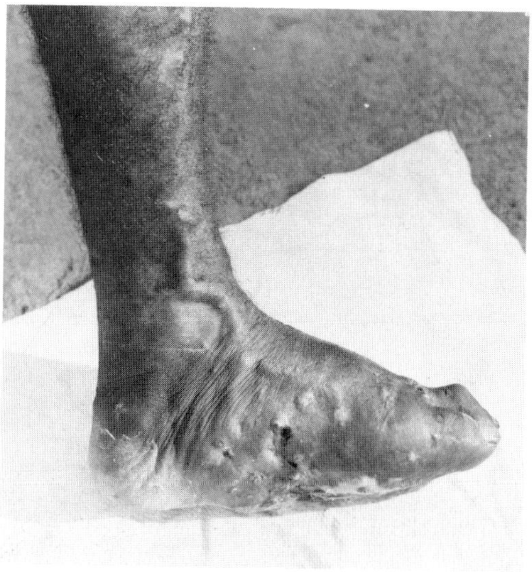

Fig. 13.1. Madura foot. #045-386-1 Armed Forces Institute of Pathology.

companied by hyperidrosis, cellulitis, lymphangitis and lymphadenopathy. The condition may be bilateral and often a secondary id-like reaction may affect the hands. Pruritis may be severe and the characteristic appearance may develop on any part of the foot that comes in contact with an irritant. Sensitizing agents may be the thermoplastic substances used in toe caps of shoes and the accelerators and anti-oxidants of rubber. People who perspire excessively are good candidates for this condition. It is believed that excessive moisture removes some of the sensitizing agents from the shoe to act as an irritant of the foot.

The toxic agents that obviously cause urticaria are believed to do so by acting on the mast cells in the dermis. Lerner and Lerner (1960) cite the triple response of Lewis in some allergic reactions as a red reaction caused by capillary dilatation, a diffuse flare caused by arteriolar dilatation and a wheal or local edema from transudates caused by increased capillary permeability. The release of histamine can be blocked by antihistamines. The antihistamines probably work by inhibition of cutaneous nerve fibers which cause pain and itching.

I have been able to isolate causative agents by patch test despite varying opinions as to its efficacy. I have found shoe polish, shoe dyes, plastic heel seats and insoles directly responsible for the dermatitis. Many patients are sensitized to the chemicals used in tanning leather, synthetic linings in shoes and rubber cements used to make shoe parts adhere in the manufacture of shoes.

Treatment. Removal of the sensitizing agent is the first step in treatment. Burow's solution soaks diminish inflammatory changes and may reduce weeping. Antipruritic medications such as calamine, and hydrocortisone cream ¼% are indicated if itching persists. Soothing protective pastes and 1 to 3% Vioform in a suitable base is helpful. In the presence of secondary infection, topical applications of antibiotics and systemic broad-spectrum antibiotics are essential. In the presence of severe allergic reactions, I prescribes diphenhydramine (Benadryl) 50-mg. capsules, 3 to 4 capsules daily for relief of itching. Tablets

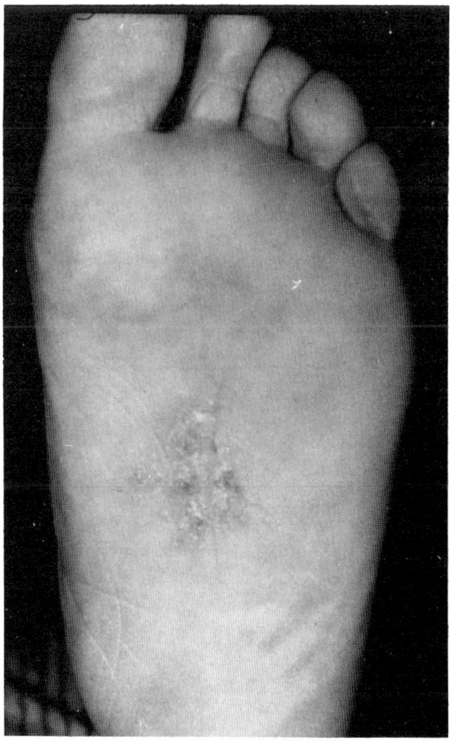

Fig. 13.2. Atopic dermatitis.

of Tacharyl HCl are helpful to relieve pruritis.

Kierland (1959), investigating pruritis, states that management comes with cure of the basic condition causing the pruritis. Pruritis may be severe in uremia even when the degree of nitrogen retention is slight. When little cutaneous reaction is noted, the pruritis may be due to a systemic reaction.

Dermatitis therapy should begin with the simplest and mildest form of treatment. If successful, the treatment should not be changed.

Local treatment consists of cool or warm, wet dressings, menthol in proper vehicles, 1 to 2% phenol in lotions, ointments or pastes. Steroids alone or in combination with antibiotics may be helpful.

Systemic treatment for pruritis may be disappointing. In urticaria, the itching may be relieved with antihistamines such as Benadryl 50 to 100 mg., 3 to 4 times daily, Dramamine 50 mg. t. i. d., Chlortrimeton, 4 mg. t. i. d., or Dimetane, 4 to 8 mg. Systemic steroids should be used in only the most severe cases with skin lesions. Acetylsalicylic acid is helpful for relief of itching. Chloral hydrate does not increase itching and can be used effectively for nocturnal itching. Teldrin (chlorpheniramine maleate), 8- and 12-mg. Spansules or capsules taken one on arising and one at night often provides 24-hr. relief from itching. The 8-mg. Spansule is suitable for children.

Vegetable-tanned shoes and inner linings or non-leather substitutes may be helpful where patients are sensitive to dichromate. Rubber insoles and dyes, fabrics that "bleed" and nickel sensitivity from eyelets may cause reactions in sensitive patients.

Weiner (1960) described a dermatitis caused by shoes with plastic uppers and rubber soles. The impermeability of the material used in construction trapped excessive perspiration in the shoes and is cited as the etiology of the dermatitis.

In the treatment of such types of dermatoses as keratosis of the soles with a variety of skin manifestations such as crusts, scales, fissures, atopic lesions, dry and lichenified skin, the podiatrist may wish to use foot baths for their soothing and beneficial anti-pruritic and keratolytic effect. Baths include use of aluminum subacetate, milk, potassium permanganate, tar, colloidal oatmeal in a starch-protein complex of oat grain in dispersible emollient oils, saline in physiologic strengths and emollient oils or lubricating soaps.

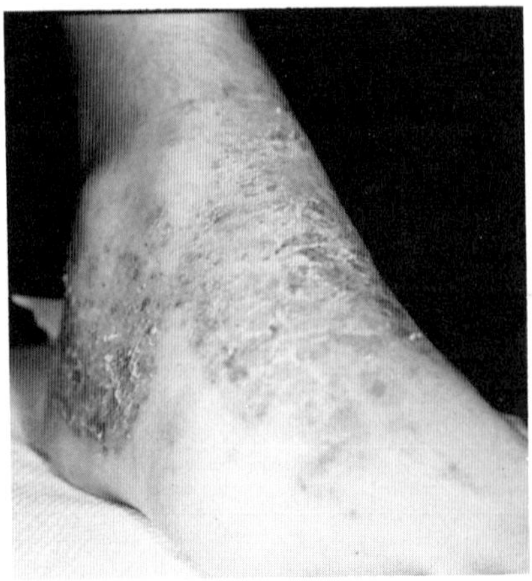

Fig. 13.3. Contact dermatitis. Heel counter and tongue of shoe.

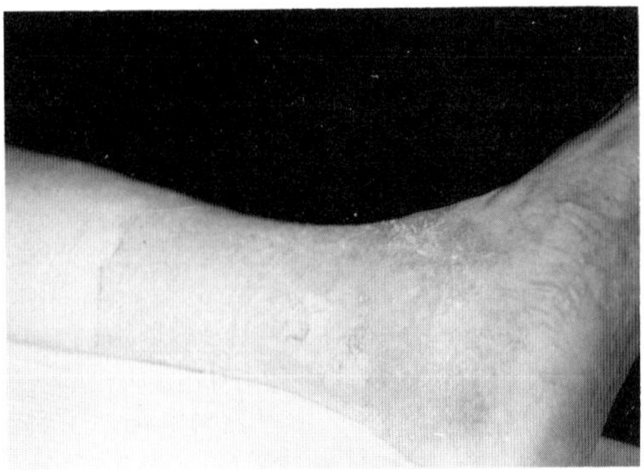

Fig. 13.4. Contact dermatitis. Note line of demarcation at upper end of stocking.

Franks (1958) advises baths for treatment of patients with dermatitis to incorporate medication and for sedation of tense patients. They are helpful in removing crusts and debris.

Jillson (1957) discusses the role of pathogenic and saprophytic fungi in causing allergic dermatitis. Intradermal skin tests are used to determine the allergen. Treatment consists of avoiding the sensitizing molds in house dust, upholstered furniture and mattresses, etc., followed by intradermal administration of dilute antigens in fixed amounts for desensitization. Extracts are injected twice weekly until the dermatitis has been cleared for several months. Booster shots can be given every 3 to 4 weeks while other dermatic treatment continues.

Fisher (1959) points out that most inexpensive shoes have a rubber thermoplastic box toe composed of scrap from old tires and girdles, etc. The rubber compound contains felt, turpentine, resin, rozin, styrene, asphalt and Carbowax as additives followed by the anti-oxidants and accelerators. He states that a satisfactory shoe should have a Celastic box-toe made with cotton flannel impregnated with pyroxylin. The lining of shoes contains rubber cement.

Trivalent chromic sulfate or hexavalent sodium dichromate used in tanning leathers is considered non-sensitizing. Fisher found a 26% sensitivity to dichromate. Perspiration will leach chemicals from the leather.

Everall and Truter (1957) could not find any basis for an antigen-antibody reaction in contact dermatitis. Existence of antibodies in epidermal hypersensitivity has not been proved nor are there antibodies in the serum.

Following a study of adhesive tape as an irritant, Ignatoff (1956) came to some interesting conclusions. The formula used in the manufacture of adhesive tape is physiologically acceptable. He states that adhesive tape reactions in ascending order of frequency are allergic, bacteriologic, chemical and mechanical. He found that less than 1% of patient's exposed to adhesive tape have an allergic response. The improper application of adhesive tape accounts for the mechanical reactions.

Montgomery and Brezak (1958) treated the pruritis of dermatitis venenata, atopic eczema and neurodermatitis on the feet with good results by using a 3% Vioform 1% hydrocortisone preparation in a cream, lotion or ointment.

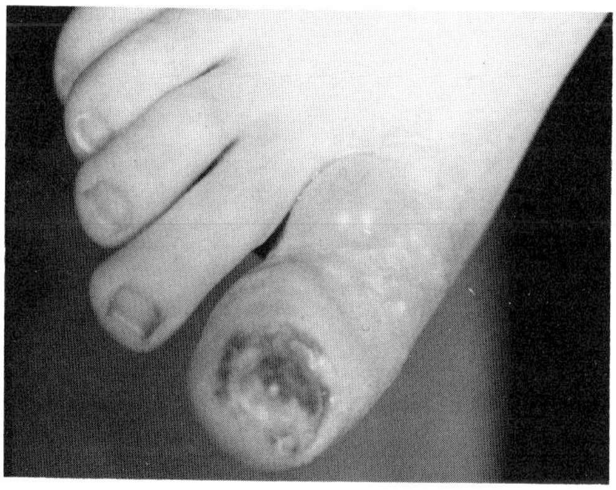

Fig. 13.5. Dermatitis venenata. Vesiculobullous lesions secondary to contact with "non-sensitizing" bandage. Patch test confirmed.

Schanberg *et al.* (1958) treated 510 patients with a variety of dermatoses with a topical steroid and a placebo. They found that "steroid therapy is effective in only a limited number of selected dermatologic patients, and is dependent on the degree of inflammation, its location and other factors."

Reyer (1957) described four cases where adhesive tape applied to the feet to relieve strain resulted in a sensitivity over a period of months which ultimately affected the periorbital skin. It was believed that pathogenic amounts of tissue protein metabolites in the circulation after relief of the spasm and painful feet resulted in this pathology.

The symptoms of atopic dermatitis are controlled by use of topical preparations such as Burow's solution, aluminum acetate, Dalibour solution or Buro-Sol to dry weeping lesions to reduce inflammation. Betamethasone valerate cream and ointments 0.1% as Valisone relieve itching and reduces inflammatory changes. Flurandrenolone cream and ointment 0.05%, also with neomycin (Neo Synalar) or as a lotion or cream in half-strength (0.025%) is helpful in controlling symptoms. Hydrocortisone cream or lotion with or without neomycin in ¼ to ½% relieves itching and controls secondary infection.

Psoriasis is characterized by silvery-white imbricated scales overlying an erythematous base. It often involves the nails with a characteristic grayish-white discoloration with pitting and subungual hyperkeratotic debris.

Pathognomonic of the disease is the presence of deep redness with overlying white scales on the elbows and knees. Pustular psoriasis ocassionally develops on the feet.

Lichen Planus may occur on the soles of the feet, although this is not the usual site. It is characterized by flat-topped, violaceous, polygonal papules. The lesions are discrete but may coalesce to form plaques. They commonly occur around the ankles, and when they develop on the soles they must be differentiated from mycotic infections.

Treatment may be by tincture or ointment serving as a keratolytic and antipruritic reducing agent. A tar tincture such as rectified oil of birch tar, 10 g.; alcohol (U.S.P.), 50 g.; ether q. s. ad 100 g.; or a hydrophilic petrolatum ointment containing epithelial cell cytotoxic substances such as podophyllum in 0.25%, 0.5% or 1% may prove effective if treatment is exercised with care. Hyperkeratoses may regress and itching is usually relieved.

Exfoliative Dermatitis is an indurated erythema of the skin which progresses to lichenification and scaling. The skin is warm and the patient experiences chills and fever. The skin itches and the palms and soles may peel with fissuring. Hair loss and nail changes may follow an acute episode in the middle-aged and elderly. Previous eczemas and ingestation of drugs may be etiologic. Systemic steroids are generally helpful.

Erythrasma is a bacterial infection of the skin most commonly manifested in the foot as an intertriginous affliction of the toe clefts. It is characterized by fissuring, scaling and maceration between the toes and is not caused by fungus or *Monilia.*

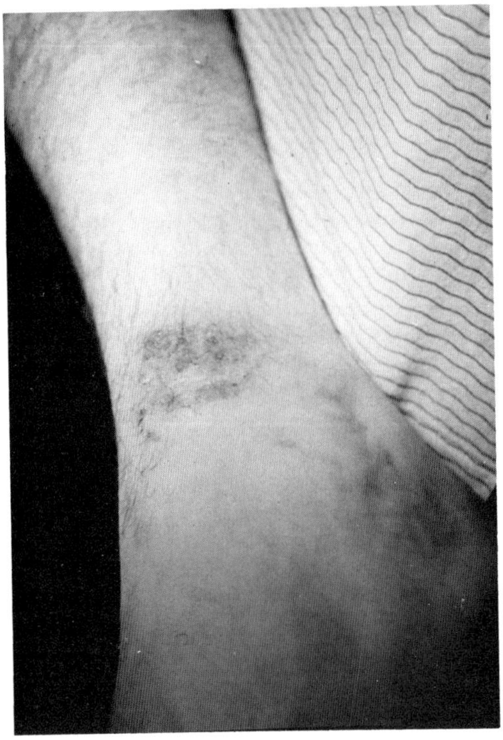

Fig. 13.6. Lichen planus.

Sarkany and Blank (1961) note that 23% of 109 normal subjects examined presented symptoms of erythrasma. Temple and Boardman (1962), in an examination of 371 university students with Wood's Light, found a 14.3% incidence of erythrasma. Bacteria were cultured from 50 of the 53 specimens examined. Clinical findings demonstrate dry, irregularly shaped, fine, red to brown scales with coral red fluorescence seen under Wood's light and by electron microscopic examinations. Smears demonstrate the presence of Gram-positive rods and filaments with granules.

Treatment. Erythromycin, especially the propionyl ester of erythromycin, (Ilosone; Erythrocin), 250 mg. 4 times daily for 5 days proved to be the drug of choice. Topical applications of soothing soaks, powders and creams are justified in controlling the symptoms. Brown (1970) approves of topical applications to relieve pruritis but has not seen beneficial results with topical antibiotics. Ointments containing phenol, menthol, camphor, salicylic acid or tar in low percentages are effective in relieving the itch.

Black Heel—Pseudochromidrose Plantaire. Kirton and Price (1965) report on 49 cases of plantar pseudochromidrose as described by Baze and co-workers from 1962 to 1964. The unusual complaint consisted of a small black patch on the back or side of the heel occurring predominantly in girls between the ages of 12 and 22. Some of the spots were circular or oval with minute round dark spots and some scattered granules of pigmentation. The condition is generally unilateral with only a single lesion occurring on a foot. The keratotic tissue can be reduced often without bleeding.

Histochemically the lesion gives a positive reaction of peroxidase, benzidine and hemochromogen proving the presence of hemoglobin. Pigment is present in the sweat ducts. Often the lesion undergoes complete spontaneous resolution and is painless. Removing trauma is essential for cure.

Neurodermatitic Reaction. Sachs *et al.* (1946) described a neurodermatitic reaction as a "pathologic process and not a disease." They stated that the reaction involves both the cutis and the epidermis. The epidermis is acanthotic, somewhat regular and with very little evidence of swelling. The middle and upper layers of the dermis present thickened walls of the arterioles and small arteries. A focal infiltration of small round and connective tissue cells are found around the vessels.

Clinically the neurodermatitic reaction resembles other dermatoses, especially nummular eczema which differs only in the presence of an intraepidermic vesicle. An exudative inflammatory process exists in both. However, discoid chronic dermatosis presents a cellular infiltration of the productive type.

Sachs *et al.* (1964) describe nummular eczema as a form of neurodermatitis. It had been described for years as a coin-shaped patch with a vesicular border and clearly pigmented center. The lesions occur on the dorsum of the hands and feet. The vesicles are small and never enlarge to the size of a bulla. Itching is common and scarring never occurs.

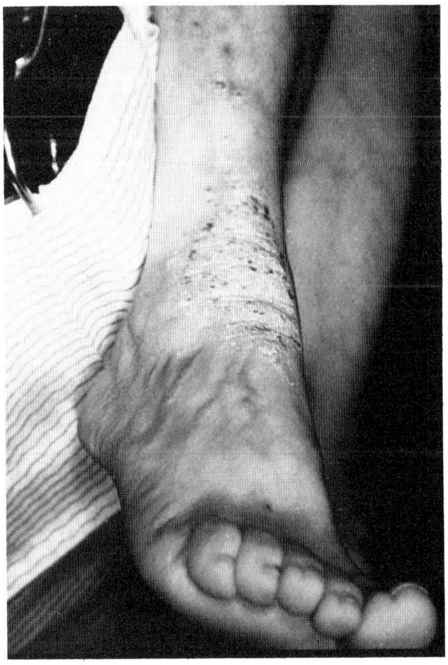

Fig. 13.7. Neurodermatitis. Note location anterior of ankle, elevated, angular margins with excoriations.

Scars. Scar tissue on weight-bearing surfaces may result from injury, lacerations, operative incisions and multiple, minimal trauma by irritants in footgear. Repair of lacerations on weight-bearing areas often cause scar tissue with a tendency for proliferation of keratoses producing painful callosities. Surgical excision of lesions on weight-bearing sites such as verrucae under the first, second or fifth metatarsals may carry with it a possibility of scar tissue formation. Ragged cuts or irritations from irregularities in shoes can produce scar tissue. Negroes may develop heavy elevated scars or keloids. Scars often develop following electrocoagulation of plantar skin lesions.

Treatment. Removal of the source of irritation occasionally diminishes the size of a scar. Dermabrasion, when properly performed, is effective. Blau (1959) recommends skin planing which provides uniformly excellent results. This is followed by use of 2% panthenol cream (Panthoderm) for several months. Generally, excision of the mass with careful fine suturing or the use of plastic strips to coaptate tissue

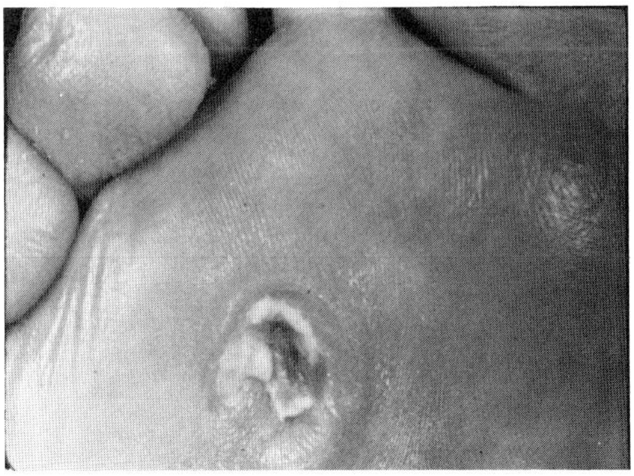

Fig. 13.8. Surgical ulceration with keloid formation following electrocoagulation of plantar wart. A "collar button" type keloid is developing.

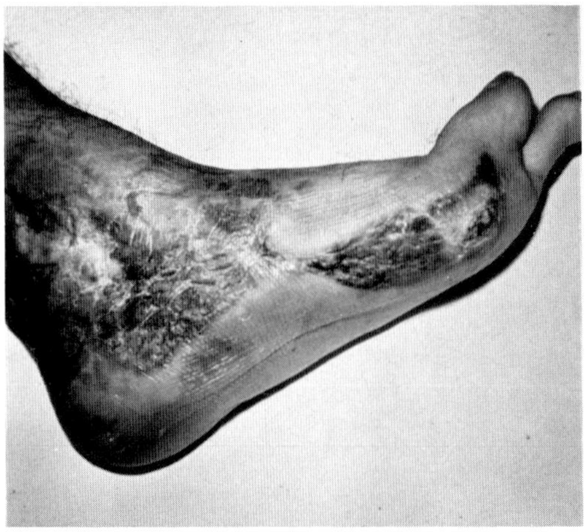

Fig. 13.9. Skin graft broken down following surgery for extensive burns. Courtesy of J. F. Yale.

eliminates scar tissue. Carbon dioxide snow has been useful. Bichloroacetic and monochloroacetic acid may destroy some scars and allow for a better repair of the affected tissue. Inunction of vitamin A and D cream helps maintain the integrity of the skin.

Dermabrasion may be very useful in removing scars, tissue pigments and helomas. Some benign superficial nevi, vascular nevi and port wine stains may be abraded. Included also are keloids, keratoses, adenoma sebaceum and skin graft sites. Planing is contraindicated if scarring is slight. Equipment should include stainless steel brushes, burrs, serrated stainless wheels and heatless stones of proper sizes, an electric motor capable of 12,000 rpm and ethyl chloride sprays. Antisepsis must be scrupulously observed since a totally aseptic technique is rarely achieved.

Treatments are given at 4- to 6-week intervals as described below. Ethyl chloride, Dermafreeze or Dermathone is sprayed over the area to be treated. Luikart (1956) suggests freezing with dichlorotetrafluoroethane to eliminate hazards of explosion. An air blower is then played over the sprayed site resulting in freezing hardness of the tissue.

The operative field should be limited to 1 to 1½ in.^{2} to prevent early thawing and to guard against damage to previously abraded tissue. Abrasion should be up and down rather than across. The field generally is bloodless and new skin regenerates.

Blau (1957, 1959) uses Dèrmathone which acts as an anesthetic and skin hardener.

Following the planing procedure, tissue will appear red, smooth and soft to the touch.

The principles to follow are to select carefully those patients amenable to plantar surgery. Remove pressure from the affected part. Follow surgical repair with 50,000 units of vitamin A daily and annoint the affected part with lanolin cream or any emollient with a lubricating base.

Intralesional injections of corticosteroids into scars may reduce their size and prevent keloid formation. The usual dosage is 0.3 to 0.5 ml. of the steroid. I have found Celestone Soluspan especially effective.

The administration of drugs sublesionally or intralesionally promises to be of great help in the treatment of many skin disorders seen in podiatry practice. Helomas, tylomas, verrucae, psoriasis, contact dermatitis and others may be amenable to this therapy.

Triamcinalone injected in combination with 2% lidocaine was suggested by Prentice (1961). A concentration of 6.25 mg./ml. was combined with lidocaine hydrochloride as the diluent. No more than 25 mg. should be injected in a 7-day period. A disposable syringe with 25 to 26 g. 3/8-in. disposable needle is used to inject into or beneath the lesion to a depth of 3 to 5 mm. Intractable psoriatic lesions appeared to undergo resolution with injections of the steroid. In Prentice's series of cases, good to excellent responses were noted in a variety of skin disorders such as dermatitis venenata, eczema, granuloma annulare, lichens planus, lichens simplex chronicus, and psoriasis of local, generalized and pustular type.

Similar injections for plantar warts may be made using vitamin A, bismuth subtartrate, benzyl alcohol, procaine or lidocaine hydrochloride, and a variety of sclerosing agents.

Locke (1961) described the techniques and use by injection of prednisolone 21 phosphate, a rapid-acting, freely soluble steroid for intralesional therapy. He recommended fanning the solution out beneath the lesion for best results in neurofibrous lesions, soft and hard corns, and tylomas.

Keratosis of the Soles. Ichthyotic dry scaling lesions may occur on the soles of the feet as a secondary dermatosis to

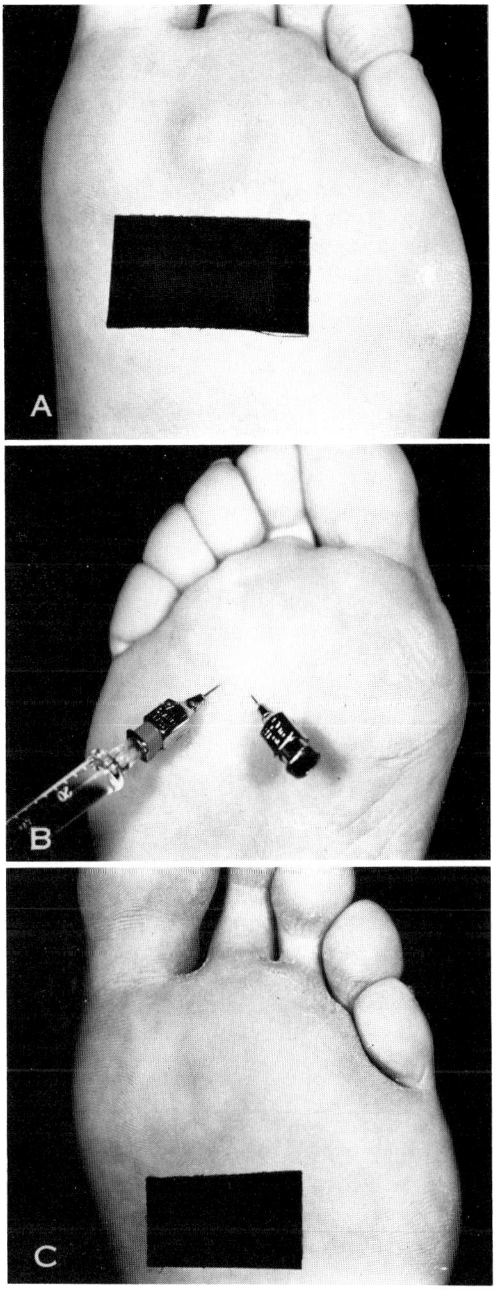

Fig. 13.10. *A*, intractable tyloma second and fifth metatarsophalangeal joints in male, age 34. *B*, needle positions for plantar injections of the anesthetic and corticosteroid. *C*, following three injections, lesion under the second metatarsophalangeal joint (one injection of 4 mg. prednisone T.B.A., two injections of 6 mg. prednisone 21 phosphate, one injection lesion under fifth metatarsal head of 6 mg. prednisone 21 phosphate). Courtesy of R. K. Locke.

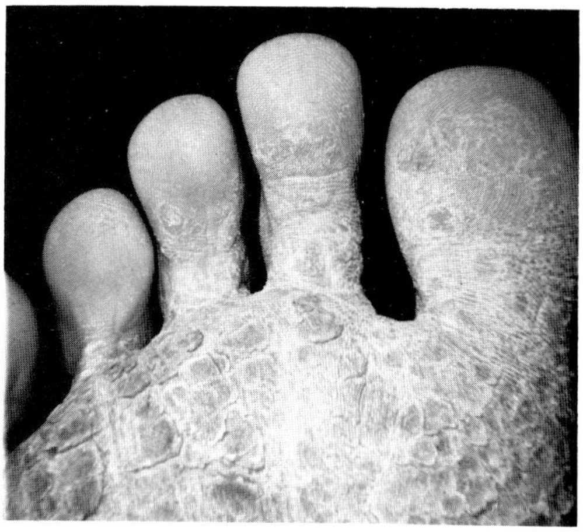

Fig. 13.11. Keratosis of the soles. Courtesy of J. F. Yale.

chemical irritants. The appearance of the scales is not unlike that of ichthyosis, a genetically-predetermined systemic dryness of the skin. Complete laboratory studies are indicated to rule out systemic disorders and the local irritants are sought out and removed. Treatment consists of local applications of keratolytic agents followed by local and systemic use of vitamin A.

Ulcerations on the Feet

Ulcerations may occur on the feet in debilitating disorders, neurotrophic or vascular disease. Destruction of tissue occurs at points of pressure. Ulcerations may be due to the exciting factors of trauma due to ill-fitting footgear, faulty foot structure, abnormal foot posture and disturbed function. The common locations for ulcers are over the bony prominences such as the posterior and plantar surfaces of the heels and the heads of the first and fifth metatarsals. Calloused areas and helomas may break down from irritation causing an ulceration which is often difficult to heal. Ulcers on the foot may also occur on the plantar surface beneath the heads of any of the metatarsals, the dorsal aspects of the toes and the distal tips and webs of the toes.

The location, shape, appearance and

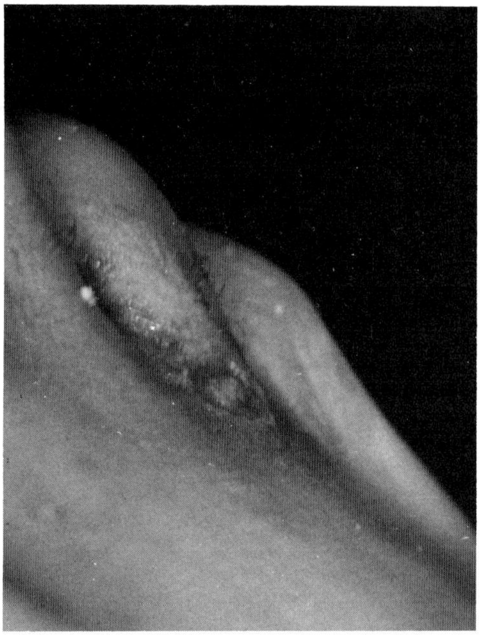

Fig. 13.12. Trophic ulcer dorsum of toe. Exposed extensor tendon.

character of the ulcerative discharge is often suggestive of the etiology. Gangrene may occur at the tips of the toes, beneath the nail plate or on the plantar surface of the great toe and about the heels secondary to ulcerations. Areas of focal gangrene are quite small and are usually seen in diabetics, arteriosclerotics and in patients with certain blood dyscrasias. They are generally localized and self-limiting but could potentially lead to widespread gangrene. One must not confuse focal gangrene with a neurovascular heloma which may be painful but less dangerous. Gangrene of the heel, leg and foot may result from trauma, burns and incisions in the presence of occlusive vascular disease.

Ulcers are usually caused by venous stasis, arteriosclerosis, thromboangiitis obliterans, impaired cutaneous sensation, neoplasms, arteriolar disease, fragility of small arteries and arterioles, infections and a host of variables. They may occur secondary to trauma and infections.

Treatment. Fox (1962) described a new therapeutic regimen for treatment of ulcers which was designed to reduce or eliminate edema and control of infection by means of oral therapy using a combination of diuretics and a suitable antibiotic. After bacterial culture and antibiotic sensitivity tests, an oral diuretic in proper dosage and a broad spectrum antibiotic was prescribed. Tetracycline, 1 g. daily for 5 days, is the antibiotic of choice.

The systemic treatment is augmented by local treatment of the ulcer. The ulcer is covered by sterile pads and an elastic bandage is applied from the foot to just below the knee. After a week, an additional test is made to find the antibiotic of choice to attack the bacteria insensitive to tetracycline. After an additional 2-week period, potassium depletion is evaluated and the continued use of the diuretic is reassessed. Henzell *et al.* (1970) note that dietary zinc sulfate 110 to 210 mg. t. i. d. promotes wound healing in the feet.

Differential Diagnosis and Treatment of Ulcers

Traumatic Ulcers. Ulcerations develop in devitalized tissues as a result of mechanical irritation such as injudicious instrumentation, pressure from ill-fitting footgear, occupational stress, sudden severe injury, or abnormal weight distribution. They are often complicated by circulatory and systemic disease such as arteriosclerosis and diabetes. In studies by Dieter and Graziano (1970) cultures of traumatic and stasis ulcers revealed offending organisms as *Staphylococcus aureus*, beta-hemolytic *Streptococcus*, *Pseudomonas*, *Proteus*, *Aerobacter aerogenes*, paracolon bacilli, *Micrococcus*, and yeast. Granuloma pyogenicum may develop in an ulcer.

Treatment. Remove the source of trauma and seek consultation for early treatment of complicating systemic disorders.

Cleanse the ulcer with hexachlorophene and debride devitalized tissue by careful instrumentation or by the use of animal or vegetable proteolytic enzymes. Walkes and Hazen (1957) noted excellent clinical results with an i.m. injection of aqueous trypsin (Parenzyme) in 44 out of 53 cases. A neomycin, trypsin and chymotrypsin ointment (Biozyme) or fibrinoly-

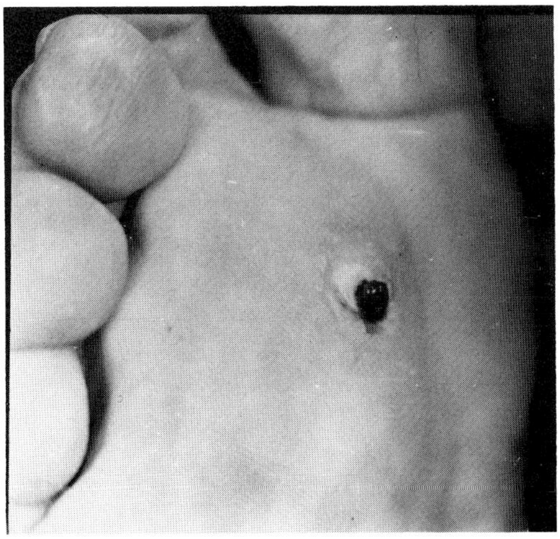

Fig. 13.13. Granuloma pyogenicum developed in an ulcer secondary to trauma.

sin and deoxyribonuclease ointment (Elase), Varidase, Panafil and Tryptar seems to be helpful in combining antibacterial as well as proteolytic action in repair of some ulcers. Improve granulation and repair by use of stimulating antibiotic enzyme topical medication. Ultraviolet radiation is helpful.

If secondarily infected, do a sensitivity test and prescribe a systemic antibiotic and local medication to combat the offending organism. In the presence of anaerobic bacteria, lavage with hydrogen peroxide is indicated when redressed. When infection is present, it is necessary to repeat sensitivity tests as new bacteria take over in long-standing ulcerations.

Construct a foot or toe prosthesis to remove undue stress from the affected part and have the patient wear an elastic bandage for adequate support. Immobilization by plaster cast will aid in repair.

Stasis Ulcers. Congestive ulcers result from devitalization of the tissues and include ulcers caused by poor venous return and bedsores. The ankles, heels and toes are commonly involved.

Treatment. In varicose veins it is necessary to assist gravitational return of venous blood by elevation of the affected extremity, bed rest and use of elastic stockings or bandages. Ligation and stripping of incompetent veins may be necessary. Skin grafts may be required to close the ulcer. Nitrofurazone dressing is helpful in protecting the skin graft.

Repair is aided by prescribing stimulating ointments such as a 0.5% water-soluble chlorophyll derivative (Chloresium) which promotes healing and reduces wound odor. Chloresium in solution (0.2%) may also be used. Garamycin, a gentamicin ointment and cream, may stimulate repair. Occasionally, there is a need for i.m. injections of proteolytic enzymes to aid digestion of debris and to stimulate repair as suggested by Corsaro (1958). A colloidal solution of denatured proteolytic enzyme (Protamide), indicated in the presence of neuritis, is used as one ampule every 2 to 5 days.

Pyogenic ulcers may be produced through invasion of the tissues by pus-producing bacteria. Unsterile instruments and careless antisepsis when treating simple skin lesions may cause pyogenic ulcers. These ulcers are often caused by breaking down of tissue from carbuncles, boils, pustules and acid therapy destroying techniques. Extension to bone from infected ulcers is not uncommon, and radiographs may be helpful in establishing a diagnosis.

Treatment. Perform sensitivity test on bacterial flora in wound to determine antibiotic of choice which may include penicillin, erythromycin, or tetracycline. Lincomycin (75 to 150 mg. by injection) is suitable where secondary bone infection is noted and where sensitivity tests demonstrate its efficacy. Local debridement and application of antibiotic enzymatic medications is helpful. Warm saline soaks facilitate drainage.

Trophic ulcers develop in peripheral neuritis, syphilis and tabes, diabetes, syringomyelia, certain paralyses, peripheral vascular disease and other debilitating diseases. The areas receiving great pressure and friction are usually sites for trophic ulcers. An x-ray examination is essential to rule out bone pathology.

Treatment. Remove pressure from affected part by judicious use of felt, foam and

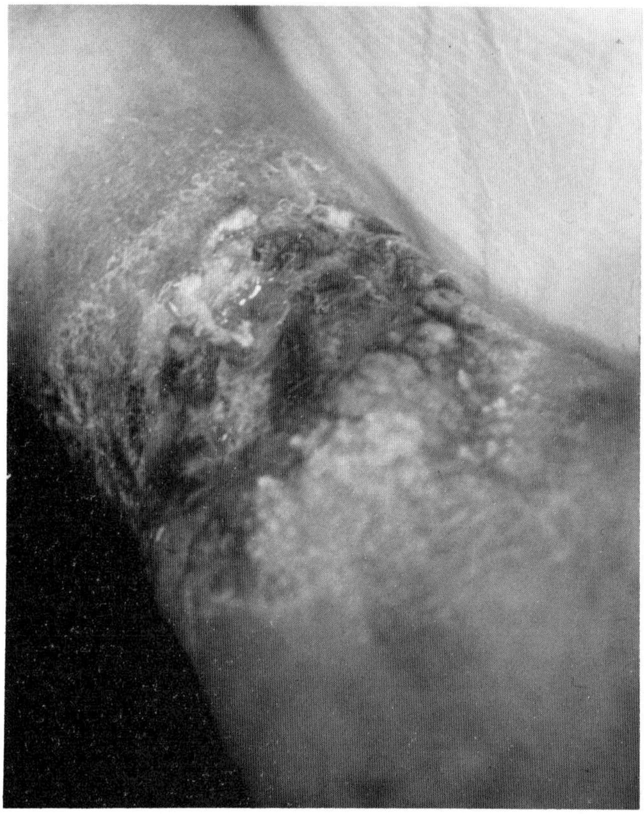

Fig. 13.14. Stasis ulcer at ankle.

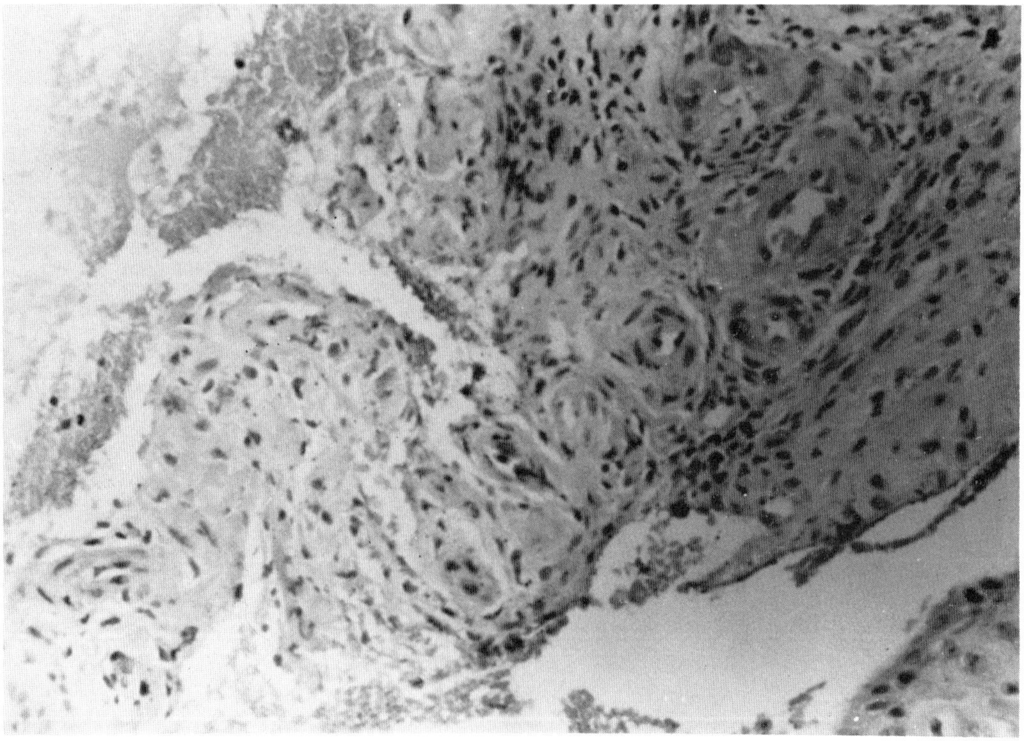

Fig. 13.15. Photomicrograph of stasis ulcer showing ulceration of epithelium (*upper left*) and vessel walls that are thick and vessels dilated (*right*). Hemosiderin pigment not evident. Courtesy J. F. Yale.

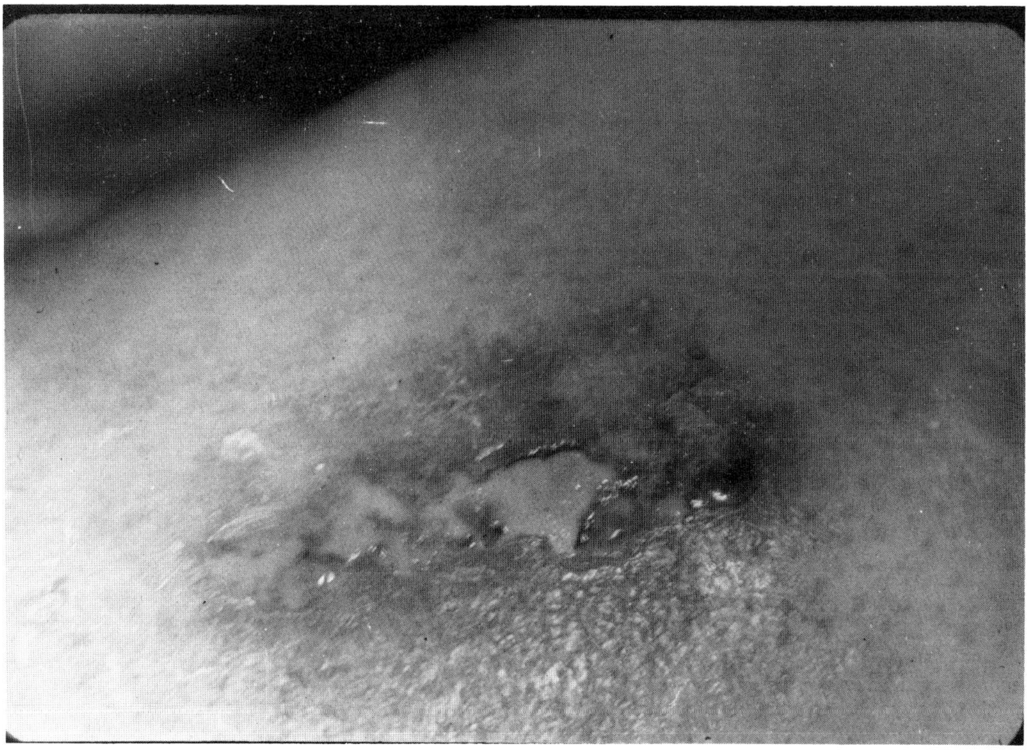

Fig. 13.16. Pyogenic ulcer.

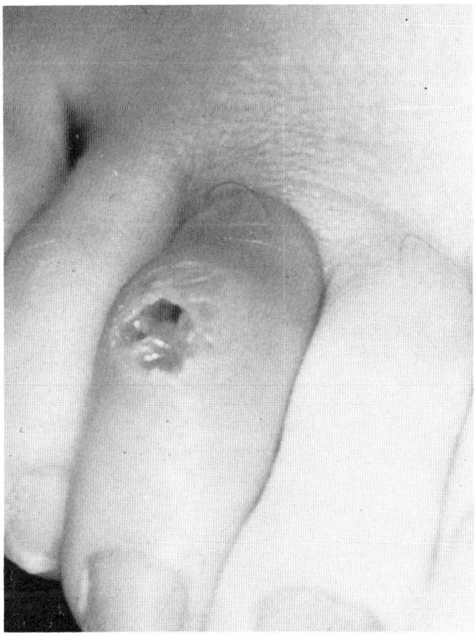

Fig. 13.17. Pyogenic ulcer. Note swelling of the infected toe.

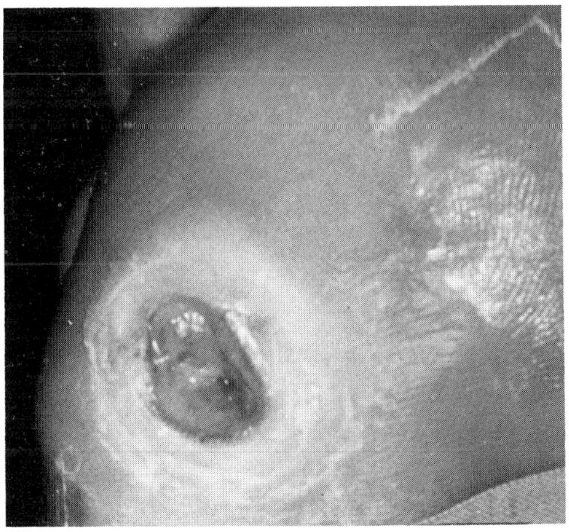

Fig. 13.18. Trophic ulcer plantar surface of the first metatarsal head.

pressure-sensitive rubber. Construct foot appliances to relieve pressure.

Correct peripheral neuritis; treat systemic diseases and peripheral vascular instability.

Bed rest with proper shielding of bony

prominences may be beneficial. Local and systemic antibiotics and enzymatic debridement may be necessary. Eisenberg (1961) recommends the application of a plaster cast for 3 weeks.

Specific ulcers are those caused by definite disease and are classed as syphilitic, diabetic, tubercular, arteriosclerotic and so forth. Cohen and Shelley (1962) described an ulceration due to Werner's syndrome in a male, aged 30, with premature signs of senility, circumscribed hyperkeratosis of the soles, tightness of the skin over pressure points and local calcification of the skin.

Treatment includes local measures to aid repair and control infection and consultation with medical specialists for treatment of the systemic etiology. Large doses of vitamin B_{12} and specific medication for the etiologic basis is helpful in repair.

Malignant ulcers are caused by unintentional damage at the time of biopsy, excess radiation, metastasis from other malignant lesions and pressure of rapidly growing malignant tumors with destruction of tissue.

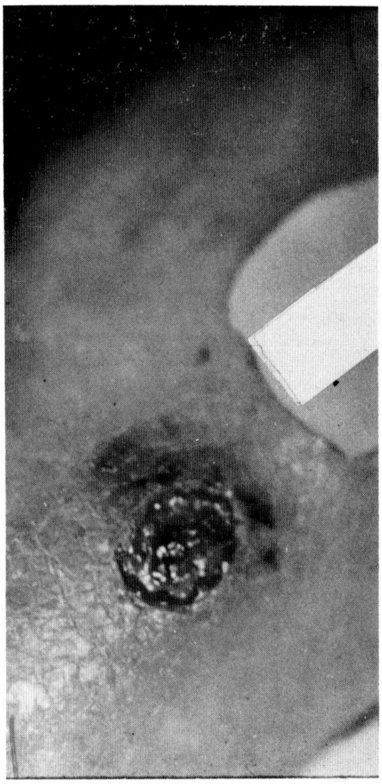

Fig. 13.21. Ulcer secondary to pernicious anemia.

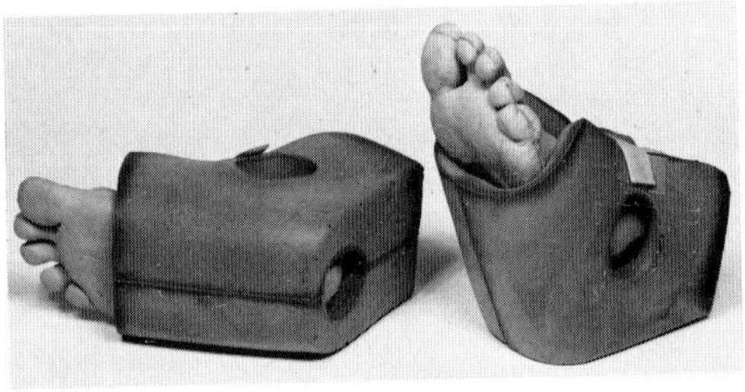

Fig. 13.19. Protection device for prolonged bed rest. Courtesy of Medical Plastics Laboratory.

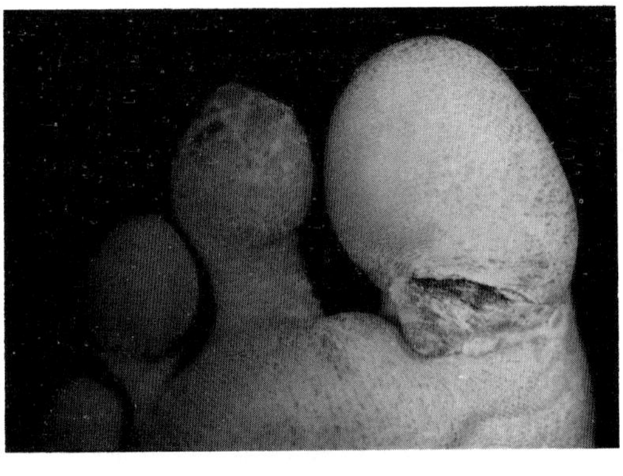

Fig. 13.20. Arteriosclerotic ulcers.

Ulcers are shallow, cupped-out lesions of the surface tissue with either an irregular, smooth or elevated border. The surface may be sloughing, granulating or fungating. When the ulcer is on the plantar surface of the foot on a weight-bearing area and penetrates to the bone it is perforating. When it is adherent to the underlying tissues, it may be malignant.

Ulcers discharge serous or seropurulent fluids. Excessive hemorrhage may indicate the presence of a superficial arteriole or possibly a vascular malignancy; chalky discharges suggest sodium biurate crystals of gouty deposits. A caseous tissue discharge is usually of tubercular origin.

Deep, indurated, adhered ulcerations may be malignant. Marked evidence of

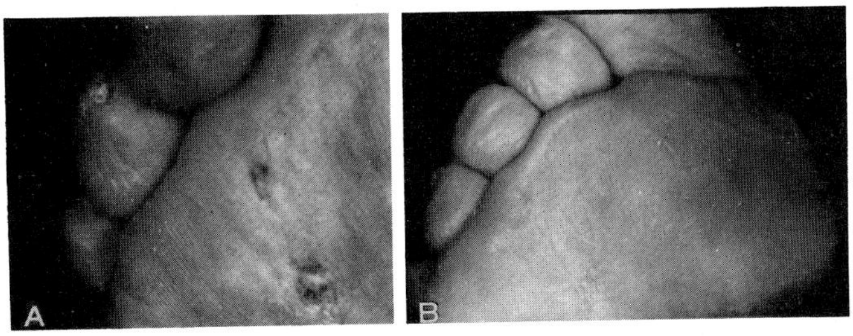

Fig. 13.22. *A*, malignant ulcers secondary to radiodermatitis following treatment of plantar warts in patient 82 years old. *B*, malignant ulcers excised. Six months postoperative.

infection around the ulcer may suggest pyogenic invasion. Sharply demarcated ulcers which are painless suggest a syphilitic origin. Marked circumscribed edema is the result of congestion.

Treatment. Limit the use of radiation on benign lesions since radiation can stimulate carcinogenesis. Early diagnosis and treatment of the underlying disorder is imperative. Surgical excision, radiation and chemotherapeutic techniques must be used early when biopsy is positive. Extensive ulcerations may require skin grafts to cover the surgical site.

Arterial perfusion with chemotherapeutic solutions are helpful in certain malignant lesions. Amputation at a high level including resection of regional lymph nodes may be life saving.

Varicose ulcers are common lesions occurring in the presence of varicose veins. Bluish discoloration of dilated tortuous veins surrounded by brownish-gray pigmentation of the skin encircling the ulcer is typical. The exciting etiologic factor is trauma to the vein or overlying tissue such as a bruise, scratch or dermatitis over a dilated, decompensated vein.

Varicose ulcers are usually located on the medial side of the leg about 3 in. above the ankle. They have been observed covering two-thirds of the lower extremity and very often involve the feet. On the feet, lesions may be seen distal and anterior to the lateral or medial malleolus caused by trauma or friction from a stiff counter. Rarely is a varicose ulcer seen on the sole of the foot.

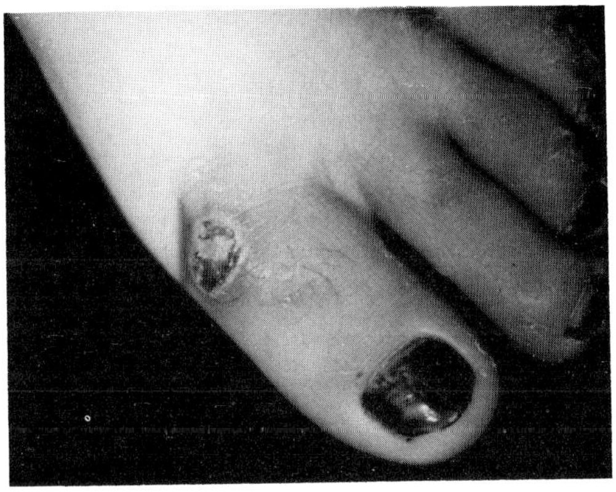

Fig. 13.23. Neoplastic ulcer. (Nail discoloration caused by silver nitrate use in the treatment of onychomycosis.)

At first the ulcers may be pinhead in size and later extend around the entire limb. These superficial lesions give off a foul-smelling serous or purulent discharge. The surrounding pigmented skin is usually indurated in long-standing cases. A local phlebitis with purplish-red discoloration and numerous telangiectasia may be evident. The margins of the sore are usually irregular and rough with a yellow surface and small pink granulations. Stagnation and congestion may cause the edematous tissues to become firm. Very often the discharge will irritate the surrounding tissue causing an eczema with intolerable pruritis, excoriations, fissuring and more ulcers.

Treatment. Early control of infection by antiseptic wet dressing and use of an antibiotic ointment is indicated. Judicious debridement of devitalized tissue by instrumentation and proteolytic enzymes may be necessary. Stimulate repair by using mild solutions of 5 to 15% silver nitrate. Destroy proud flesh using silver nitrate stick 50%.

Oxycycline and hydrocortisone in a spray is helpful in controlling infection and moisture. Even compression of limb by pressure bandages from behind the toes to below the knee or elastic stocking from behind the toes, with closed heel and of midthigh length may be used.

A venous heart dressing may be helpful. Silver nitrate as indicated is used on the ulcer following mechanical or chemical debridement and control of infection. Stimulating ointments, such as ichthammol 10 to 20%, zinc oxide, half-strength or Scarlet Red Ointment may be applied. If the ulcer is infected, do a sensitivity test and prescribe accordingly. Enzymatic debridement, antibiotic ointments and nitrofurazone may be used topically. Systemic protolytic enzymes are helpful early as are systemic antibiotics of choice. Cover the ulcer widely with a sterile gauze pad. Use a 2-in. thick sponge rubber pad on gauze and compress firmly over the ulcer by bandaging. Elevate the extremity and apply elastic bandage or elastic stocking. Change the dressing every 3 to 5 days.

Gelatin-like flexible compression casts are applied according to directions by manufacturer (Gelocast bandages, Unna's boot). Bandages are changed weekly or more often if necessary.

Such activity as walking with compression dressings supplies a physiologic environment. The contraction and expansion of leg musculature against the bandage provides a local hyperemia which aids in repair of the ulcer.

Saphenous ligations, geographic incisions, tying off or stripping of veins, and injections of sclerosing agents may be used in recalcitrant cases. Skin grafts may be necessary where healing is stagnant.

Diabetic ulcers occur in known diabetics and unknown diabetics on an area of the foot receiving abnormal trauma or friction.

The cause may be ill-fitting shoes or hose, irritating chemicals such as corn remedies, extremes of heat and cold and the usual self-inflicted wounds resulting from injudicious instrumentation. Faulty weight distribution may cause abnormal pressure on certain parts of the foot.

The points receiving greatest pressure are the plantar surface of the first and fifth metatarsal head, other depressed metatarsal heads with superimposed

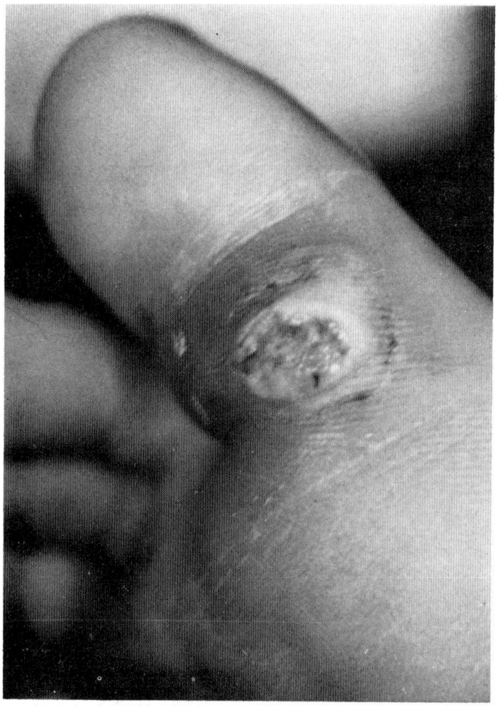

Fig. 13.24. Diabetic ulcer with infection and cellulitis.

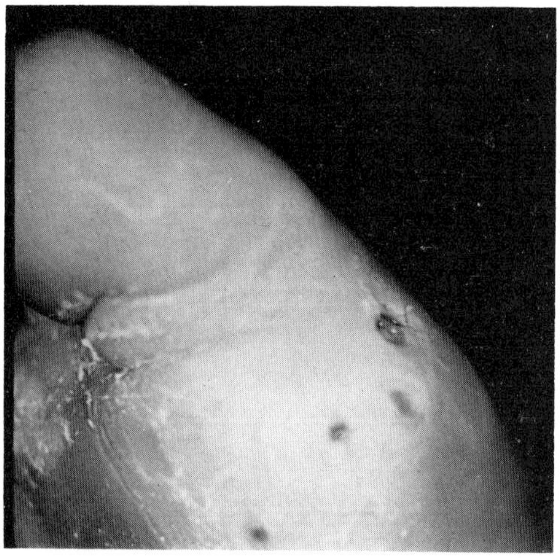

Fig. 13.25. Multiple connecting sinus tracts undermining the skin in a diabetic patient.

luxation of the corresponding toe, the medial aspect of the first metatarsophalangeal joint and the lateral aspect of the fifth metatarsophalangeal joint, the posterior aspect of the heel, the borders of the toenails and the distal ends of the toes.

The ulcer has a red margin and the skin appears spongy. It is very slow and insidious in onset. Its progress is usually discouraging while the margins appear undermined. A callus often overlies the ulcer on the plantar surface and the discharge is serous and watery. A urinalysis and fasting blood sugar and a good case history will confirm the diagnosis. The patient may be arteriosclerotic and peripheral neuropathic symptoms are common.

Treatment. The patient must be under an internist's care for diabetic control at all times. Bacterial cultures and antibiotic sensitivity tests, identification of the bacteria and selection of the proper antibiotic and control of cellulitis is imperative. Footgear must be prescribed to support and accommodate the feet. Functional and structural deformities must be corrected, accommodated or protected by prosthetic devices.

Remove pressure from ulcerated areas by felt padding or accommodative removable appliances. A Ripple-soled shoe may be used by cutting away the "Ripples" on the spongy outer sole beneath the ulcer to protect the lesion. The ulcer is suspended between ripples.

Mild wet dressing of saline solutions (1 tablespoonful of table salt to each quart of water) serve as a soothing, non-irritating antiseptic lavage and application of antibiotic enzyme ointments allows for proteolytic debridement. Judicious debridement of devitalized tissue may be necessary. Sterile loose dressings are applied and carefully observed for possible irritation.

Use necessary internal and local medication to stimulate circulation. Cyclandelate (3,3,5-trimethylcyclohexylmandelate) has proven to

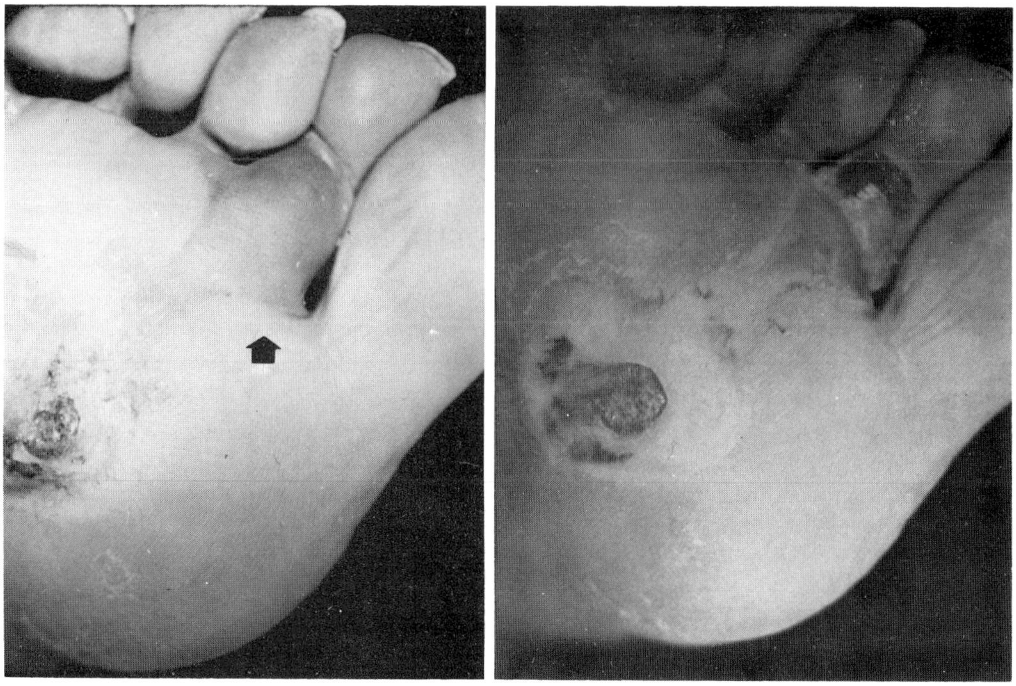

Fig. 13.26. Sinus tract in diabetic patients. Note infected callus and extension by way of least resistance distally to plantar surface of the second toe (*left*). Fig. 13.27. Incision and drainage of diabetic abscess (*right*).

be helpful in diabetic and ischemic ulcers. Systemic broad-spectrum antibiotics may be necessary to control cellulitis. Instructions for diabetic foot care and cleanliness should be given.

Frank and Silver (1962) found that ulcers in the presence of a neuropathy were best treated by excluding antibiotics and wet dressings. Instead they substituted a light cradle with a 25-watt bulb suspended 20 to 25 in. from the part and maintained a temperature of 90°F.

Collens and Vlahos (1962) recommended dilute solutions of triiodide complex which releases free iodine. The solution consists of 0.5 g. of KI dissolved in 100 ml. of water with 1.0 g. crystalline iodine (I_2) added. They presented five cases in which gangrenous parts scheduled for amputation responded well to this treatment when the antimicrobial solution was used as wet dressing and injected into suppurating sinus tracts and sloughing tissue daily.

Rakow (1967) recommends the use of the solution in a variety of ways, e.g., placing the iodine solution on a drain loosely packed into a sinus tract. It may also be applied directly into a tissue slough. A sterile pad may be saturated and sandwiched between two dry sterile pads, applied to the wound and allowed to release nascent iodine. Dressings should be changed daily. Rakow further notes in his experience that vasodilators and anticoagulants have not proved successful in treatment of diabetic ulcers.

Perforating ulcers occur at points of pressure and usually in individuals between the ages of 40 and 60. They are characterized by a perforation from one tissue surface through to the opposite surface.

Alcoholism, diabetes, syphilis and arteriosclerosis are the most common predisposing causes. Pressure from a corn or callus over the first and fifth toes and their respective metatarsal heads, pressure and friction on the heel and ends of the toes are direct causes. The ulceration is deep-seated, covered with heaped up callus and perforated by the avenue of a sinus through to the opposite skin surface, e.g., from plantar to dorsal.

It is believed that the combination of mechanical pressure, vascular instability

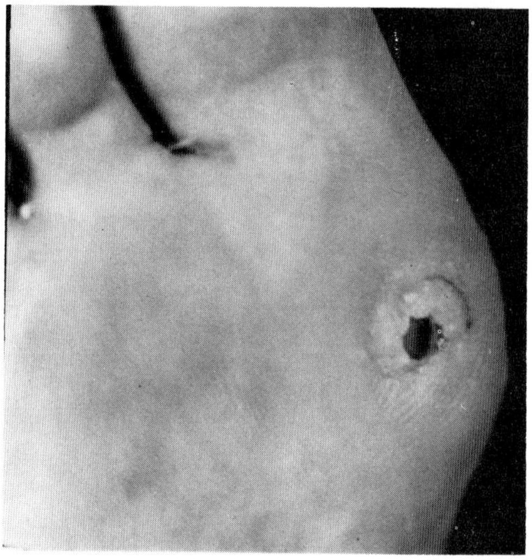

Fig. 13.28. Perforating ulcer secondary to arteriosclerosis. Exposed flexor hallucis longus tendon.

and neurogenic disorders may cause perforating ulcers.

Treatment. Remove devitalized tissue mechanically and by enzymatic debridement, e.g., streptokinase-streptodornase (Varidase), fibrinolysin and deoxyribonuclease ointment (Elase) and neomycin, trypsin, chymotrypsin ointment (Biozyme).

The proper antibiotic ointment is dependent on sensitivity tests. Identification of bacterial flora is mandatory. Insert Penrose drains and use warm saline dressings. This may be followed by iodoform gauze packings. Protect the ulceration from trauma by judicious bandaging and appliances.

Consult the internist for treatment of the etiologic basis for development of the perforating ulcer, e.g., diabetes, arteriosclerosis or peripheral neuropathies.

Skin graft may follow wide excision of ulcer.

Bone disintegration at the distal ends of the toes rescembling osteomyelitis is capable of "almost complete reconstruction" according to Pogonowska *et al.* (1967).

Syphilitic ulcers are painless, typically gummatous lesions often found at the head of the first and fifth metatarsals. The plantar surface of the hallux interphalangeal joint is a favorite site of many ulcers of all types. The usual location is on the upper two-thirds of the thigh and the anterior surface of the leg. It may be perforating and have a cadaverous appearance.

The ulcers are a pale grayish-white covered by a heavy parchment-like tissue. Often there are multiple lesions which coalesce with clearing on one side and destruction at the other. The edges are pigmented and depressed toward the center and the resultant scar is thin and pliable. These ulcers have a punched out appearance with sharply cut, undermined edges and a ragged base. They may be circular, semi-circular or serpiginous in shape and the margins are indurated and sharp.

Very often a regional adenopathy, skin rashes of macular, papular and erythematous lesions, a positive V.D.R.L. test and rapid healing with the therapeutic use of potassium iodide is characteristic of this type of ulcer which can be treated in the same way as a perforating ulcer.

Tuberculous Ulcers occur in tuberculous individuals with a history of tubercular abscess in the subcutaneous tissues and bone.

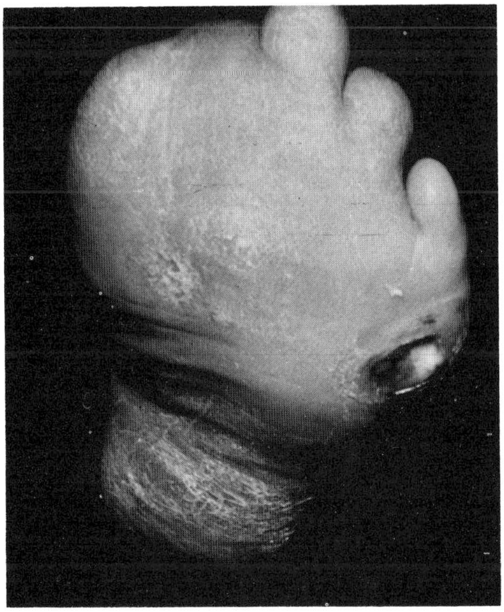

Fig. 13.29. Charcot deformity with secondary syphilitic ulcer head of fifth metatarsal. Courtesy J. F. Yale.

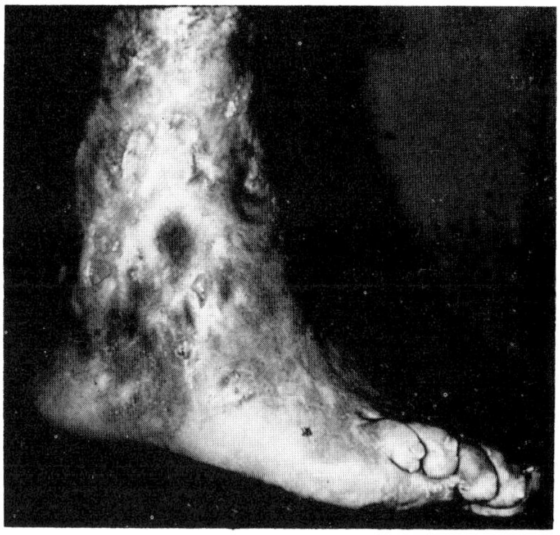

Fig. 13.30. Syphilitic ulcers. Gummatous lesions on anterior of leg and dorsum of foot.

Objectively, the skin is undermined for some distance around the margins of the ulcer. The surface is pale, granulations are small and areas of caseation necrosis are characteristic. The discharge is thin and scanty while parts about the ulcer are livid and mildly tender. No evidence of increase in temperature is noted and the biopsy may provide histologic changes that will provide a clue to the diagnosis of tuberculous ulcer.

Treatment. Systemic treatment of tuberculosis is mandatory. The patient should have bed rest. Daily foot bath in solutions of hexachlorophene are helpful in preventing secondary infections.

Excision and curettage of necrotic bone with sterile dry dressings relieve the ulcers.

Infective ulcers affecting the toes, soles and the heels are the most common kind found in the feet. A strong proprietary medicine for helomas and tylomas, injudicious cutting of corns, calluses, and nails; or unsterile debridement of a blister may cause an infective ulcer. This type of ulcer is the same as pyogenic ulcer. Objectively, the ulcer is small, deep and bounded by a heavy, tough slowly growing skin. A purulent exudate is evident.

Treatment. Sensitivity tests of bacterial flora are indicated. Use of local medication and internal antibiotics depends on the type of bacterial invasion. Rest of the affected part and liquid diets aid in control and repair of the infected ulcer.

Hazay (1960) suggested injectable trypsin as an adjunct to treatment with antibiotics. Inflammation is reduced readily by this method.

Luft (1960) studied the reactions to parenteral enzyme therapy and made the following observations, "Trypsin and chymotrypsin, oral and parenteral, are excellent drugs for use in inflammatory conditions of the lower extremities." Luft further notes that allergic or anaphylactic reactions are not uncommon. This reaction was preceded by local swelling at the site of injection. The generalized reaction varies from malaise to severe anaphylaxis. Frequent signs are urticaria, respiratory distress, conjunctivitis, nausea, abdominal cramps and vomiting. Epinephrine 1:1000 should always be at hand for immediate use if a reaction occurs.

Local antibiotics such as neomycin for Gram-negative bacteria and bacitracin for Gram-positive bacteria, or polymixin combined with chymotrypsin, streptokinase, ribonuclease and other proteolytic enzymes are helpful. Chymoral-100 is taken orally four times daily, Orenzyme or fibrolytic enzyme (Papase) may relieve swelling and inflammation associated with infective ulcers.

A broad-spectrum antibiotic of choice helps to limit and clear up the infection. Penicillin, erythromycin, tetracycline, Chloromycetin, cephelexin monohydrate and a host of other efficient antibiotics may be helpful.

Fibrinolysin and deoxyribonuclease combined may be mixed with 50 to 100 ml. of sodium chloride solution to make a solution for treatment of the infected ulcer. Strips of gauze are soaked in the solution, applied to the wound for about 6 hr., and then removed along with the necrotic tissue. This procedure is followed until healthy granulations appear in the wound.

14

Onychology

Structure and Function of the Nails

The nails are horny, elastic, transparent tissue on the dorsal distal ends of fingers and toes formed by intimately adhered keratotic cells similar to the cells of the epidermis.

The nail proper is composed of a nail body which is convex on the outer side and concave on the under surface with a distal free edge and two lateral edges. The two lateral edges described anatomically are medial or tibial and lateral or fibular, respectively. This plate rests on the nail bed. The nail plate is imbedded posteriorly into the dermis. It is covered by a soft tissue known as the unguinal fold at its posterior aspect as it lies in an unguinal groove. The cells in this groove are not horny and are called the matrix. The eponychium is a thin layer of skin overlying the matrix.

The matrix is thickened and raised in a series of longitudinal ridges. It is from this matrix tissue that the nail is developed, produced and grows forward. The matrix is pink in color and is a specialized, highly vascular tissue corresponding to the mucous layer of the skin. It is readily visible when the nail plate is removed.

Toenails protect the vascular anastomoses at the ends of the toes and are subject to trauma from ill-fitting footgear, local pathologic processes and systemic disease. The nails are affected by the same pathology which affects the skin from which they are differentiated.

Common Nail Disorders

Krausz (1970) reported a nail survey of 10,900 podiatric patients with a total of 6754 nail disorders. This study indicates that at least 61% of those patients examined for podiatric problems have some nail disorders. The four most prevalent problems reported by Krausz were onychocryptosis, 1765; onychauxis and onychogryposis, 1493; onychophosis, 1334; and onychomycosis, 551. Each of these may be a precursor to secondary infection and even subsequent loss of limb in the diabetic or the patient with peripheral vascular disorders.

Onychocryptosis is a condition in which the free edge of the nail has penetrated the periungual layers and has become embedded in the soft tissues. Usually the etiology involves trauma, a diseased nail, ill-fitting footgear or injudicious cutting of the nail. Occasionally the nail lip is hypertrophied and is forced into the nail edge. Occasionally a subungual exostosis elevates the center of the nail forcing the margins down. Secondary infection and profuse granulations or proud flesh are common. An ischemic hyperesthesia may develop at the site of greatest nail pressure in peripheral vascular disorders. I have treated several infants from 2 to 12 months old suffering from onychocryptosis.

A subungual heloma may develop at the distal third of the nail plate from trauma or pressure of a short shoe or seam in an open-toed shoe. The nail plate appears discolored and is elevated from the excresence in the nail bed. Pressure from the dorsum of the nail plate against the subungual mass produces pain.

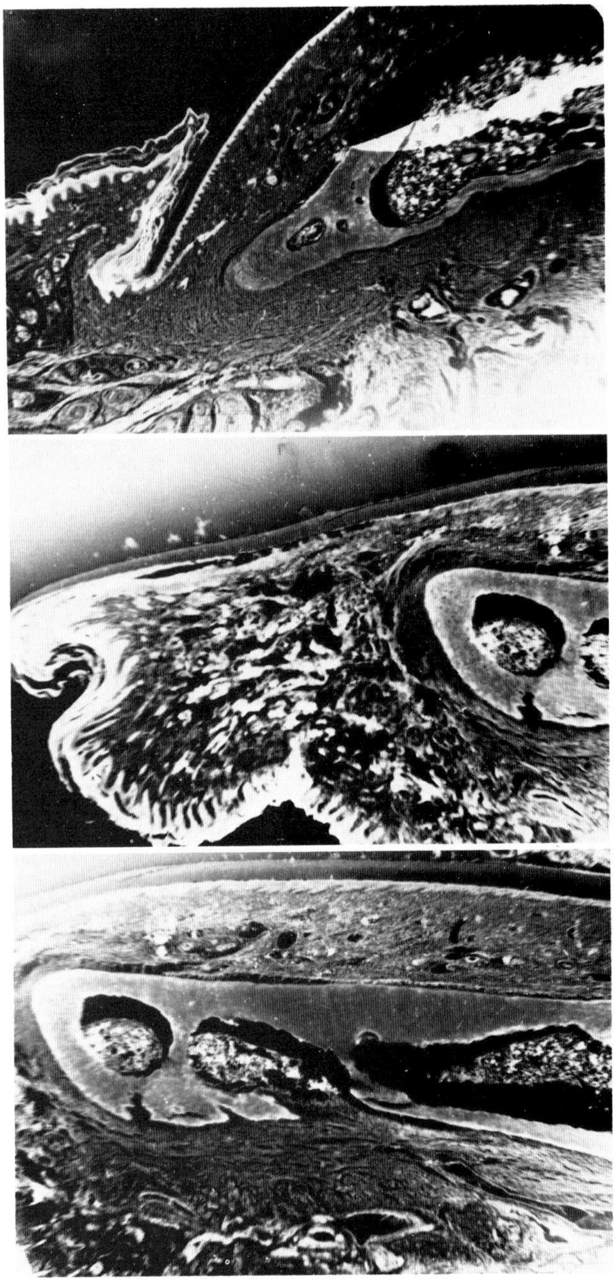

Fig. 14.1. Cross-section of the toenail. Note part of nail plate, lateral nail fold, papillary ridge of bed and a section of the phalanx. Fullterm fetus, stillborn. Courtesy of C. E. Krausz. (*Top.*)

Fig. 14.2. Longitudinal section of the toenail. Note that the plate has reached the distal end of the toe in this fullterm fetus. Courtesy of C. E. Krausz. (*Center.*)

Fig. 14.3. Most of nail body is observed. Courtesy of C. E. Krausz. (*Bottom.*)

Often the painful lesion is an onychophosis or callus in the nail groove. When a nail groove is calloused, lateral digital pressure causes pain. A yellow, gray to white, hard, horny, flat or deep keratotic mass may be in evidence beneath the nail plate. Reduction of the callus by sharp curettage and advice on footgear is necessary.

Treatment of the ingrown toenail depends upon the extent of the pathology. Unlike treatment in the past, therapy today is highly specialized and varies according to whether the condition is uncomplicated or complicated.

Uncomplicated onychocryptosis occurs when there is penetration of the nail groove or lip by an offending portion of an essentially healthy nail caused by injudicious cutting of the nail or by trauma to the lip. The lip may be forced into the nail by shoe pressure or by a blow, or, the nail may be forced into the groove or nail lip. The resultant pressure on soft tissues may create a tyloma or heloma in the nail groove or along the side of the lip. A slight contusion or small ulceration or abrasion is very often found in these cases.

Treatment is aimed at relieving pressure. Assuring the proper fit of shoes and hose is essential. Removing the offending portion of the nail by careful specialized techniques of splitting or sharp curettage may be necessary. Packing the nail groove as described below keeps the nail away from the traumatized tissues.

If callus is present, the nail groove is packed with a 15 to 25% salicylic acid ointment and cotton. In 3 to 5 days and with judicious curettage, the tyloma and debris are removed. If necessary a new salicylic acid pack is applied. If the entire tyloma has been removed, care is taken to keep the nail free from the groove.

Packs are constructed from cotton, gauze, felt, Celastic, latex, resins, dental acrylic, adhesive plaster, plaster of Paris, foam rubber, and a variety of other substances. Sulci protectors and toenail wiring have been used extensively in England with a degree of success. All of these have been tested and proven to be effective in keeping the nail from penetrating the groove.

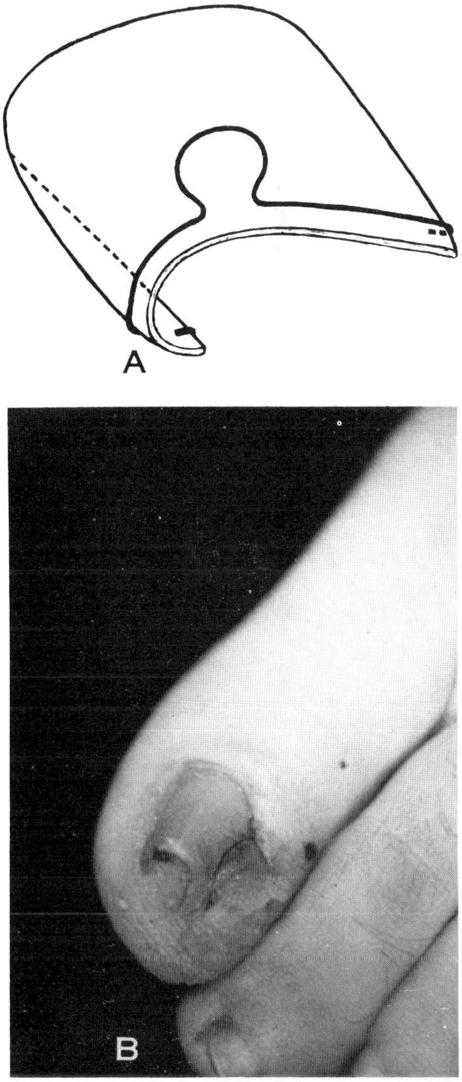

Fig. 14.4. *A*, toenail wiring for correction of ingrown toenail. Courtesy of Ross Fraser. *B*, complicated onychocryptosis in which wiring would not be appropriate. Granuloma in nail groove overlapping nail border.

Sanders (1955), Sivitz (1953) and Mogull (1954) cite the advantages of using acrylic to protect and pack nail grooves.

The pack is placed in the groove with or without a soothing ointment or cream. The packing material is placed underneath the lateral margin of nail to lift it up and away from the nail bed and groove. It is carried out along the cutting edge of the nail to separate the edge from the groove and nail lip. The packing is removed at intervals and new packs are applied as needed.

If an ulceration is found in the nail groove, it is treated as necessary before packing. Goldy and Steinberg (1956) have described the etiologic factors in multiple-infected onychocryptosis and stress the need for laboratory studies, bacteriologic evaluation and often complete physical examinations to clarify the etiology.

Complicated onychocryptosis requires all the skill of the professional. Multiple infections may be challenging. The pathology varies from deep ulcerations in the grooves, profuse granulations, granulomas, infections, paronychia and distortion of the nail plate. Hypertrophy of the lips of the nail where the edges of the nail are incurvated at their margins and are incapable of being reversed, may be a complicating factor along with or secondary to other pathology.

The accepted treatment for complicated onychocryptosis is as follows: local anesthesia is produced by nerve block or field block. The podiatrist must be sure to remove a large enough section of the offending plate to allow for drainage. The nail plate is split by a nail splitter and/or straight edged nail forceps directly back to the eponychium following the nail striations. The eponychium is elevated and a nail splitter is carried back through the nail matrix. The splitter is forced back gently until all resistance is lost. The sectioned portion of the nail is freed from its attachments by a sharp nail splitter and is gently extracted with a hemostat. A drain may be inserted and analgesics and antibiotics prescribed for pain and to avoid inflammatory and infectious changes. Such wet dressings as dilute boric acid solution, saline, aluminum subacetate, potassium permanganate or nitrofurasone are indicated. Follow-up care may necessitate use of systemic or local antibiotics.

If profuse granulation is present, radical treatment rather than use of palliative astringents and cauterizing agents facilitates earlier repair. I prefer to use a sharp tissue forceps when excising the profuse granulation, and then touch up the capillary bleeders with a concentrate of silver nitrate stick or electrocoagulating current. To leave the granulation prolongs postoperative care and slows down repair.

Radical correction of complicated ingrown toe nail. When the nail is inverted from its base forward, and is, in the judgment of the podiatrist, a chronic offender, radical surgical procedures should be attempted. Radical surgery consists of removing offending portions of the nail, and nail bed and matrix. Plastic surgical repair of lip anomalies may also be necessary if the nail lips are chronically enlarged.

Specialized Corrective Techniques. DuVries (1933) describes the technique of removing a longitudinal wedge from the hypertrophied nail lip and suturing down the elevated enlarged lip without disturbing the matrix. I have found this valuable in selected cases of hypertrophy of the unquilabia.

The Winograd Technique for Correction. In another technique (after Winograd, 1929), used for many years with fair results, the nail is split back from the distal edge through the nail plate and matrix to isolate the offending portion of the nail. A scalpel is placed through the split of the nail and carried back through the eponychium down to the bone to about ¼ in. distal to the distal interphalangeal joint. It is then carried forward to and through the soft tissue at the distal end of the nail plate. A semi-elliptical incision is then carried from the proximal to distal end of the first incision to include the matrix, nail plate and nail lip. The section removed should be wedge-shaped. The wound is debrided with special attention to removing all of the visible matrix. The margins are underscored and the tissues apposed for closure by sutures. Some operators suture only the posterior fold; others carry sutures through the entire wound including a single suture through the nail plate. If a suture is to be used through the plate one must place a hole in the plate before attempting to force the suture needle through. This, of course, facilitates better union and protects the needle from damage. Sutures are removed between 7 and 12 days postoperatively.

Since the need for sutures is questionable

and their use in an avascular area results in considerable postoperative pain, the closure may be facilitated by use of Steri-Strips instead of suturing material. This technique is less painful, allows for more rapid healing and is most effective in minimizing scar tissue. I have performed various modifications of the Winograd technique to correct complicated ingrown toe nails in hundreds of cases. Results have been excellent.

I prefer the technique developed by Frost (1962) and described below.

The Frost Technique for Correction. Under a 0.5% lidocaine toe block, and with a tourniquet around the base of the toe, the nail is split longitudinally along its entire length by following a longitudinal ridge or striation just within the beginning of the arc and the incurvation as indicated by the solid and broken dark lines (Fig. 14.5).

A scalpel is laid in this channel, and a vertical incision is made down to the phalanx for the entire length of the nail to about 1/16 in. beyond each end of the nail plate (Fig. 14.6).

At the proximal end of this incision, another incision is made at right angles to it, just beyond the proximal end of the nail, and just through the skin down to the adipose tissue layer (Fig. 14.7).

The corner of this skin triangle is grasped, and a scalpel is used to free it from the adipose tissue to form a full thickness skin flap (Fig. 14.8).

With this flap retracted to one side, another longitudinal incision is made, as indicated by additional black line (Fig. 14.9), about 1/16 in. external to the edge of the nail and parallel to the first incision to the same depth. Nearing the tip of the toe, the depth of the incision is decreased and the line of the incision is turned to meet the first incision.

The distal point of this segment is grasped with forceps and an incision is made down to the phalanx. This segment of tissue is removed (Fig. 14.10) from the dorsum of the phalanx by sharp dissection.

The nail root area is inspected for glistening white fragments of matrix which, when found, are removed by sharp dissection (Fig. 14.11).

The flap is repositioned (Fig. 14.12) and the tourniquet is removed. Three Steri-Strips are applied. The area will bleed profusely for a short time, but in about 5 min. a coagulum will form. A piece of Telfa, paraffin wax mesh or Adaptic is applied over the wound followed by three 2- x 2-in. gauze squares and a firm circular dressing of 1 in. Kling bandage.

The patient is ordered off his feet for 48 hr., when the dressing, stiff with coagulated blood, is removed. The patient returns for redressing in 10 days at which time the Steri-Strips are removed. Cut-out shoes are worn until regular shoes can be worn comfortably.

J. Yale (1970) delivered a paper before the Military Society of Orthopedic Surgeons at West Point on the success achieved in keeping soldiers ambulatory by using a phenol-alcohol technique for correction of the "ingrown toe nail." The technique he described is a refinement of the techniques utilizing phenol as originally proposed and reported by Boll (1945), and improved by Nyman (1956), Suppan and Ritchlin (1962), Kleiman (1964), Green (1964) and others who have also lectured on this effective method of toe nail surgery. Although the actual surgical approach varies with individuals, the objective—destruction of the matrix—is the same. I have found this technique to be successful in private practice.

This chemosurgical technique described involves the permanent eradication of the toenail matrix. In over 500 cases of ingrown toenail treated by the podiatry service at Fort Ord over the preceding 2 years, it has proved to be of tremendous value. The procedure, performed under local anesthesia on an ambulatory outpatient basis, is done in the face of local infection without the utilization of systemic antibiotics. With specific application to the military, soldiers treated with this technique are able to return to limited duty the same day and to full duty within 1 week.

The Phenol-Alcohol Technique for Correction. The procedure outlined below is for an infected ingrown toenail at the medial aspect of the right hallux.

After preparation of the toe for surgery,

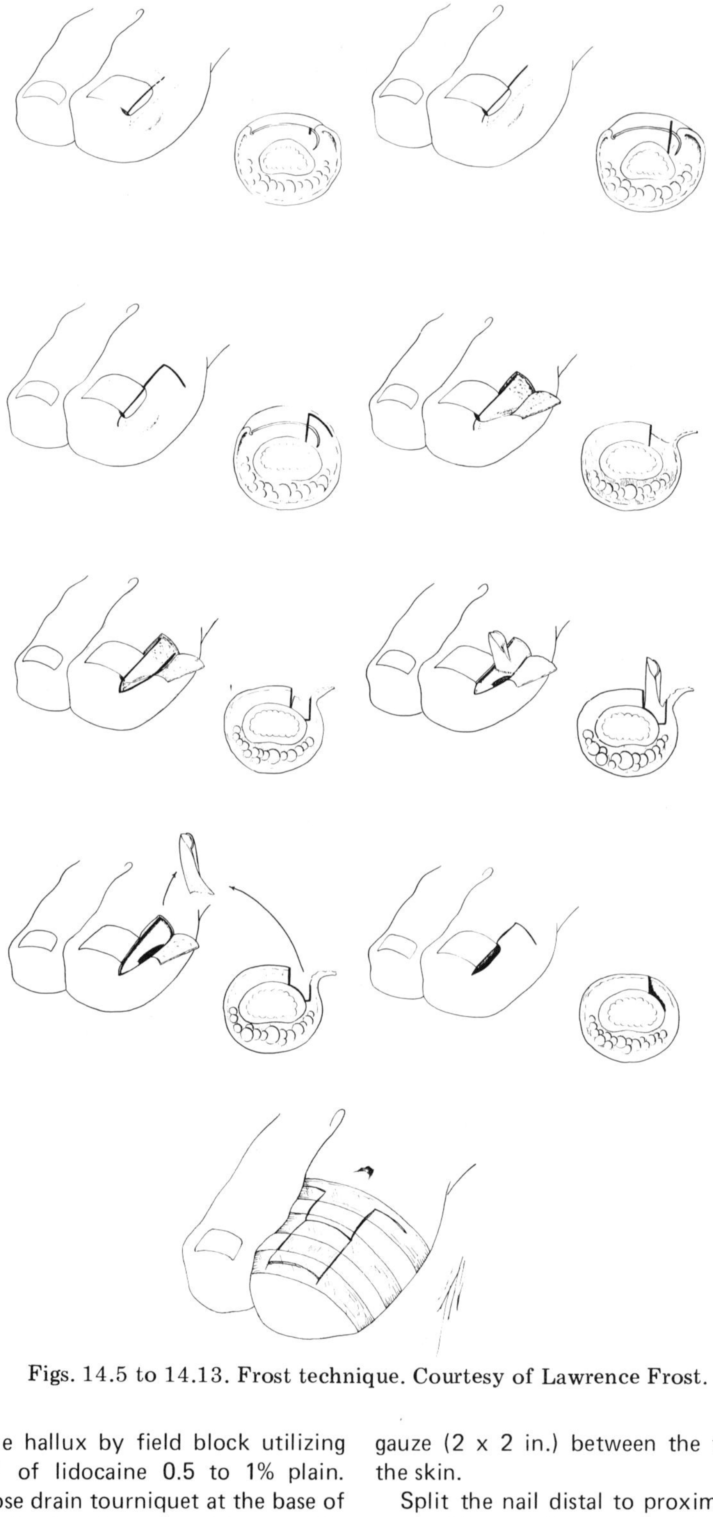

Figs. 14.5 to 14.13. Frost technique. Courtesy of Lawrence Frost.

anesthetize the hallux by field block utilizing about 1.5 ml of lidocaine 0.5 to 1% plain. Apply a Penrose drain tourniquet at the base of the toe with the first hemostat. Use a sterile gauze (2 x 2 in.) between the tourniquet and the skin.

Split the nail distal to proximal beneath the eponychium following the linear nail lines approximately 1/6 to 1/8 in. lateral to the medial nail border. Excise the offending nail spicule toward the main nail body with a hemostat clamped onto the entire spicule below the eponychium.

Curette the enlarged nail groove and matrix below the eponychium. Excise any exuberant granulation tissue present with the toenail nipper.

Remove most of the cotton from a cotton applicator stick. Dip the tip of the stick into the bottle of 88% phenol without getting too much phenol on the tip. Apply the phenolated tip to the nail groove and matrix from distal to proximal beneath the eponychium for 1½ min. taking care that the phenol does not run across the posterior nail wall. Remove the first applicator stick, sponge the area, and apply the second applicator stick in the same manner for a period of 3 min.

Flush the surgical site with isopropyl alcohol.

Apply a Neosporin-G cream dressing to the surgical site utilizing two sterile gauze pads, 2 x 2 in., and toe stockinet. Remove the tourniquet and apply ¼ in. tape to the base of the toe to anchor the dressing.

There is very little postoperative discomfort. Twelve Zactirin tablets (plain) or Emperin No. 3 are prescribed for postoperative pain to be taken q. i. d. if needed. The first redressing is done in 4 to 7 days. A serous drainage, the result of the chemical burn, is noted and lasts from 3 to 6 weeks. During this period, the patient is instructed to keep his foot dry.

It is imperative that fresh phenol be used and that the procedure be accomplished under strict

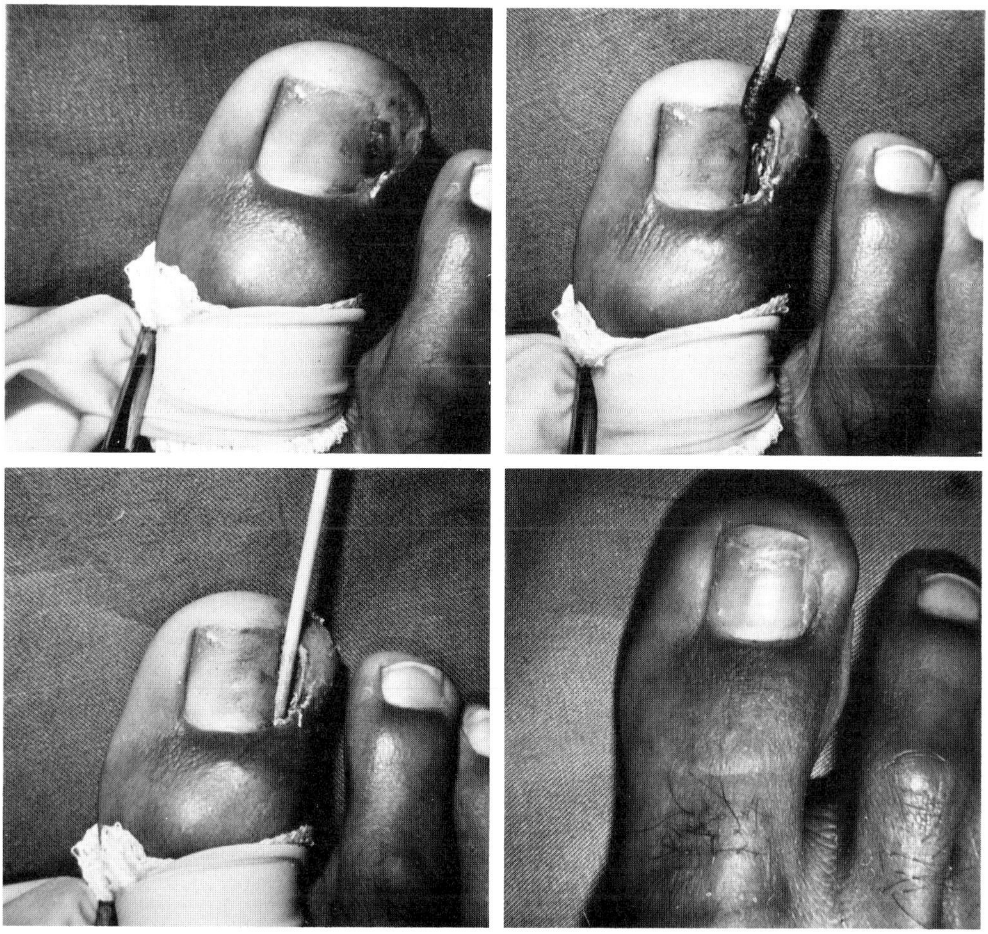

Figs. 14.14 to 14.17. Phenol alcohol technique for correction of ingrown toenails. Courtesy of J. F. Yale.

hemostasis. Because of the phenol's neurolytic effect, a minimum of postoperative pain is experienced. If an infection exists the predominant organism cultured is staphylococcus coagulase positive. In infections caused by betastreptococcus, cellulitis has remained localized to the infected toe. Recurrence rate has been minimal. Postoperative x-rays reveal no periosteal or subperiosteal changes. Care must be taken to avoid a chemical eponychia caused by the careless application and spread of the phenol. This would result in the formation of transverse lines in the form of sulci (Beau's lines) which progress forward with the growth of the nail.

Negative Galvanism. Polokoff (1935 and 1961), Rubin and Weiss (1964) and Dyer and Cohen (1955) report on the use of negative galvanism for correction of incurvated nails. Gardner (1958) notes that there is little postsurgical pain and rarely infection in this use of negative galvanism. The foot is prepared for surgery and toe block or field block anesthesia is instituted. The offending border of the onychocryptosis is split from the distal end through the matrix. The plate and matrix are gently removed and hemostasis is affected by tourniquet or by digital pressure. A wet, warm, saline-soaked, positive electrode 4 x 4 in., is placed on the calf and a blunt sabre-shaped blade is fitted into a holder connected to the negative pole. The blade is placed in the nail groove and the negative current raised to 5 milliamperes. The blade is worked along the nail groove and into the matrix area alternately for about 10 to 15 min. Hydrogen bubbles exude from the contact area of the needle. An ointment dressing is applied and the wound is treated as a burn for a few days. Treatment is enhanced by enzymatic debridement of the necrotic tissue.

Electrocoagulation using a high frequency current is also used to destroy matrical tissue.

Onychotripsy. Perrone (1970) developed a nail matricectomy by use of a low-speed, high-torque air motor. He believes that the onychotripsy is accomplished with a minimum of surgical trauma and less pain when the air motor is used. The section of nail is removed by nail splitter (onychatome) under local anesthesia. A Busch burr is used in the chuck handpiece and placed on the eponychial envelope. Careful onychotripsy erases the nail matrix. One must develop a touch and feel of tissue through the burr and handpiece. The technique is rapid and postoperative care is minimal. The site is kept dry and a coagulum forms.

The Trephine Technique. Steinberg (1954) introduced a new instrument and technique for surgical correction of ingrown toenail. The instrument has a trephine-like annular cutting head. In this procedure, the toe is anesthetized and prepared for surgery. A nick is made at the distal nail margin about 1/8 in. from its embedded border and an incision is made at the junction of the posterior and lateral eponychium or the posterior corner of the nail. The incision should be extended to the tubercle at the base of the phalanx and angulated slightly toward the affected edge of the toe. The incision is undermined by blunt section. The trephine engages the nick in the nail and is gently forced back in a boring fashion to include the nail, nail lip, nail bed, profuse granulations and fibrous connective tissue. The head of the instrument should advance to a point under the skin in the region of the matrix. The instrument is held perpendicular to the bone at this point and the sharp edges at its end sever the tissues that are engaged in the trephine. This includes the aforementioned tissues and the matrix.

Sterile sulfanilimide powder is dusted into the wound. The posterior section of the wound is closed by clip or Steri-Strips. The free edge of the nail in the wound is excised to remove a possible irritant from the site of wound healing.

A dry dressing is applied and the usual measures for wound repair are followed. Healing is usually rapid. Steinberg reports success in 100 cases in 1956 and to date can record thousand of cases successfully treated in this manner.

Onychauxis and Onychogryposis. Onychauxis or club nail is an overgrowth or hypertrophy of the nail in any or all of its dimensions. The affected nail assumes a dirty brown, yellow, gray or black color, while the surface of the nail becomes horny and claw-like. The great toe is the most commonly affected either by trauma, fungus infections, pressure from ill-fitting shoes and hose, nutritional disturbances, eczema, psoriasis or circulatory diseases. The nail bed may also be hypertrophied from the pressure of the thickened nail plate. Calluses and often helomas are found in the thickened nail bed beneath the free tibial, fibular and distal margins. Callused nail grooves may become extremely painful.

Onychogryposis is a deformity of the nail accompanied by hypertrophy beginning at the matrix and extending either laterally, medially, forward and downward over the end of a toe, or upward and backward to press into the dorsum of the foot. If the etiology is systemic, all the nails are involved, if traumatic, only one or two may be affected. The palliative and surgical treatment prescribed for onychauxia is suitable for onychogryposis. It is usually necessary to reduce this type of nail with a diamond burr and utilize curettage to straighten out the margins.

Palliative treatment consists of cutting, high-speed drill grinding and debridement of the nail under aseptic conditions. One must constantly be aware of the presence of septic subungual debris. The reduced nail and exposed nail bed are covered with an antiseptic analgesic and emollient dressing to relieve tenderness. Results are excellent. If the subungual tissue is callused or if a heloma is present, the use of a 25 to 40% salicylic acid ointment or plaster applied for at least 3 days loosens the tissue for a better and more successful debridement at the next visit

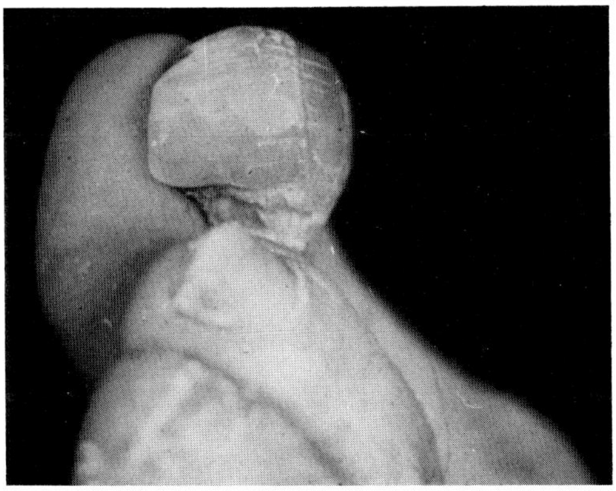

Fig. 14.18. Onychauxis.

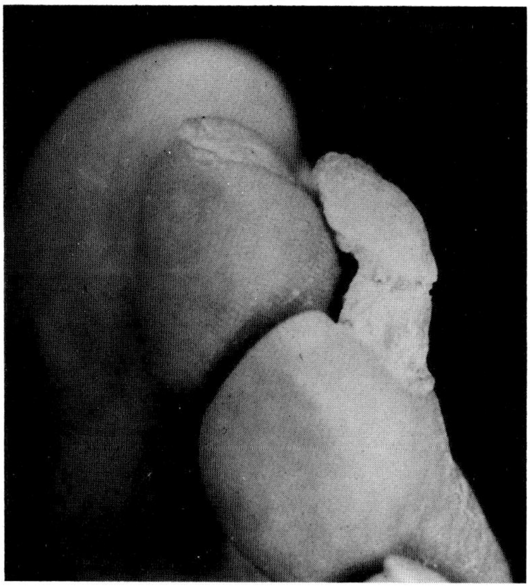

Fig. 14.19. Onychogryposis.

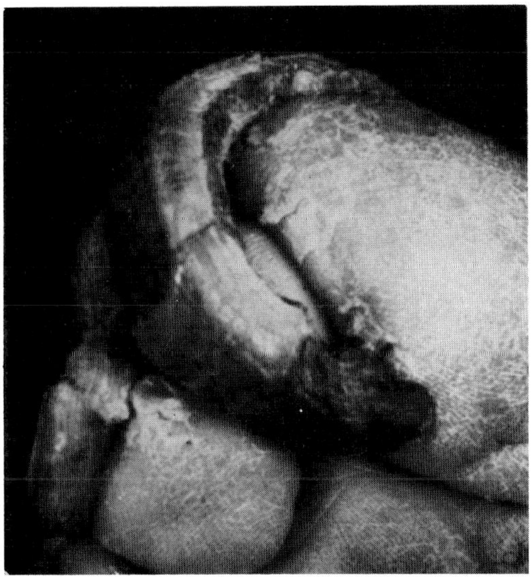

Fig. 14.20. Onychogryposis. Overlapping distal end of hallux causing pressure pain plantar surface of toe.

when the patient returns for curettage and further debridement.

Surgical treatment is instituted where the risk is good. Removal of the entire nail plate under nerve block anesthesia is often indicated. This is accomplished by using a flat or semi-curved instrument and running it from side to side beneath the nail plate to separate the plate from the bed. Upon loosening the

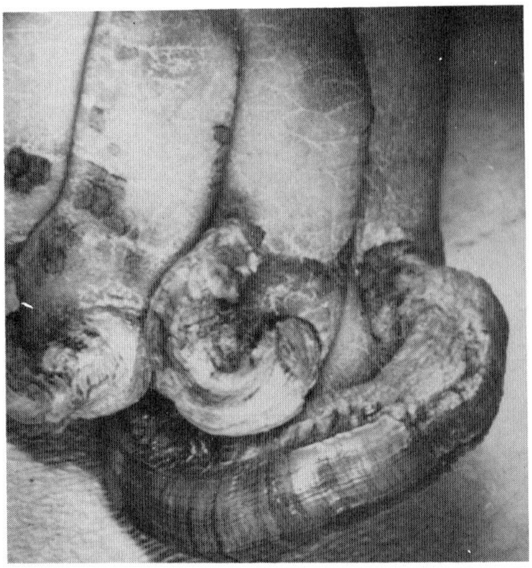

Fig. 14.21. Onychogryposis.

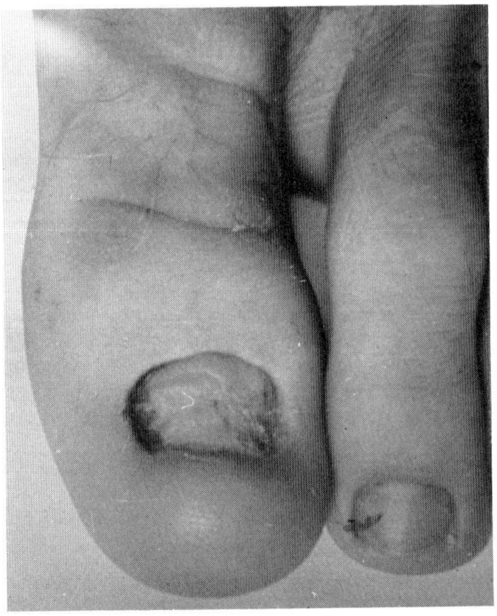

Fig. 14.22. Excision of hallux nail *in toto* followed by phenol and alcohol. Postoperative result—5 months.

entire plate it is easily separated under the posterior fold and extracted with a slight twist of the Allis forceps or hemostat. The bed and posterior fold are swabbed first with concentrated 88% phenol for 3 min. and then with 70% alcohol. Drainage is prolonged with this technique but results are generally good when the nail is redressed periodically with dry bandages or antiseptic medications.

Another technique for radical removal of the nail plate entails removing the distal two-thirds of the distal phalanx of the toe together with the nail. While this is effective, cosmetic results are poor.

Basically, the technique is as follows: Complete toe block anesthesia is effected. An incision is made starting at the level of the dorsal medial aspect of the toe about ¼ in. distal to the interphalangeal joint. The incision is carried forward below the medial nail lip, around the distal end of the toe to meet a similar incision from the lateral side. Another transverse incision is made over the dorsum of the toe to connect the incisions. The soft tissues including the nail plate, nail bed, subcutaneous tissue and nail folds are dissected back, staying close to the bone, removing the section as outlined above from ¼ in. anterior to the joint forward. The distal two-thirds of the distal phalanx is resected by bone forceps and filed smooth. The plantar flap is brought up over the remaining bone and sutured.

Zadik (1950) advocated obliteration of the hallucal nail bed without shortening of the distal phalanx.

Kaplan (1960) developed a technique to completely eradicate the club nail, minimize postoperative pain and provide a good cosmetic effect. Of over 500 cases which had been operated, 359 were followed, with not a single reoccurrence of the hypertrophied nail. Kaplan's technique is described below.

Following induction of anesthesia by complete toe block and adequate hemostasis, the handle end of a Bard-Parker scalpel is forced under the nail separating it from the nail bed and removing it completely by blunt dissection. The site is given a complete surgical prep and a tourniquet is applied. Two linear incisions about 1.5 cm in length are made on the medial and lateral aspects of the toe following the nail fold lines proximally to just short of the interphalangeal joint and including the posterior eponychium. The eponychial skin is sharply and superficially dissected back to expose the matrix. A third incision is made at the distal end of the toe joining the distal ends of the medial and lateral incisions connecting the nail folds. The distal end of the incised tissue is grasped by Allis forceps and dissected back on the distal phalanx to include the nail bed and matrix beneath the previously elevated eponychium. All loose tissue and bony exostoses are removed by bone rongeur and the retracted eponychial flap is sutured back in place with one suture of 3-0 silk on each side of the medial and lateral incisions.

Owens (1962) described a technique for complete removal of onychauxis. The technique consists of a modified Winograd operation to excise the inverted medial and lateral margins of the nail. This is followed by total excision of the remaining nail plate and bed with the matrix back to the base of the distal phalanx on its dorsal surface. The flaps are sutured back to the lateral skin margins and the center heals by third intention. The technique is similar to Kaplan's but allows for excision of nail lips.

Jones (1965) used a full-thickness graft from the dorsum of the foot to the denuded dorsal surface of the toe for closed postsurgical healing and no disfigurement of the hallux.

Whitney (1968) following total avulsion of the nail plate rescrubs the foot with hexachlorophene. Frost incisions are carried back from the nail grooves and laterally just proximal to the distal interphalangeal joints. These are lifted back by sharp section to expose the medial and lateral aspects of the matrix. The central posterior fold is dissected back exposing the entire matrix. The total matrix is then excised by sharp section and all remnants and bony irregularities are removed. The flaps are folded back and sutured with 4-0 silk. The end of the eponychial central flap is sutured to the nail bed. The entire operative site is carefully bandaged, following apposition of the tissues.

Onychomycosis is commonly caused by *Trichophyton mentagrophytes*, *Trichophyton rubrum* and *Candida albicans* and it may destroy the entire nail or cause secondary infections. The clinical characteristics may vary from slight scaling in the lateral folds of the nail to thickening and opaqueness of the plate with the distal portions becoming powdery.

Pardo-Costello (1960) found that about 18% of nail problems are due to onychomycosis. White and Laipply (1958) present 708 cases of onychomycosis studied microscopically. They conclude that the presence of spores or hyphas, especially in subungual keratin or the nail plate is indicative of onychomycosis. Staining with the periodic acid Schiff reaction technique revealed fungi twice as frequently as did other methods in their series.

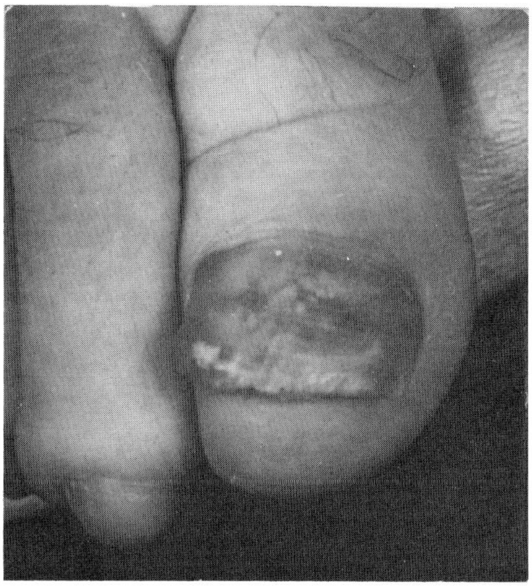

Fig. 14.23. Onychomycosis. Brown, gray, yellow discoloration of hallux nails with subonychial debris were present.

Fletcher (1959) and others had difficulty in culturing for positive identification of fungus infections of the nail. Studies revealed that identification was possible through clinical observations; *Trichophyton gypseum*, circular white plaques with scaling; *Trichophyton rubrum*, dry, lusterless, scaling, streaked, raised from bed and epithelial debris under nail plate which is discolored brownish-yellow, with worm-eaten appearance spreading back to matrix; *Candida (Monilia) albicans*: the only member of its genus that infects nails. Paronychia is the common sequela to Candida infection. The nail plate is soft and a light colored yellow and white. The subungual tissue is moist and purulent. Removal of the nail plate often reveals an ulcerated nail bed.

Treatment of onychomycosis is most difficult. Perseverance in both the doctor and patient are required for successful treatment. Reduction and removal of the objective nail pathology is essential for best results. Treatment may be either radical or palliative.

Palliative treatment is accomplished through mechanical debridement such as grinding, cutting and curettage of the gray, yellow-brown diseased nail tissue. Destruction of the diseased nail by 40% salicylic acid plaster is helpful. Fungicidal solutions and ointments are applied daily to the nail bed. Commonly used topical medications are borotannic complex, salicylic acid, undecylenic acid, sodium propionate and ammoniacal silver nitrate. Ultraviolet light and x-ray therapy may also be used. Periodic reduction by the podiatrist follows. Home care may consist of scrubbing the affected nails nightly with hexachlorophene followed by application of a fungicide. Anti-mycotic therapy for prevention of skin activity should be a part of the over-all regimen.

More radical procedures consist of complete avulsion of the toenail, destruction of matrix with concentrated phenol followed by use of penetrating fungicides on the nail bed. Whire (1950), Bereston (1950) and Peck and Klein (1951), however, do not feel that use of fungicides alone has been effective.

Another technique of proven value is the reduction of the diseased nail as much as possible followed by debridement. The remaining nail is further reduced by the application of a 40 to 60% salicylic acid plaster or ointment. The acid is applied first by isolating the infected nail with adhesive, then the acid is placed in the aperture of the adhesive overlying the nail. The patient returns in 4 to 6 days and debridement continues followed by additional acid treatment. When the entire nail plate is reduced and the nail bed appears pink, fungicidal therapy is administered in the form of undecylenic; proprionic acid compounds or borotannic acid compound. Frequent changes of solution are desirable. Complete surgical removal of the nail plate and application of fungicidal solutions is also effective treatment.

Hendler (1954) describes the fungi most frequently infecting nail tissue. *T. gypseum* and *T. mentagrophytes* shows the initial lesion as a white superficial patch on the posterior nail fold. This progresses to inflammation and destruction of tissues surrounding the plate and results in a yellow, lusterless, opaque and often friable nail. Subungual hyperkeratosis and dystrophic changes develop but rarely is paronychia a complication. Infections of *T. gypseum* are difficult to treat successfully. Reducing the thickness of the nail periodically by using a high-speed drill followed by sharp curettage may be helpful. Adjunctive fungicides applied to the diseased nail daily prevents and often cures the condition.

In *T. purpureum* (*T. rubrum*), the lesion develops slowly and insidiously at the lateral border of the nail. Yellow and/or white streaks coalesce and subungual hyperkeratosis is prominent. The plates become thin and brittle. An "Id" reaction may develop. Paronychia is absent. Rosenfield (1955) states that in his experience treatment of *T. purpureum* gives poor results with frequent reoccurrences.

In *C. albicans*, onychia and paronychia are common. Pain may be slight to severe with evidence of infection. The posterior fold is red and spongy to touch. On incision, seropurulent discharge may be noted. The nail plate may be elevated and loose yet firm in texture. *C. albicans* often responds well to treatment.

Locke (1955) discusses the etiologic basis for onychomycosis and establishes some interesting data. Predisposing factors causing onychomycosis are direct trauma, multiple minimal trauma and contamination by instruments. Short, narrow shoes may result in contact with infected shoe lining and leather.

Jaskoski *et al.* (1962) established, from 70 fungus specimens cultured on Sabouraud's agar, that only 3 of 30 identified species were pathogenic; the remaining 27 were soil contaminants.

The hallux nail is the most commonly affected nail, yet the fourth and fifth toenails are often affected through trauma. Subonychial hemorrhage often acts as a culture media for fungi and should be avoided. Onychia and paronychia may be secondary infections where tinea pedis is the exciting factor.

Mogull (1957) developed a technique of debridement of the infected nail and removal of infected nail borders followed by the construction of an acrylic nail plate. The color of the acrylic is matched to the nail; several serrations are made in the nail plate and the acrylic is applied to conform to the shape of a new nail. Wet cellophane is placed over the new acrylic plate. When the acrylic is hardened the new nail is shiny. It can be buffed and shaped. An interesting observation by Mogull is that the new nail forming beneath the acrylic takes on a healthier look. I have also observed this change in several cases where an acrylic nail plate covering a diseased nail for several weeks resulted in marked improvement of the diseased nail.

Ignatoff and Bleiberg (1958) note that onychomycosis occurs in about 15% of all mycotic infections, although it often is the consequence of dermatophytosis. They found that the following procedure was most effective in treating onychomycosis. Thorough burring down of infected nail should be accomplished. Occlusive dressings of 60% salicylic acid ointment should be applied weekly. After 4 to 10 weeks, debridement results in a clear, pink nail bed. A chemical compound with strong fungistatic qualities, a borotannic complex, is applied twice daily. This topical application (Onycho-Phytex) consists of a molecular fusion of borates and tannates in a penetrating vehicle of ethyl alcohol.

As the new nail grows, all dystrophic and diseased nail is removed. The fungicidal solution is used twice daily.

I have recognized that debridement and curettage increased the rate of repair only when the judicious use of chemicals served as part of the treatment regimen.

In an unusual case of ocular keratitis accompanied by onychomycosis and corneal dystrophy, Spoor (1967) reported that the attending ophthalmologist and dermatologist concluded that an allergic reaction keratitis was the etiologic basis for the eye problem. Griseofulvin was the medication of choice and its continued use was necessary to prevent recurrence of the keratitis.

In a study of the treatment of 25 subjects with onychomycosis, Jaskoski (1969) found that 76% either showed no improvement or the condition persisted. He ascertained from his study that the more effective results are predicated on longer periods of treatment with borotannic complex combined with the use of oral griseofulvin.

Frost (1960) describes encouraging results in a series of 36 cases treated by atraumatic avulsion of the nail plate followed by daily use of a borotannic complex.

Goldberg (1960) notes that clipping and abrasion, "enhances the process of recovery" when using oral griseofulvin 250-mg. tablets q. i. d.

Strahs (1962), following thorough debridement of the nail bed, used a lacquer formulation of Chloranil in treating 25 cases of onychomycosis.

Feldman (1960, Walker (1960), Maibach and Kligman (1960), Carpenter (1962), Reiss and Kornblee (1963) and Dix and Sloan (1966) disagree as to the treatment time necessary to cure onychomycotic infections with oral griseofulvin. Dix and Sloan also conclude that the borotannic complex alone was more effective than when combined with griseofulvin orally.

Other Diseases and Deformities

Inflammation of the matrix may produce nutritional or trophic disturbances of the nail plate. This is evidenced by a deep rubor behind the eponychium accompanied by swelling, elevated temperature and pain. Secondary infection resulting in destruction of the matrical cells may follow.

Treatment depends on the etiology. Whether multiple minimal trauma from footgear, sensitivity to allergens or invasion of bacteria are the causative agents, they must be sought out and treated.

Eczema. Generalized eczema may present dystrophic changes in the nails. The eczemas must be handled judiciously to prevent chronic deformities of the plate. Although the nail may become corrugated, if it repairs well the corrugations disappear. Deep discoloration, splitting and brittleness may occur. Paronychia and secondary inflammatory changes around the nail are often seen in acute eczematous states.

Treatment. Early incision and drainage is indicated in paronychia. The eczema is calmed by use of saline soaks, aluminum subacetate wet packs and combinations of nystatin, neosporin and corticosteroid creams or lotions. Avulsion of the entire nail plate is indicated to facilitate drainage.

Onychia is an ulceration or inflammation of the matrix of the nail and is usually of bacterial origin. Psoriasis of the nail is also a common cause of onychia. Typical signs of infection are present to assist in the correct diagnosis. Treatment involves incision and drainage with the use of local and systemic antibiotics.

Paronychia, an inflammation of tissues around the nail, may be caused by trauma or by abrasions about the nail or in the nail grooves. It is pyogenic and often exhibits staphylococcus, streptococcus and colibacillus on examination. All the signs of infection and the lesion which becomes noticeable 24 to 36 hr. after primary insult establishes the diagnosis. Krausz (1950) noted that in a series of 278 nail cases, only 0.5% had the symptoms of paronychia. This percentage is based on screening patients with a variety of nail conditions. In my experience the percentage of infected nails that exhibit paronychia is much higher.

Treatment. Paronychia is best treated by removing the entire nail plate to allow for drainage. The use of local antibiotics and wet saline dressings usually proves to be successful therapy. In cases of cellulitis and lymphadenopathy, a sensitivity test governs the type of antibiotic best suited to combat the infection.

Psoriasis. Several nails may be affected by psoriasis. The nails become dry and lose their luster. The process usually starts at the distal margin of the plate and works back to the nail root with the

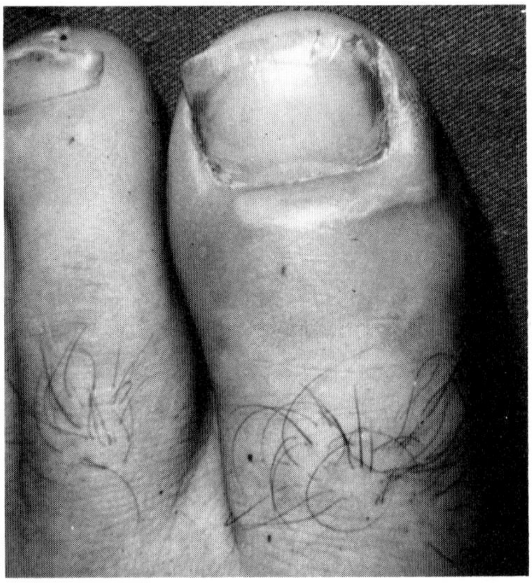

Fig. 14.24. Pyogenic paronychia. Courtesy of J. F. Yale.

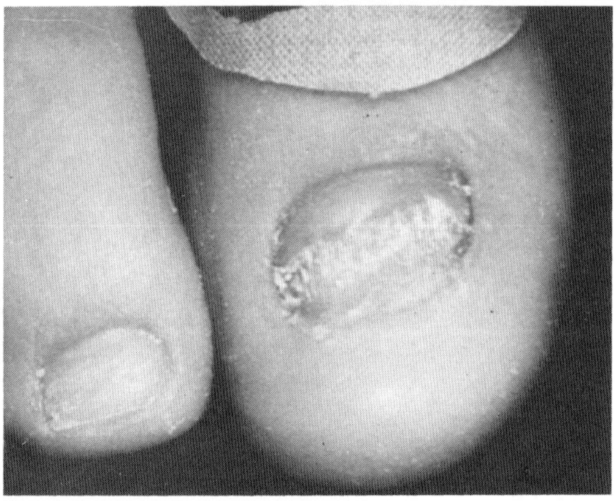

Fig. 14.25. Psoriatic toenails. Note distal margin irregularity.

formation of thick, friable, yellowish brown, corneous material between the nail plate and bed. Small, circular "thimble-like" pitting concavities develop at the loose margins of the nail plate. These pits and grooves result from previous damage to the matrix from the psoriatic inflammation. Discoloration of the nail bed, onycholysis and subungual keratosis develop from the nail bed or hyponychial involvement in advanced psoriatic nail disease (Zaiss, 1969). Psoriatic arthritis may effect the interphalangeal joints in the presence of severe skin disease and psoriatic nails.

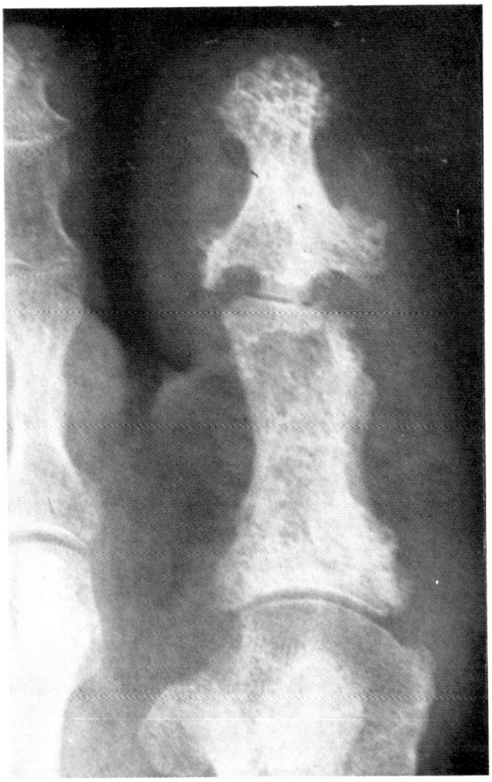

Fig. 14.26. Psoriatic arthritis. Courtesy of *Clinical Foot Roentgenology*, Baltimore: The Williams & Wilkins Company, 1966.

The nail becomes separated from the nail bed and may break, split or fall off. In mild cases accompanied by typical psoriatic skin lesions, small punctiform depressions in the nail plate are noticed early. There is a decrease in the growth potential. Generally, the patient presents skin lesions on the extensor surfaces of the elbows and knees. A red base appears with an overlay of silvery-white imbricated scales.

Palliative treatment for psoriasis of the nails may be advisable. Grinding the nails down by high speed drill and removal of debris by curettage is beneficial. The application of fungicides to prevent secondary mycotic infection is advisable. Applications of mineral oil, cod-liver oil and vitamin A cream keep the nail plate smooth following periodic debridement. Very often the treatment of choice is total excision of the nail plate without matricectomy so that a better nail may develop.

Onychoclavus. Johnson (1962) describes onychoclavus as being a special type of onychophosis occurring on the tibial or fibular edge of the fifth toenail. An onychophosis may develop in any of the nail grooves as a secondary complication of shoes with pointed toes or from pressure of deformed nail margins. Johnson notes the rotation of the fifth toe on its long axis resulting in trauma of weightbearing on the dorsolateral aspect of the nail. A clavus develops at the nail margin receiving pressure of weightbearing from a tight shoe. The distal interphalangeal joint is hammered or flexed. The lesion is a gray to brown, circumscribed, waxy-looking mass.

Treatment. A conservative treatment is reduction of the excrescence, repeated application of a 25% salicylic acid ointment, subsequent debridement of the remaining clavus and proper shielding. A sinus tract may develop in the nail bed at the site of a clavus. A radical or surgical approach that sacrifices the nail and the distal phalanx may be necessary.

Exostoses are removed at the margins of the middle phalanx. This is accomplished by two elliptical incisions around the nail distally and dorsally placed to provide a plantar flap and total removal of the matrix, nail plate, clavus and distal phalanx.

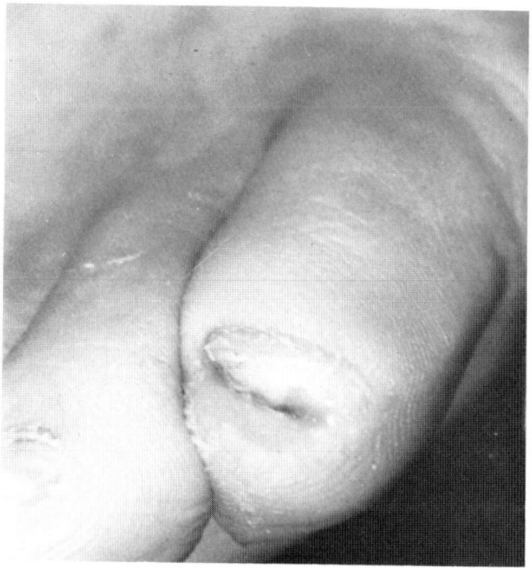

Fig. 14.27. Sinus tract distal end of nail bed.

Subungual Granuloma Pyogenicum. Ross (1955) notes that granuloma pyogenicum, when described by others, has been located at the margins of the nails. When it occurred under the nail plate it was usually described as onychia. Comparative studies suggest the correct terminology as subungual granuloma pyogenicum. Das Gupta (1965) records 34 cases of subungual melanoma that were operable and Eicheholtz and DeAngelo (1965) demonstrated squamous cell carcinoma with invasion to the bone following old subungual infections.

I have seen hundreds of cases of subungual granuloma pyogenicum secondary to multiple minimal trauma, direct trauma to the hallux nail and injudicious debridement of subungual debris. Often a subungual exostosis is an etiologic factor.

Treatment of this soft pedunculated mass of moist, vascular, often infected tissue, is performed under local anesthesia. The nail plate and necrotic tissue are removed by sharp section and the base is cauterized with an electric needle or silver nitrate concentrate. If an exostosis exists, this should be removed.

Digital Calcinosis in Nail Sulcus. Frost (1957) reports a case of digital calcinosis at the proximal end of the fibular nail sulcus. The nail was mildly incurvated. The mass was a small hard immobile nodule covered by an adherent, cornified, yellowish epithelium. Dorsoplantar and mediolateral x-ray views revealed a nodular calcified mass lateral to the middle third of the distal phalanx. Pathologically the bone was arranged in a circular fashion and represented a calcification of a previously existing cyst structure. No cartilage matrix was recognized. This could represent local ossification as a result of trauma, trichinosis, epidermoid cyst or foreign body. Excision is the treatment of choice.

Subungual Exostosis. The presence of an elevated nail plate with or without discoloration, a thickening of the nail bed and pain on digital pressure may be evidence of a subungual exostosis. Subungual heloma, tyloma, granuloma, ulceration, glomus tumor or enchondromas and intramedullary cysts must be ruled out by careful clinical, laboratory and radiographic examinations. It is believed that most subungual exostoses represent an ossifying form of fibrocartilaginous metaplasia caused by multiple minimal trauma.

Treatment. Surgical excision is the treatment of choice. Toe block anesthesia is induced and

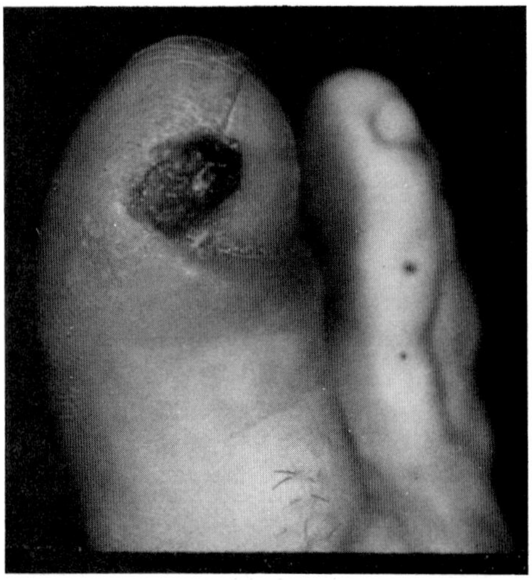

Fig. 14.28. Granuloma—onychocryptosis.

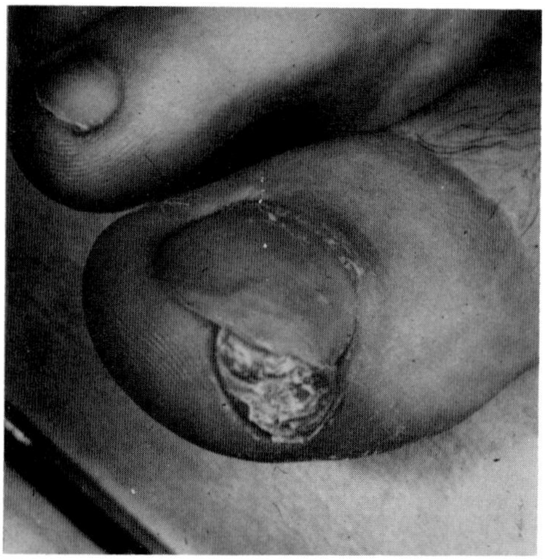

Fig. 14.29. Subungual heloma overlying exostosis.

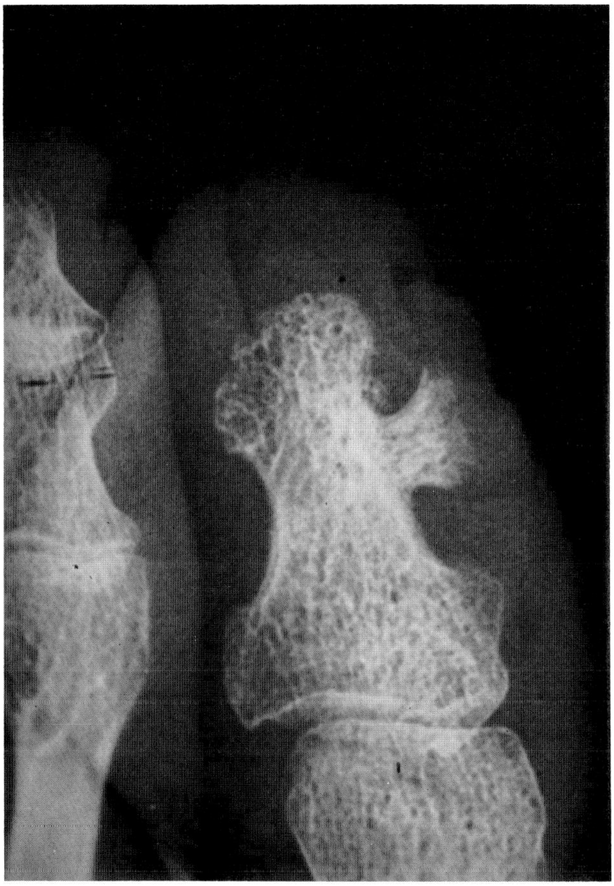

Fig. 14.30. Subungual exostosis. Courtesy of *Clinical Foot Roentgenology*, Baltimore: The Williams & Wilkins Company, 1966.

an elastic tourniquet is applied for hemostasis. The affected nail plate is gently separated from the nail bed with a minimum of trauma and the exostosis is exposed. This is removed with bone forceps and curettage. A sterile dressing of antibiotic ointment is applied and the wound is allowed to granulate in with subsequent redressings of stimulating ointments. On occasion a complication of all nail surgery may result in the development of an inclusion cyst.

Sandel (1958) believes the fishmouth type of incision to be too traumatizing resulting in sloughing and occasional gangrene. I have used this procedure without incident for many years.

Wichman (1967) describes a simplified version of subungual exostectomy. Following the usual sterile preparation for surgery, a transverse incision about 1/4 in. long is made at the distal end of the toe. The dorsal surface of the phalanx is explored blindly by inserting a 1/8 in. wide dental chisel to chip off prominent surfaces. This procedure is completed using a cross cut rasp to file the bone smooth. Bleeding is encouraged to flush out the wound. The patient is ambulatory and no sutures are necessary. Similar approaches have been used by Polokoff and Probber with excellent results. Their raspostectomy and osteotripsy techniques have provided good to excellent results in hundreds of cases.

Objective Signs of Systemic Disorders

Dermatitis Exfoliativa. In dermatitis exfoliativa, nail lesions are common. The nails become deformed and thickened,

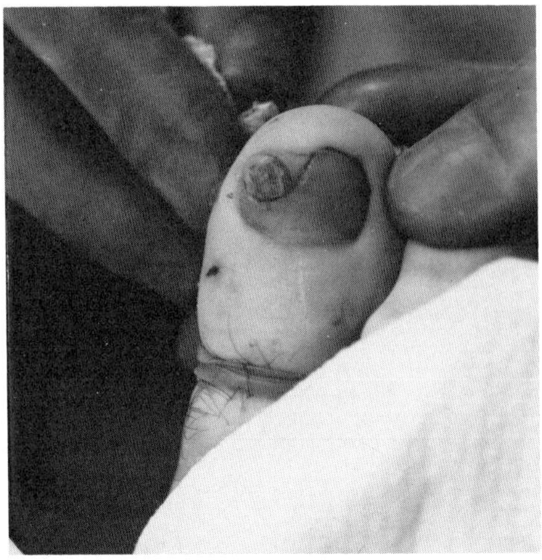

Fig. 14.31. Subungual exostosis. Note overlying excresence. Courtesy of D. Mowbray.

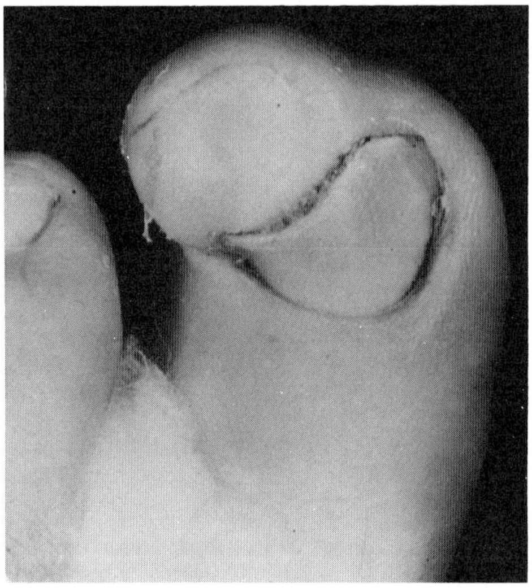

Fig. 14.32. Chondroma distal end of hallux.

lose their color and develop underlying hyperkeratosis. The nail loosens and may be lost completely. The thickened nail is reduced by drill, scalpel or sharp curettage. Emollient creams are prescribed to maintain the texture of the skin.

Ichthyosis. In ichthyosis a marked hyperkeratosis develops under the nail, the periungual tissue is scaly and the nail plate is often deformed. Onychauxis and onychogryposis with discoloration are common. Debridement and vitamin A by topical application is indicated.

The matrix is radiosensitive and becomes thinned, friable, discolored and atrophied with injudicious over-exposure to the x-ray. The surrounding skin may be pigmented, wrinkled and atrophied as in ichthyosis. A history of treatment by x-ray should differentiate the problem.

Pemphigus. In pemphigus the changes taking place in the skin affect the growth of the nail. Dystrophic changes, discoloration, pitting and transverse sulcus formation may result from inflammatory

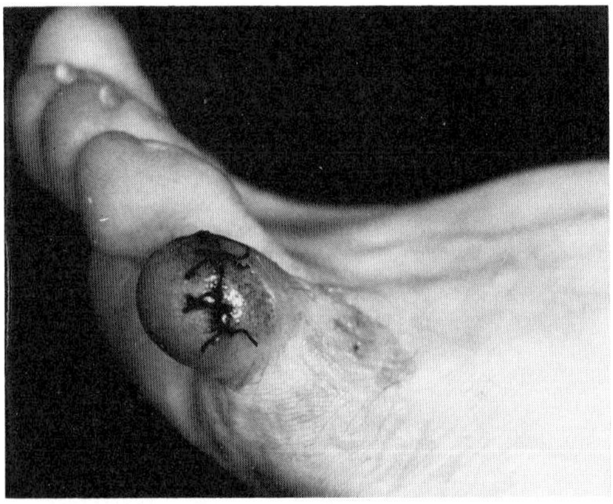

Fig. 14.33. Total excision of nail and distal one-third of fifth toe. Subungual exostosis.

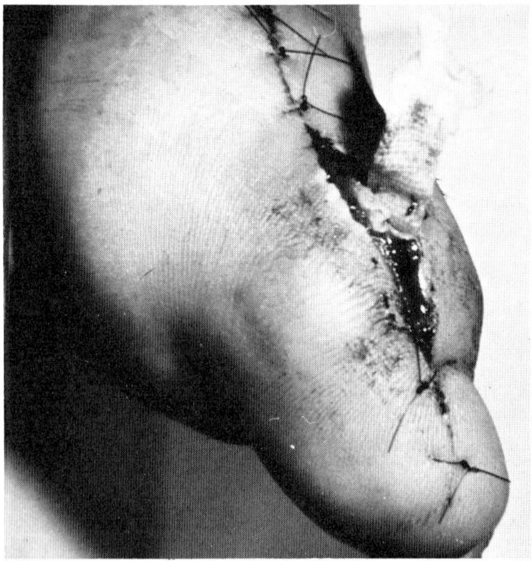

Fig. 14.34. Inclusion cyst. Complication of nail surgery. Excision of inclusion cyst.

changes, edema and faulty nutrition around the matrix. Contact dermatitis caused by sensitivity to detergents or nail polish may cause thickening of the nail, brittleness and cracks. Oils, tar and greasy substances may cause discoloration.

Transverse lines in an atrophic nail which is shiny and bent over the ends of the fingers and rarely on the toes is seen in **sclerodactylia**. This must be differentiated from trauma-induced lines.

Elephantiasis. In elephantiasis, the skin is thick, corneus and hyperkeratotic. The nails develop a raised free border, atrophy and become otherwise deformed with spicules implanted in the nail bed. The color varies from gray through brown to black. Curettage and reduction of nail borders by drill help prevent secondary infections.

Syphilis, being the great imitator that it is, may produce almost any objective characteristic that nails are heir to. The nail plate often presents Beau's lines, and infections in the adjacent tissues are common. Early treatment by an internist, however, reduces the possibility of permanent nail damage and other sequelae of advanced syphilis.

Onycholysis or loss of the toenail is seen in tabes dorsalis and hyperthyroidism and may also occur in severe trauma and hyperidrosis. Treatment is systemic. The distal nail plate gradually separates from the nail bed and progresses proximally resulting in a white nail caused by air entering the subonychial space.

Koilonychia is characterized by a thin lusterless nail plate with central bending in spoon-like fashion and usually occurs in cases of hypochromic anemia. Stanley (1956) states that it also accompanies thyrotoxicosis and may develop in certain occupations exhibiting toxic reactions. It is not found in severe pernicious anemia. Cases have been found where koilonychia has responded to correction of an underlying polycythemia vera. Bergeron and Stone (1967) report a suggestion of autosomal dominant genetic transference affecting males and females alike in a study of 12 members of a family. The presence of secondary infection requires excision of offending borders of the deformed nails.

Black nails are the result of subungual hemorrhage and should be differentiated from melanocytic and pigmented changes in the nail bed and matrix. Higashi (1968) noted that most pigmented changes in the nail were due to an increase in the number of melanocytes due to such factors as inflamma-

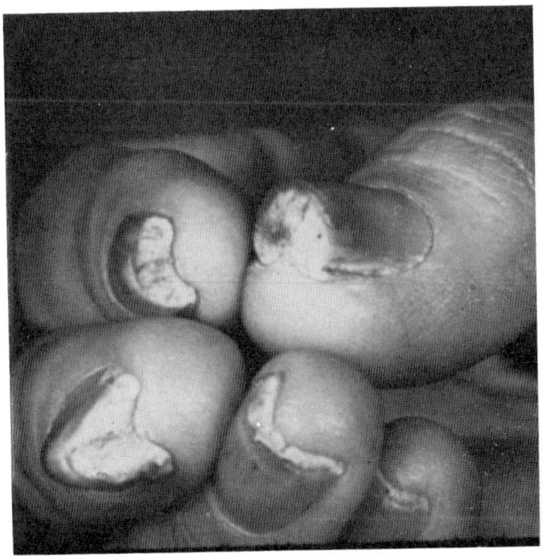

Fig. 14.35. Pachyonychia, fingernails. Courtesy of C. Krausz.

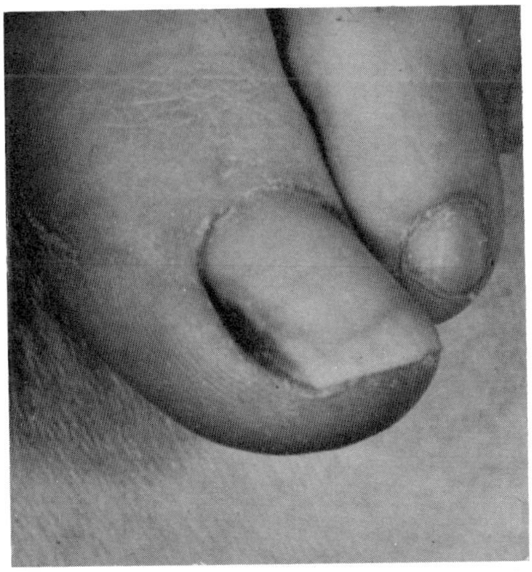

Fig. 14.36. Pigmented nevus at nail border.

tion, irradiation and metabolic disturbances.

Bodine (1967) described **subungual coagulum** as a dark red mass with vertical dark lines running along the long axis of the nail caused by multiple minimal trauma and capillary fragility. Often following trauma, a massive hemorrhage lifts the nail plate up from the bed. Early release of pressure by drilling an opening through the nail plate is indicated and repair is then usually uneventful. Failure to drain the blood may result in an accumulation of a dark blood clot which serves as an excellent focus for bacterial and mycotic infection.

The presence of pigment and an ulceration in the nail bed must be differentiated from a subungual melanoma by biopsy and histologic examination (Pack, 1967).

Beau's Lines. In Raynaud's disease or other vasospastic and circulatory disturbances, Beau's lines may be seen on a cyanosed nail plate. The cyanosis remains; distortion and atrophy of the nail takes place and gangrene eventually destroys the tissue. A peripheral vascular surgeon must be consulted early when the podiatrist finds evidence of circulatory disorders.

Anemia and Vitamin Deficiency. Grayish, thinned nails with longitudinal striations may be due to anemia. The symptoms subside with appropriate treatment with folic acid and vitamin B_{12} or with iron therapy and the blood picture improves. Brittle, ridged and furrowed nails may improve with administration of vitamin B_2 and vitamin D.

Endocrine Disorders. The hypothyroid myxedematous patient may present brittle, thin, white-spotted, striated nails in addition to the typical dry, scaly myxedematous skin. The protein-bound iodine is watched as treatment progresses. Adequate systemic treatment by an internist relieves podiatric symptoms.

A loss of lunula is noted in hypopituitary disease. Hypogonadism may produce a watch-crystal type or thinned, transparent nail plate. Patients with hyperthyroidism or hyperpituitarism exhibit shiny, well-developed nails. In hyperthyroidism the nail plate may become soft from excessive perspiration. Hyperpituitarism may result in the nails appearing convex from side to side and proximal to distal edges.

Onychatrophia is a diminution in the normal development of the nail in size, thickness or texture. The nail may appear thin, brittle, pitted in the center or spoon-shaped and is often separated from the nail bed. Paronychia or onychitis may cause vascular or nutritional disturbance to the matrix causing onychatrophia. Inflammatory skin disorders, nervous disease, trauma and constitutional disorders may be etiologic. The nail may develop a longitudinal split such as in the systemic disorders—cerebral paralysis, tabes, syphilis, tuberculosis, congenital familial dystrophy, thyroid diseases, circulatory diseases and chemical poisonings. Systemic treatment is necessary and local palliation prevents infection.

Anonychia is a congenital absence of matrix and complete lack of development of a nail plate.

Pulmonary diseases, kidney disorders or congenital cardiac problems may cause hyppocratic nails which are club-like and thick, light gray to dark brown in color, and convex from side to side and from the proximal border to the

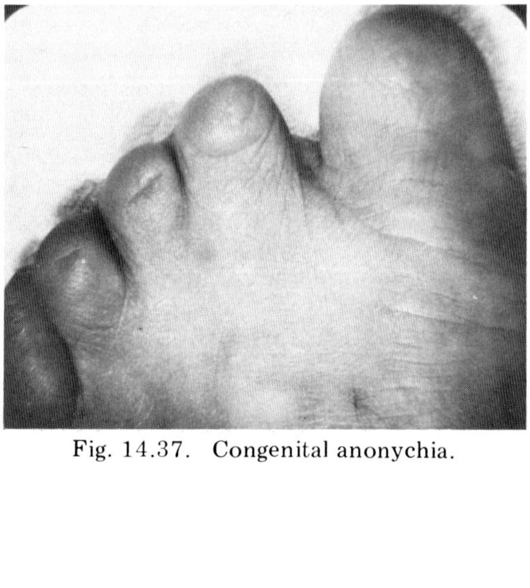

Fig. 14.37. Congenital anonychia.

distal end.

Arthritis. The nails may pit in acute rheumatic disturbances. A dry, brittle nail with subungual keratosis is seen often in chronic arthritic lesions.

Quincke's pulse is alternate redness and pallor of the nail plate produced by the capillaries in the nail bed. Heat increases this pulsation. Blanching occurs with each diastole of the heart. When this pulse pressure is so great as to be visible one must consider the possibility of aortic valvular insufficiency, rheumatic heart disease or arteriovenous fistula, and the patient should be referred to an internist for diagnosis and treatment.

Arterial Disease. In vasospastic arterial disease, the cuticle is widened and the nail fold thinned. There is a blending of the nail fold, cuticle and nail plate which return to normal after sympathectomy. Severe ischemia is the usual cause of extremely painful nails that are not deformed. Treatment is aimed at the etiology and pathology and surgical intervention is frowned upon in vasospastic disorders.

15

Tumors and Cysts

The lesions discussed here are those that can be tentatively interpreted by clinical examination and later corroborated by laboratory study. Tumors and cysts involving bone are beyond the scope of this text and the author recommends the study of *Clinical Foot Roentgenology* for their interpretation. All masses removed from the foot should be properly evaluated clinically and macroscopically and by microscopic examination. Careful history-taking is essential if full appreciation of the pathology is to be realized.

There are exciting physical, chemical and biologic factors which precede the development of tumors. Tumors are autonomous new growths that must be differentiated from inflammatory disorders regenerative processes and repair mechanisms. They may be progressive and unlimited in their growth.

DuVries (1959) differentiates benign from malignant tumors by noting that benign tumors have a capsule; if they are removed, they should not reoccur. Their blood supply is generally poor and they do not adhere to adjacent issue. Their outline is smooth, even or regular and they do not metastasize. The cells of a benign tumor are adult; growth is slow and their influence on life is negligible. Malignant tumors have the opposite characteristics: they are composed of embryonic cells and can be fatal if not removed in their early development.

Nickel (1958) states that if malignancy is suspected, primary surgical excision is the treatment of choice. Operation may be too late if the patient must wait for a microscopic report. Malignancy may be presumed if a nodular elevation develops on a flat mole and there is crusting and oozing, if there is satellite pigmentation, if a red halo develops around a nevus, or if there is spontaneous bleeding and accelerated growth. Nickel also notes that malignant melanomas may show none of these changes and thus he strongly recommends biopsy of all treated lesions.

Levene (1959) studied the relationship of pressure to the dissemination of melanoma. Five hundred eleven lesions of the foot were seen at Christie Hospital, Manchester, England. Melanomas commonly found in females all appeared in the arch areas of the foot while squamous cell carcinomas and hyperkeratotic lesions were on the metatarsal and heel areas. Angiomas extended from plantar to dorsal areas. The squamous cell lesions were more common in males.

Foreign Body Granuloma. When a minute foreign body penetrates the skin—as frequently occurs in the feet—an initial overlying lesion of hyperkeratosis may develop. The lesion becomes nodular resulting in pain that requires complete removal for relief. Very often the granulomatous lesion is enveloped by a firm fibrous capsule resulting in a cystic degeneration.

Treatment. The treatment of foreign body granuloma is aimed at removing the foreign

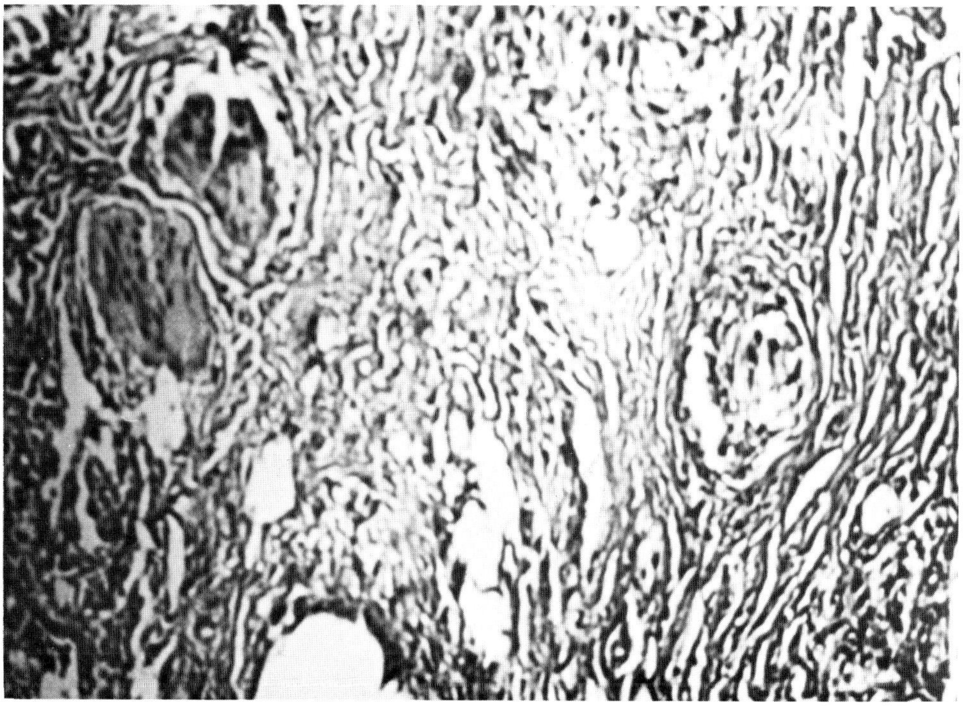

Fig. 15.1. Foreign body granuloma. Note crystalline material. Foreign body giant cells visible with about 22 and 19 nuclei showing, respectively. Note collagen surrounding cells.

body and the pathologic tissue surrounding it. This may be accomplished by the use of field block anesthesia with Xylocaine 1% and 1:100,000 epinephrine and completely excising the entire granulomatous mass including its capsular attachments. Closure is aimed at closing the gaping space with sutures followed by the use of compression bandages.

Granuloma Pyogenicum. These lesions commonly occur at the margins of the nails or in the nail grooves and on nail lips. They may develop at any site on the foot. They resemble an infected angioma but are differentiated by their soft red to brownish color, vascular, sharply demarcated, pedunculated and sessile growth. Growth is rapid. These granulomas are caused by irritation of the skin, by an offending portion of nail, or self-inflicted trauma. Sensation may vary from severe pain to painlessness. Rome (1958) says the granulomas bleed readily and often suppurate with no tendency to heal. The lesions measure from the typical 1 cm. to 4 or 6 cm. in size. Entrance of staphylococci into a small opening is thought to be the causative factor.

Treatment of pyogenic granuloma consists of early correction of the localized infection with antibiotic therapy. Healing is enhanced by removing the offending portion of the nail to diminish continued irritation. In most instances it is advisable to use toe block anesthesia followed by removal of 1/3 of the offending border of the toe nail. This is accomplished in a deft manner to minimize the trauma to the nail bed and the posterior nail fold. Complete excision of the granulomatous mass is followed by either electrocautery of the granulomatous base or the use of a silver nitrate stick while the patient is still under anesthesia. Treatment is continued in an effort to resolve the proliferation of the previously irritated cells.

Benign Multiple Acanthoma. Steinberg calls attention to a condition, which he calls "benign multiple acanthoma," found in multiple recurrent ingrowing toe nails in young people. He reports

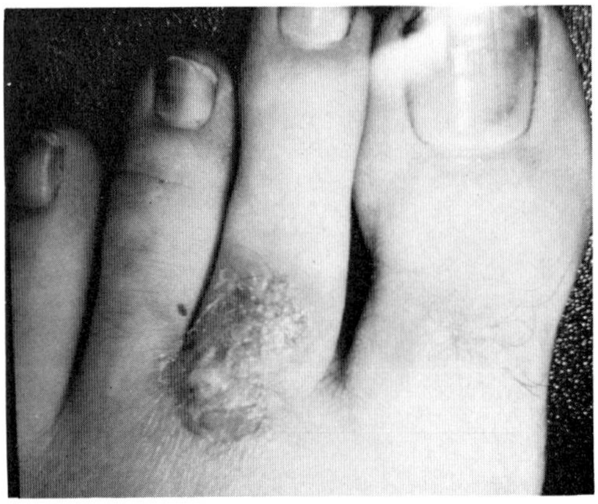

Fig. 15.2. Granuloma pyogenicum. Slightly elevated moist red granulation tissue on the dorsum of the second toe.

cases to substantiate his findings and cites the following diagnostic criteria: persistent recurrence involving two or more toes; bulbous tissue formation on the distal nail flap, usually on both sides of the toe; muco-purulent exudate with a characteristic biopsy; little or no deformity of the matrix; familial tendency; less pain than usual ingrown nail; firm tissue which does not bleed as freely as granulation tissue.

Treatment. Toe block anesthesia is instituted and the offending border of the nail including the bulbous formation on the distal nail flap is removed. The patient is placed on wet saline soaks to calm down the inflammation and to cleanse the muco-purulent exudate from the affected part. This is then followed by the use of electrodesiccation on the affected part or the application of a silver nitrate stick to diminish the activity of the cells. If muco-purulent exudate persists, sensitivity tests are made to aid in selecting proper medication.

Profuse Granulation. A self-inflicted nail groove infection or irritation of the nail lip by a poorly cut or developing nail may result in abrasion of the nail lip or groove causing a superficial ulceration. With further irritation the tissue reacts with excessive proliferation and profuse granulations envelop the nail border. These granulations are bright red, shiny, raw, oozing vascular tissues. They form a granuloma when left alone and untreated.

Treatment. Profuse granulations are best removed under local anesthesia. The excision of the entire granular mass plus the application of silver nitrate to the base is indicated. The patient should be followed-up at intervals of 3 to 5 days for the purpose of establishing whether the profuse granulations are under control. If any evidence of the development of granulation tissues persists, the presence of a foreign material or irritant should be suspected. Removal of a foreign body or matrical tissue in the nail groove is mandatory for correction of this disorder.

Granuloma Annulare. This dermatosis, commonly found in children, generally involves the dorsum of the feet although it can occur on any part. An annular nodular lesion, red-brown in color, may enlarge by peripheral spread. The center clears as the margin spreads. This condition is otherwise asymptomatic and is frustrating to treat.

Treatment. Intralesional injections of tri-

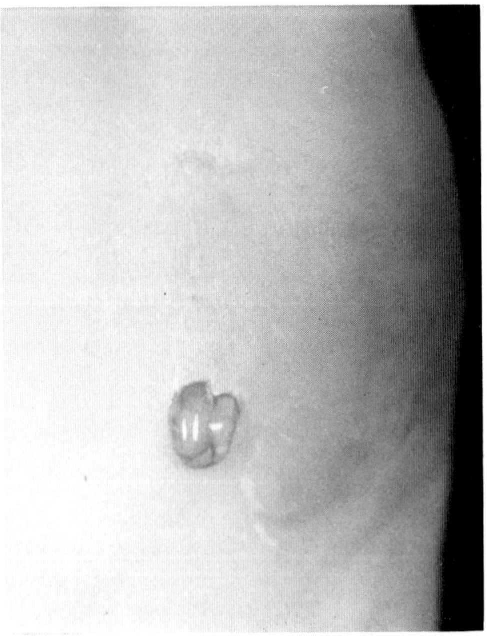

Fig. 15.3. Granuloma pyogenicum plantar surface of the foot.

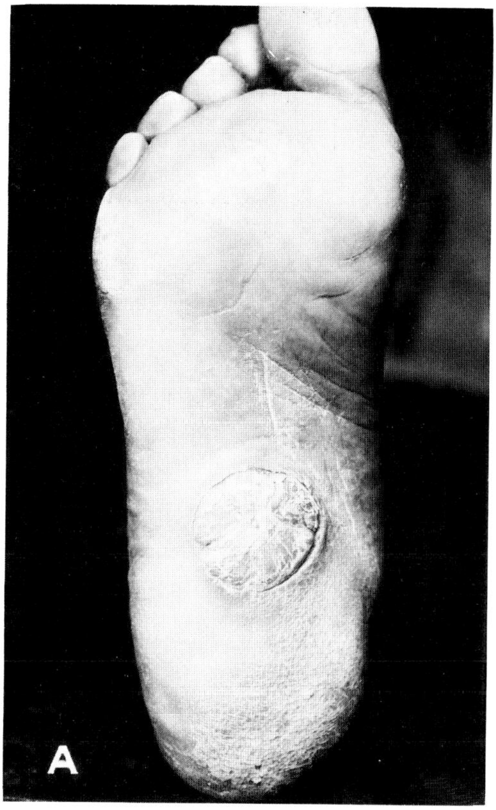

Fig. 15.4A. Nodular subepidermal fibrosis. Courtesy of M. Blass.

amcinalone have been helpful. Often procaine injections and even biopsy result in clinical cure. Vitamin D may increase the activity of the lesion. Silver *et al.* (1961) found that trauma to the lesion appears to be followed by involution. When lesions occur in other parts of the body, the patient is referred to a dermatologist for treatment. A psychogenic etiology must be considered.

Nodular Subepidermal Fibrosis. This benign lesion is also known as a histiocytoma. It is a hard, firm nodule found in the dermis and attached firmly to the epidermis. The overlying skin has a shiny, red-brownish appearance. This is believed to be scar tissue secondary to a scratch, bite or other irritation of the skin. Steinberg described a plugged duct porokeratotic cyst that must be differentiated from a verruca and a nodular subepidermal fibrosis. A moat at its circumference is one of the differential features and it is histologically different.

Treatment is surgical removal of the nodule.

Fibroma. A fibroma is a firm benign nodular, clearly circumscribed and palpable mass of fibrous connective tissue capable of developing in any tissue derived from mesenchyme. Histologic examination will corroborate the clinical impression. A fibroma may be found in combination with several tissues such as in a neurofibroma, fibrolipoma and angiofibroma.

Lipomas are soft lobulated masses of enlarged lipoid cells with an increase in fibrous stoma. The size of a lipoma remains constant and does not enlarge like a bursa that has been irritated and inflamed.

Keloids are large, heavy scars commonly occurring in Negroes. The scars stand out from the skin and are composed of large amounts of fibrous connective tissue simulating benign tumor formation. The scars are disfiguring and commonly affect function when occurring on parts that normally are freely movable. Callus tissue often develops in scar tissue causing pain on pressure. I have seen several keloids develop following destruction of warts by electrodesiccation. The resultant lesion is an intractable keratosis.

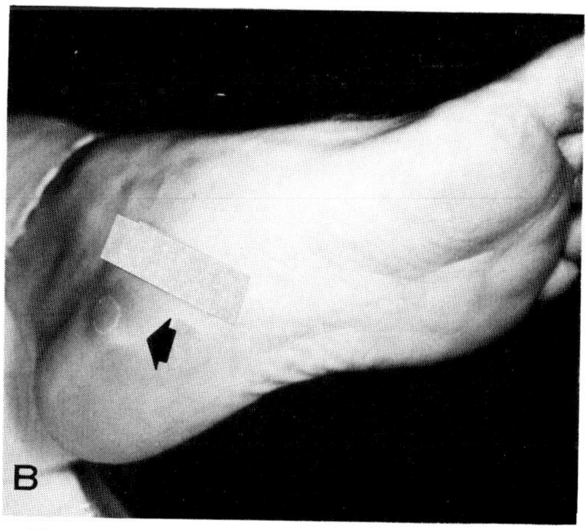

Fig. 15.4B. Fibroma. Medial plantar surface of the heel.

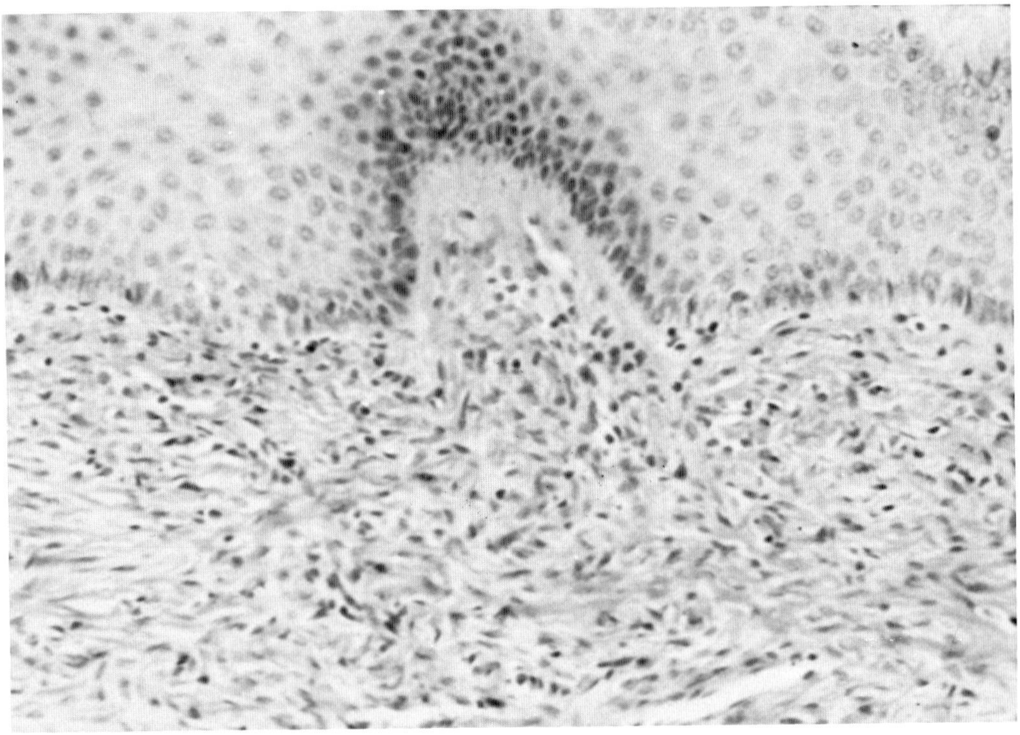

Fig. 15.5. Photomicrograph of dermatofibroma. Note the proliferation of fibroblasts and capillaries pushing up the epidermis and distorting the basement membrane. Courtesy of J. F. Yale.

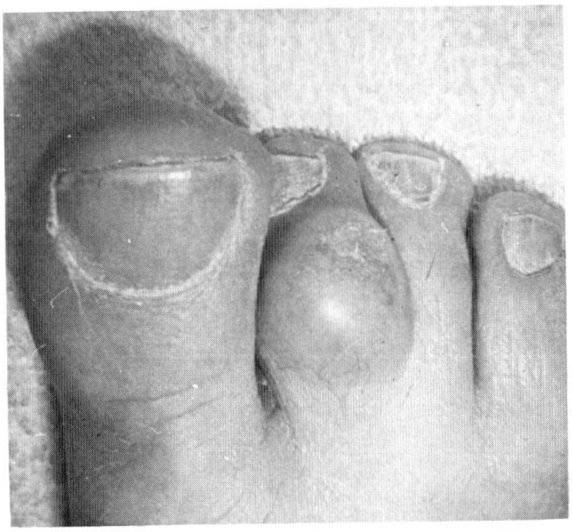

Fig. 15.6. Fibroma. Courtesy of J. F. Yale.

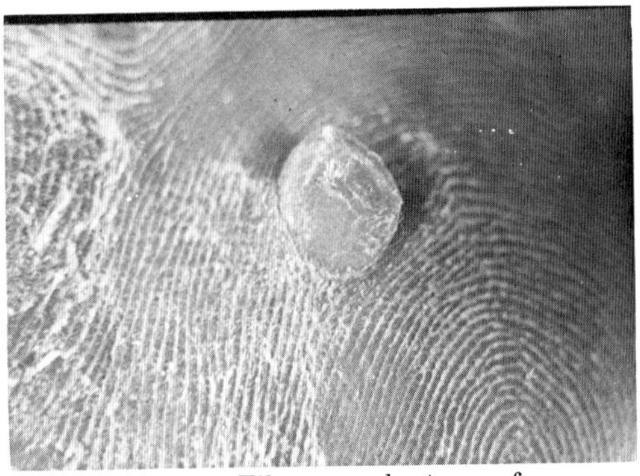

Fig. 15.7. Fibroma, plantar surface.

Treatment. Keloids are reduced in size or softened by the use of x-ray, ultrasound or chemotherapy. On occasion, the use of Dry Ice over the affected part can result in destruction of the keloid and the removal of the hyperplastic scar tissue. Scars may be removed by the use of a negative galvanic current. Some investigators have noted that the injection of vitamin A into the keloid has resulted in relief of pain and eradication of the scar. Periodic reduction by 40% salicylic acid plaster is effective when combined with other treatment as outlined above. Monochloroacetic acid has proven successful in the slow destruction of keloids.

Benign angioma may be found in the skin, subcutaneous tissues, the skeletal muscles or the tendon sheaths, bones or joints. Deep-seated angiomas may cause considerable pain, but when they are superficial they remain painless until irritated by extrinsic factors. Angiomas vary in size from a few millimeters to the involvement of a complete extremity. The foot is the most frequent site for angioneuroma or glomus tumors. Kaposi's sarcoma frequently originates in the feet and should be differentiated from angioma.

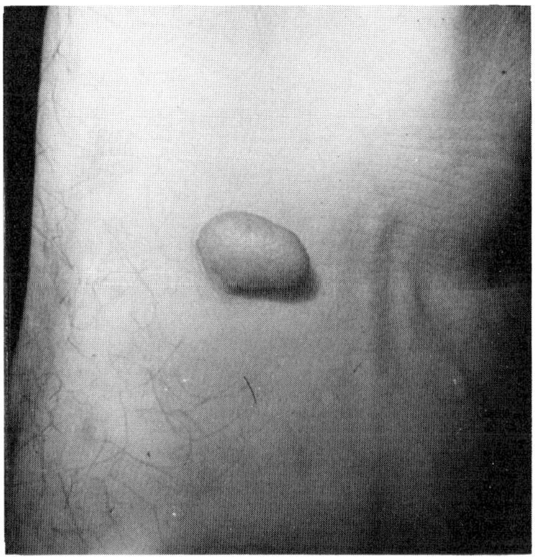

Fig. 15.8. Fibroepithelioma, dorsum of the foot. Firm, fibrous, elevated mass about 0.7 cm. in diameter with smooth shiny capsule.

The classification of the various types of angioma has been difficult because of different growth rate, histiologic appearance and confusing etiology. Oughtersan and Tenant categorized vascular tumors in three groups. The first group consists of the vascular malformations such as arteriovenous fistula, vascular nevi, and arterial, venous and lymphatic angiomas, and vascular blastomas. The second group was made up of the glomus tumor and angioneuromyomas. The third group consists of the Kaposi's idiopathic multiple hemorrhagic sarcoma.

The nevi of vascular growths may vary in size from a few millimeters to large, tumorous masses. Combinations of vas-

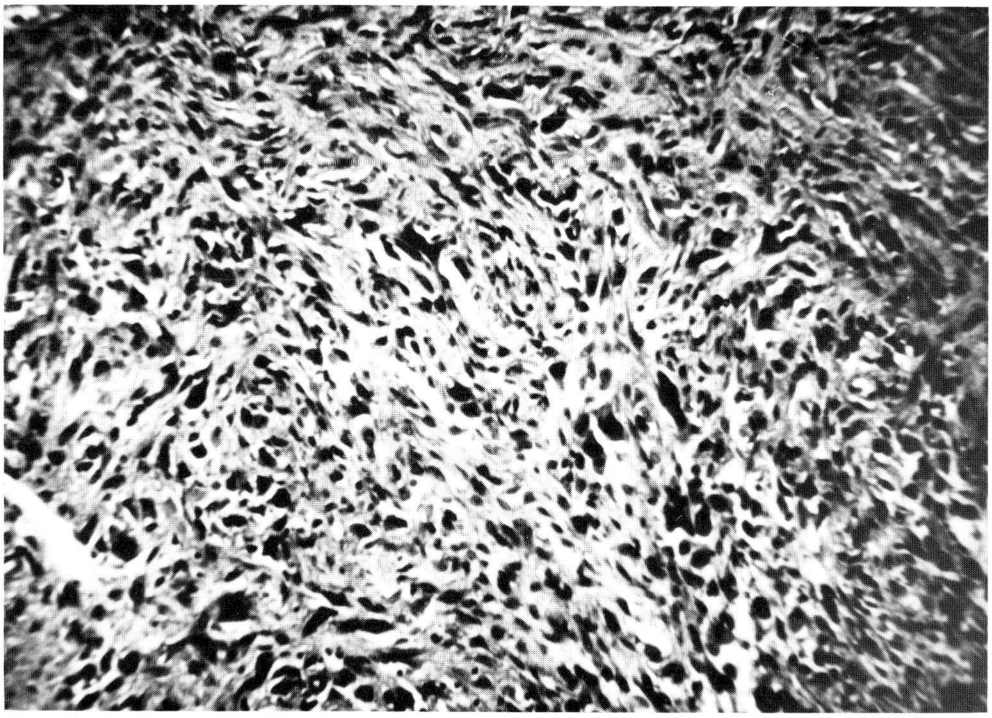

Fig. 15.9. Plantar fibroma. Dense fibrous stroma with dark-staining nuclei and little collagen replacement. Courtesy J. F. Yale.

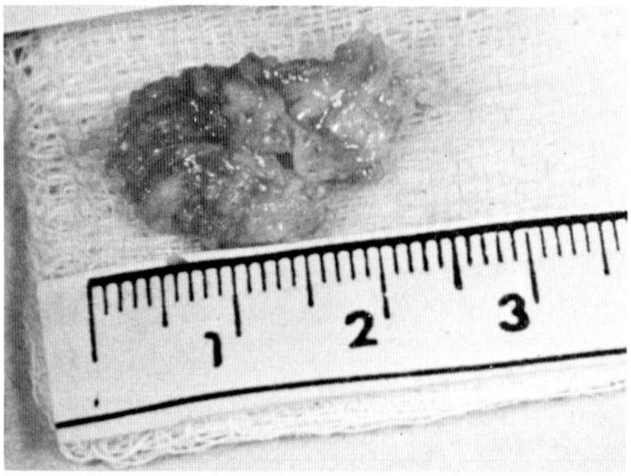

Fig. 15.10A. Fibroma, gross specimen.

cular growths may result in marked distortion of the lower extremity.

Treatment of angiomas depends on the location and degree of involvement. Treatment may vary from simple destruction by use of chemosurgical destruction or electrosurgical procedures to the extensive destruction or removal of the diseased parts by radical surgical intervention. X-irradiation may also be used.

Cutaneous Mucous Cysts of the Toes

J. Yale (1967) in a review of the literature and following experience with the diagnosis and treatment of cutaneous

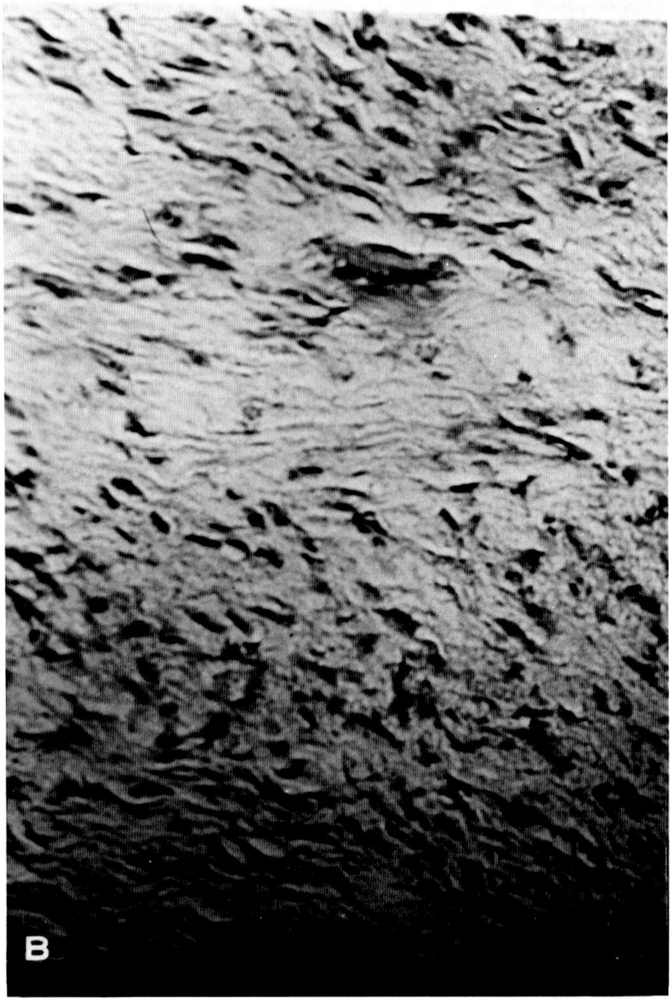

Fig. 15.10B. Fibroma. Old areas of cellularity have been lost and replaced with collagen. This lesion was removed after having been present for many years. Courtesy of J. F. Yale.

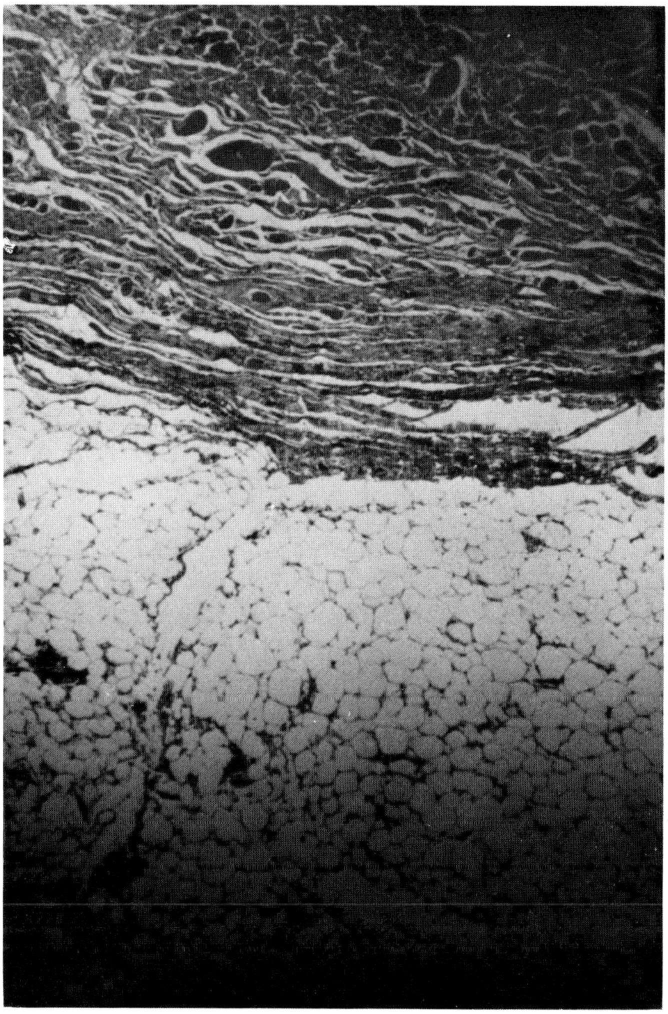

Fig. 15.11. Photomicrograph of normal skin and subcutaneous tissue. No evidence of inflammatory changes. Note junction of normal fat cells with the subcutaneous collagen and nuclear atypia as compared with Figures 15.9 and 15.10B. Courtesy of J. F. Yale.

mucous cysts described the lesion as follows: "Cutaneous mucous cysts are soft or fluctuant, rounded or oval, translucent lesions which sometimes are reddish in hue occurring on either side of the mid-line, over the distal interphalangeal joints of the fingers and toes. They range in size from 3 to 12 mm. in diameter.... In their early state they are covered by a thin, smooth, shiny epidermis. Older lesions may be verrucous in appearance. A straw-colored viscid material may ooze from a ruptured lesion... only to fill again without obliteration in 2 to 4 weeks. They commonly occur closer to the toe nail than to the joint."

According to J. Yale, cutaneous mucous cysts must be differentiated from inclusion cysts, sebaceous cysts, fibromas, ganglia, knuckle pads over joints, Heberden's nodes, xanthoma or giant cell tumors of the tendon sheath, blebs, verrucae, helomas, vesicles or bullae due to friction, osteochondromas, rheumatic nodules, periungual abscesses and hemorrhagic blebs. He concludes that "the refractory nature of these lesions to intra-lesional steroid therapy and the poor surgical results

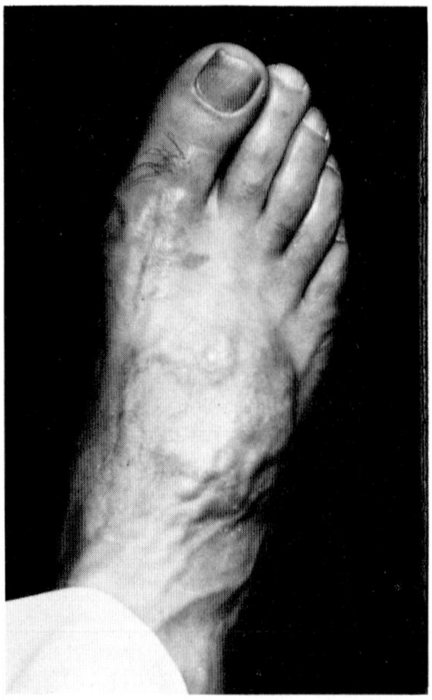

Fig. 15.12. Diffuse lipoma. Courtesy of D. Mowbray.

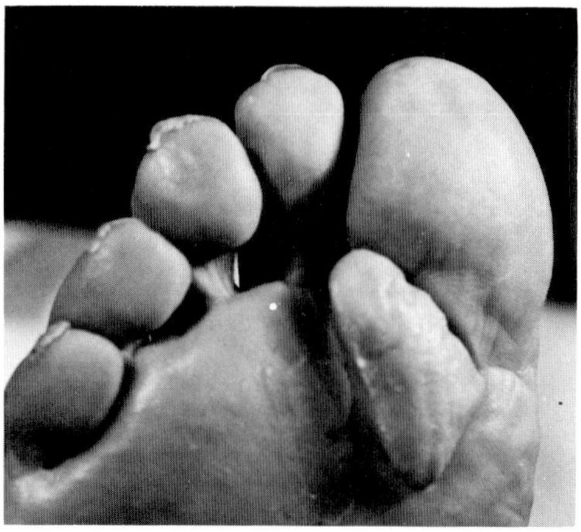

Fig. 15.13. Fibrolipoma. Courtesy of D. Mowbray.

reported in the literature make the eradication of these lesions difficult. It would seem that a better treatment is needed."

Nevi. The surface of a nevus is smooth and the growth consists of small dark pigmented red vascular dilations.

It is essential to remove nevi that show evidence of itching, crusting, increase in pigment or size, elevation, ulceration or rapid growth and hemorrhage. Wide excision and the careful utilization of plastic surgical techniques are essential. It is wise to have all lesions so removed evaluated microscopically by a pathologist. According to Fergusion (1955)

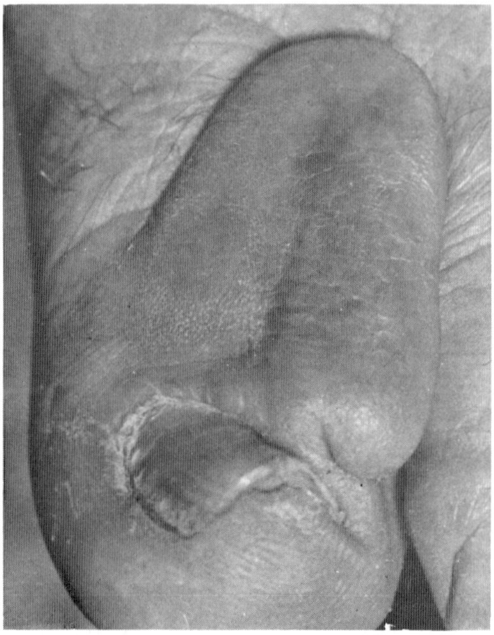

Fig. 15.14. Keloid on hallux.

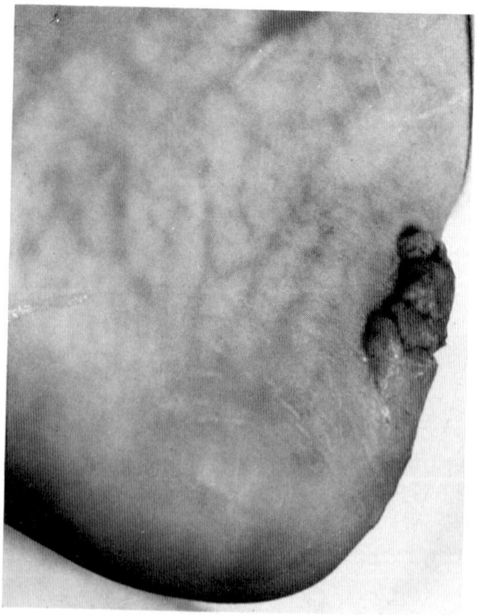

Fig. 15.15. Keloid, posterior of heel. Courtesy of D. Mowbray.

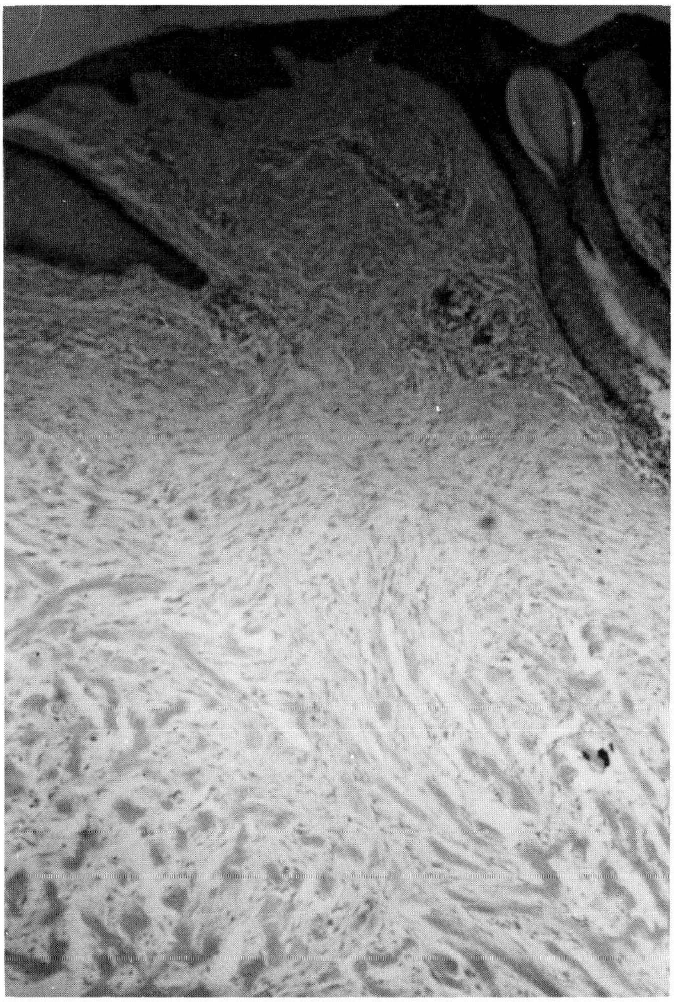

Fig. 15.16. Photomicrograph of a keloid. Hypertrophic fibrous reaction. Bundles of collagen fibers in subcutaneous tissue. Courtesy of J. F. Yale.

there is evidence that 50% of malignant melanomas arise from pre-existing nevi. Heller (1958) notes that it is good prophylactic medicine to remove nevi on the foot where they are subject to multiple minimal repeated trauma.

Hemangioma Simplex. These lesions are elevated and often pedunculated with an irregular surface and a varied color from bright red to dark red.

It is essential to evaluate these lesions both microscopically and macroscopically. In the event the lesion shows evidence of rapid growth or the development of hemorrhage it is essential that it be removed. Removal is affected by wide excision and closure with fine suturing material. Compression dressings are applied.

Cavernous Angiomas. These growths are typical of hemangioma simplex on a larger scale. The color varies from red to cyanotic blue depending on the size and depth of the lesion. Cavernous lesions are connected by vascular channels to the deeper blood supplies. Sometimes only a trace of blue is seen beneath the superficial skin over a wide area. They are spongy tumors, elevated and purplish red. They are fully developed at first but do not undergo involution like many growths noted at birth.

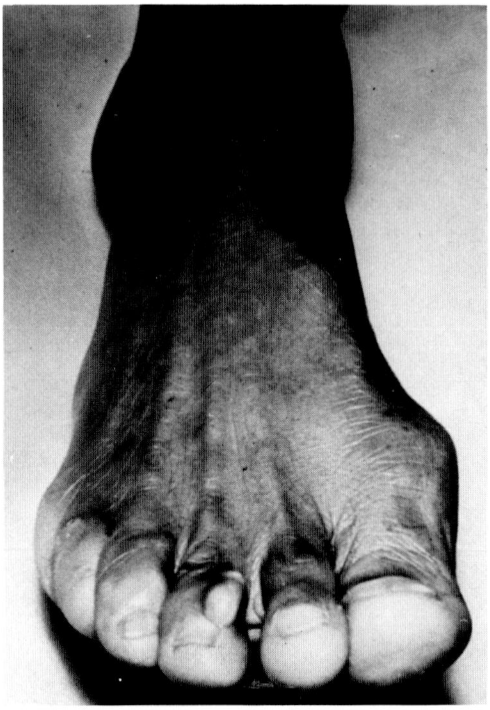

Fig. 15.17. Cutaneous mucous cyst, third toe. Courtesy of J. F. Yale.

The podiatric surgeon can allow these lesions to go untreated unless the patient complains of some discomfort. If removal is necessary great care should be taken because of the ability of these lesions to spread into the adjacent tissues and the deeper blood vessels. X-irradiation may shrink the lesion sufficiently to give adequate relief.

Angioblastoma. Despite their malignant clinical and histologic appearance, angioblastomas do not metastasize. These vascular tumors are nodular, and are red or bluish-red. Multiple lesions are often present. The larger lesions often ulcerate and become locally invasive and destructive.

Treatment consists of wide surgical excision of the lesion and adequate microscopic evaluation to differentiate it from Kaposi's idiopathic multiple hemorrhagic sarcoma.

Glomus tumors are commonly found in the extremities and beneath the nails of the feet. They are composed of

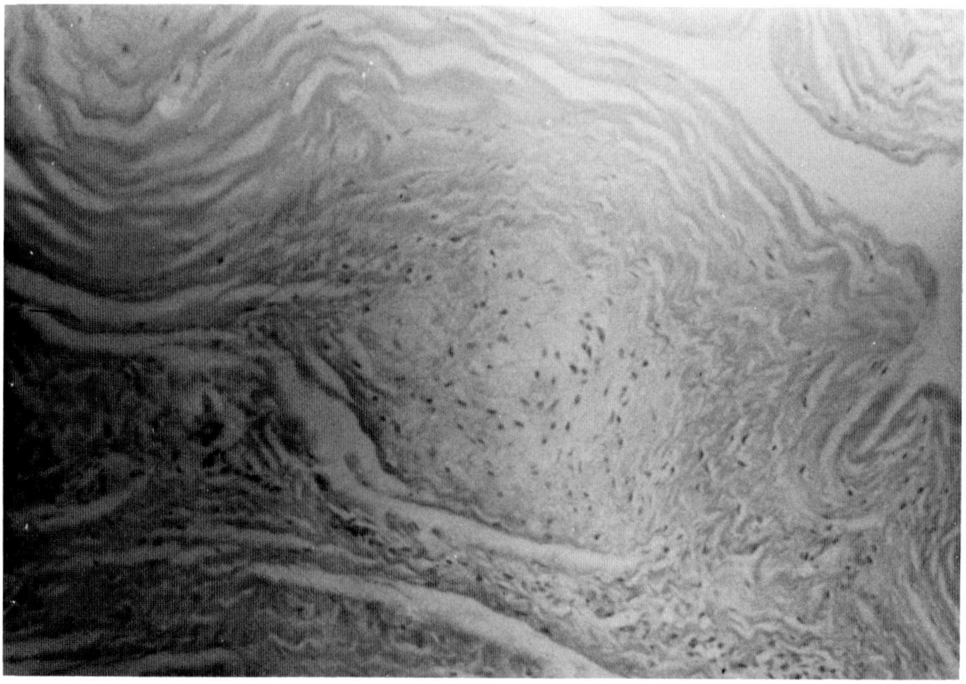

Fig. 15.18. Microscopic structure of cutaneous mucous cyst. Late stage of evolution. Cyst ruptured and remnants of the cyst wall are obscured. Courtesy of J. F. Yale.

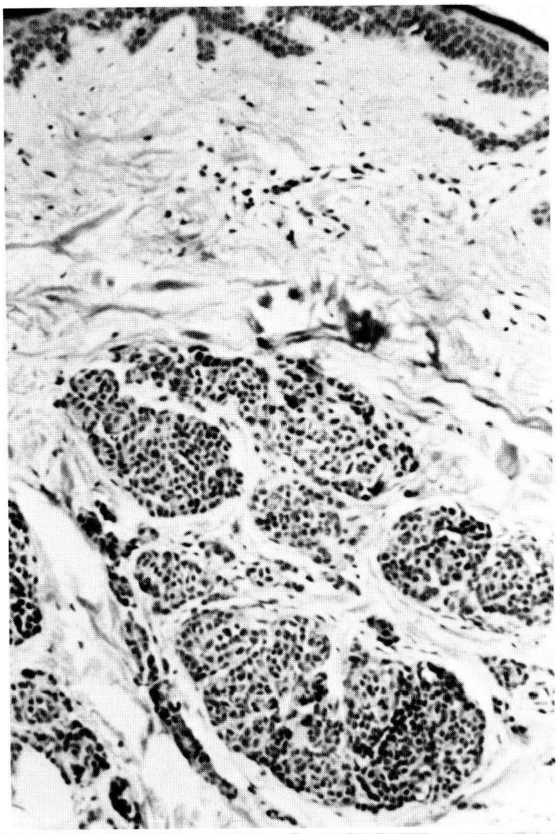

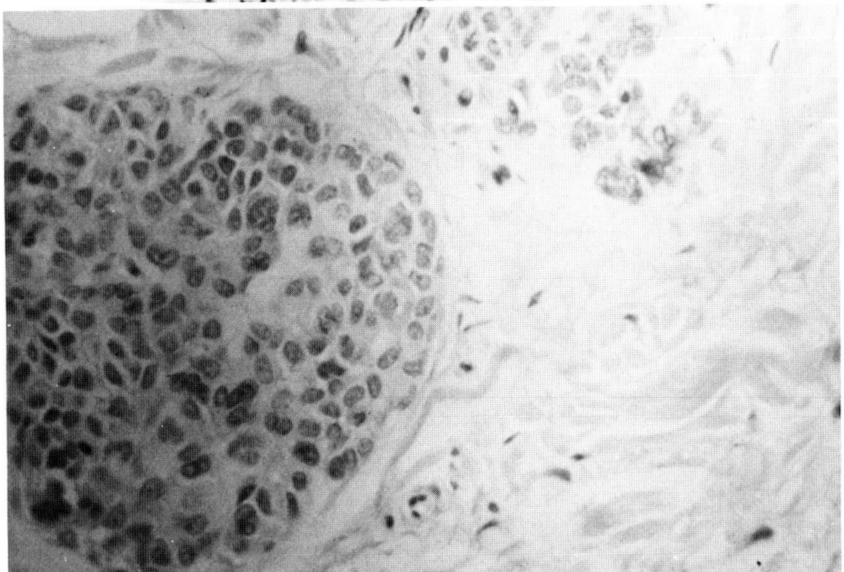

Fig. 15.19. Intradermal nevus, low power. Islands of proliferating nevus cells. Courtesy of J. F. Yale (*top*). Fig. 15.20. Intradermal nevus, high power. Note cluster of proliferating nevus cells (*bottom*).

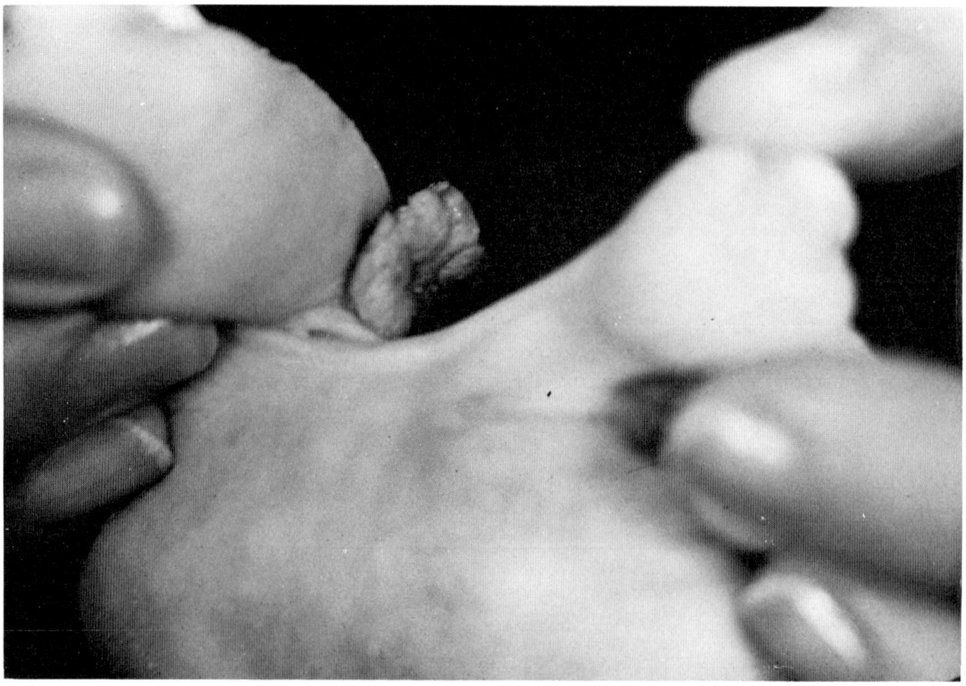

Fig. 15.21. Interdigital hemangioma.

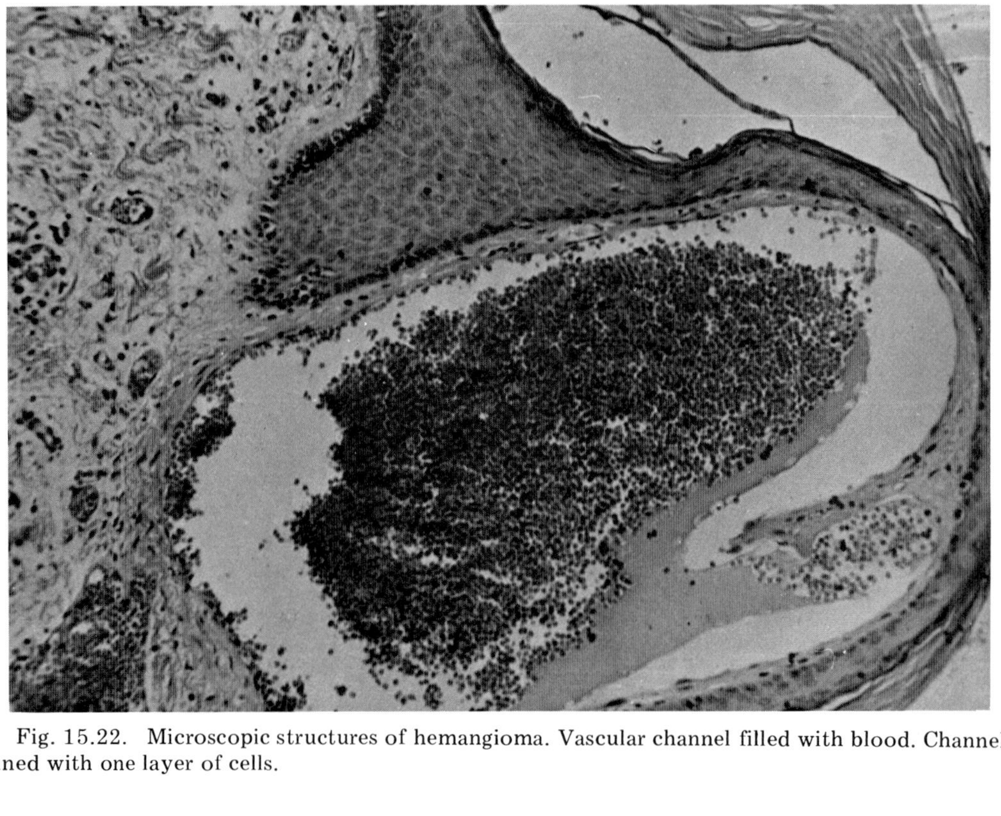

Fig. 15.22. Microscopic structures of hemangioma. Vascular channel filled with blood. Channel lined with one layer of cells.

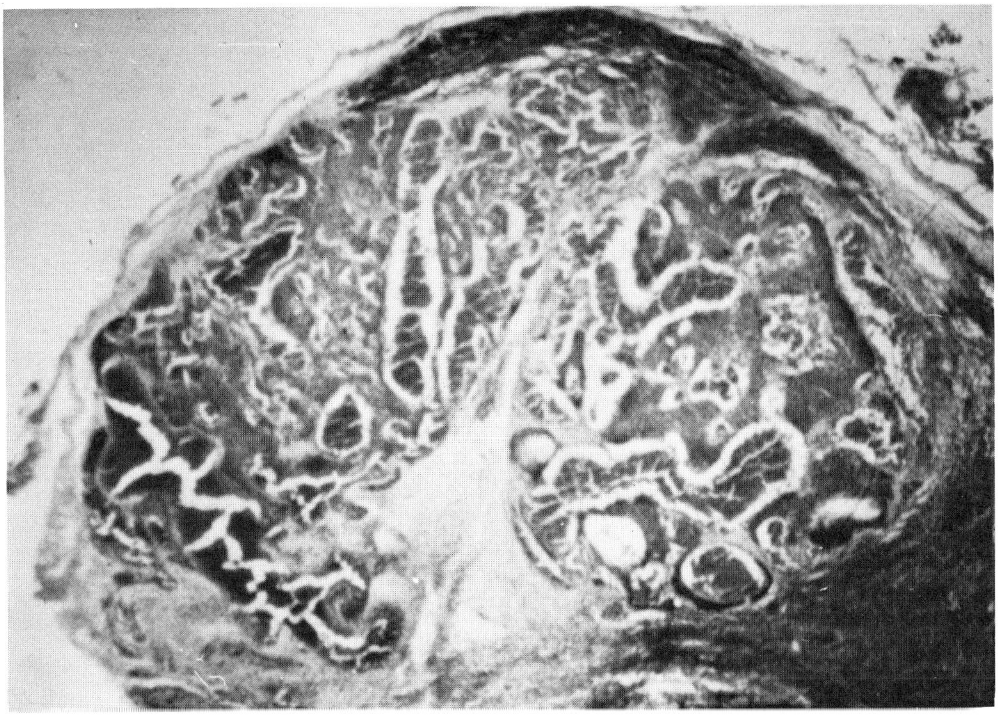

Fig. 15.23. Photomicrograph of glomus tumor. Small vascular channels surrounded by glomus cells.

muscle, nerve and vascular tissue, originating from the neuromyoarterial glomus in the nail bed. The tumor is red or bluish-red and is found in sites where granulomatous tissue development frequently occurs. Glomus tumors are small and can be diagnosed clinically by their slow growth, and characteristic color and by the characteristic loss of normal color reaction beneath the nail. The glomus tumor is often painless but can be extremely painful with pain radiating back into the foot. There may be very little evidence of pathology despite severe pain. As pain increases, it varies from a stabbing to burning and excruciatingly sharp pain often out of proportion to the size of the lesion. Plotnick (1960) states that the tumor may pulsate and skin temperature may increase.

Sandel (1966) described unilateral multiple glomus tumors occurring in the fourth intermetatarsal space and one posterior to the cuboid on its inferior surface. Surgical excision and microscopic examination corroborated the clinical appearance of glomus tumor. Sandel states, "the cardinal point to remember in diagnosing glomus tumor is that its pain is far in excess of any other condition normally found in the part under consideration."

Freed (1965) described a glomangioma that appeared on the mediodorsal aspect of the fourth toe. It presented itself clinically as a small, freely movable, sessile-shaped, subdermal mass. The tumor develops from the end-organ of the arteriovenous anastamosis. Marked hemodynamic effects may accrue. Freed notes that the prompt removal of the entire glomus plexus produces intermediate relief of the severe pain.

Microscopic examination reveals a well-encapsulated lesion. The growth must be differentiated from pyogenic granuloma and profuse granulations so common about the nail grooves and lips.

Treatment consists of wide excision of the lesion followed by the use of electrodesiccation or radiation therapy to the base. It is essential that all glomus tumors or suspected lesions be examined microscopically. A radiograph of the toe to rule out a subungual exostosis is helpful. If there are bone changes involving the distal phalanx it is good judgment to remove the entire nail, the tumor, nail bed and the distal third of the distal phalanx.

Sebaceous Cysts. Clogging of the passage of sebum as it exudes from the sebaceous gland results in the formation of a sebaceous cyst. The growth is circumscribed in the dermis and encapsulated by a dense, shiny, white, fibrous tissue containing a cheesy, soft material.

Treatment. The surgical excision of a sebaceous cyst is the only successful treatment for these lesions. Semi-elliptical incisions are made around the suspected lesion. The lesion is followed down to its origin in the dermis and subcutaneous tissue to which it may have extended. The adjacent tissue is explored for additional lesions. Closure is made in the usual manner; however, if the sebaceous cyst is large, closure should be effected with subcutaneous sutures prior to skin closure. Compression bandages are indicated.

Inclusion Cysts. These cysts may originate from embryonic misplaced epidermoid tissue. The walls of these cysts are firm and often contain hair, matrix or other foreign bodies.

I have surgically removed shiny white firm cysts beneath deep-seated excrescences. On several occasions the small cyst was removed from the deep-seated excrescence commonly called heloma neurofibrosum. These lesions are very common on the ball of the foot beneath areas of extreme pressure and irritation. It is not unusual to find more than one mass in and about the affected part. Inclusion cysts are a common postsurgical complication following nail surgery arising 2 to 6 months following radical excising of an ingrown toe nail. The tissue beneath or adjacent to the previous skin incision scar becomes red, elevated and often pointed.

Treatment. Incision and drainage followed by excision of the entire white glistening capsule is the treatment of choice.

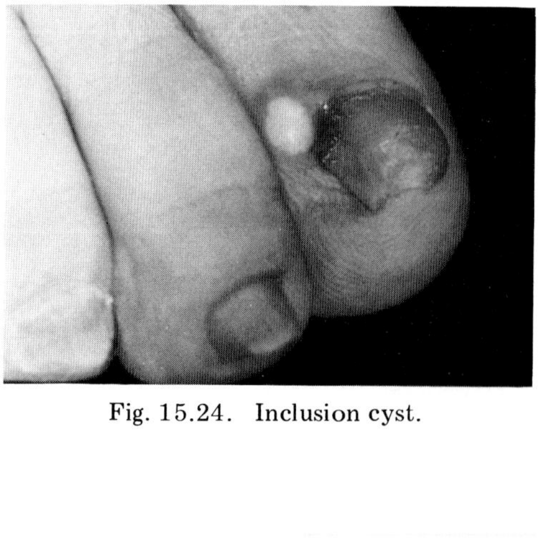

Fig. 15.24. Inclusion cyst.

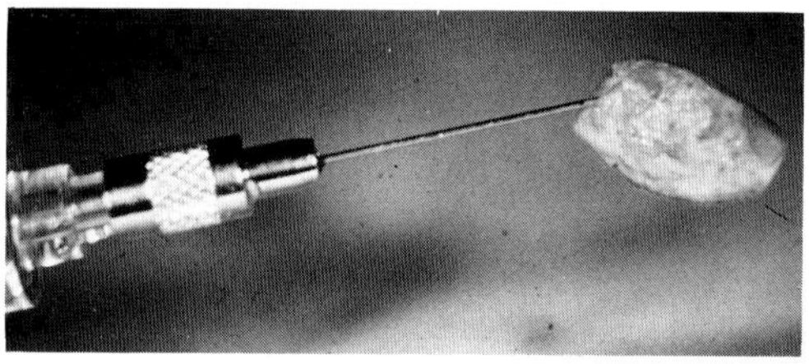

Fig. 15.25. Inclusion cyst surrounded by reactive fibrosis due to chronic irritation of connective tissue.

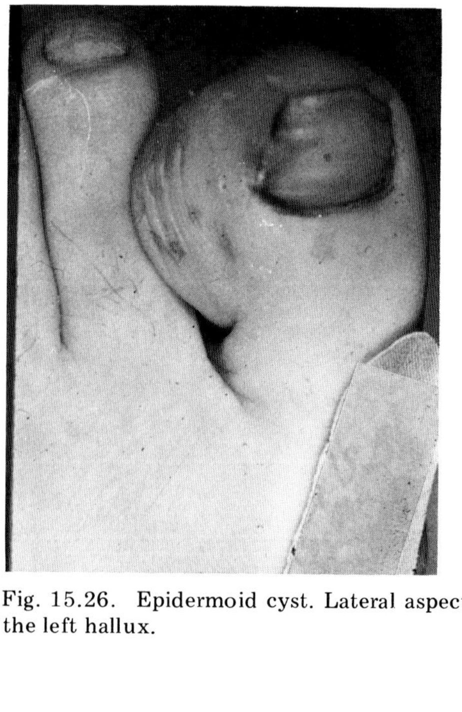

Fig. 15.26. Epidermoid cyst. Lateral aspect of the left hallux.

Kaposi's Sarcoma. Kaposi's idiopathic multiple hemorrhagic sarcoma is most common in males and on the dorsal and plantar surfaces of the feet. The initial lesion is a soft and vascular rare malignant tumor thought originally to be caused by trauma. As the growths enlarge, they coalesce to form red, reddish-brown or bluish-black lesions that become indurated and often mildly hyperkeratotic. The vascular nodules may involute and leave atrophic pigmented scars. The slow development with remissions and regressions are bilateral and symmetrical and often spread to involve the lymph glands, spleen, liver and lungs. The extremities may become swollen, hard and distorted presenting pigmented, atrophic scars. Patients usually die within 2 to 10 years after onset. Early detection before it spreads to the vital organs may save the patients's life as Kaposi's sarcoma in its early stages is radiosensitive.

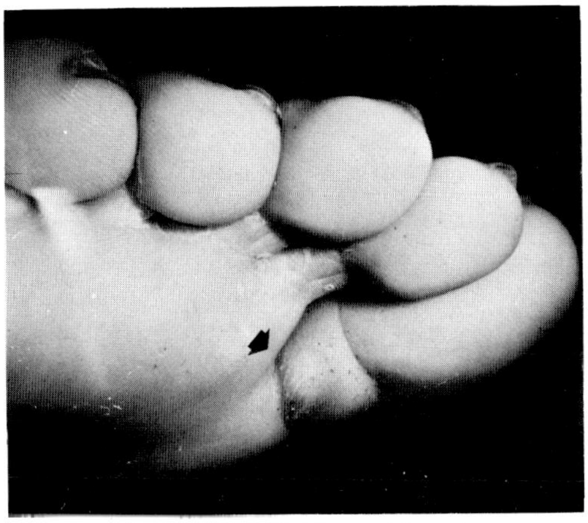

Fig. 15.27. Epidermoid cyst.

Yale and Yale (1966) discuss two cases of Kaposi's sarcoma. In one of these cases the sole of the foot presented several nodules. One of the lesions was 2 cm. in diameter with a large fungating mass, overlying a smaller, malodorous, necrotic base. Medial and posterior to this lesion were lesions of 1 cm. and 0.5 cm. diameters with rough corrugated

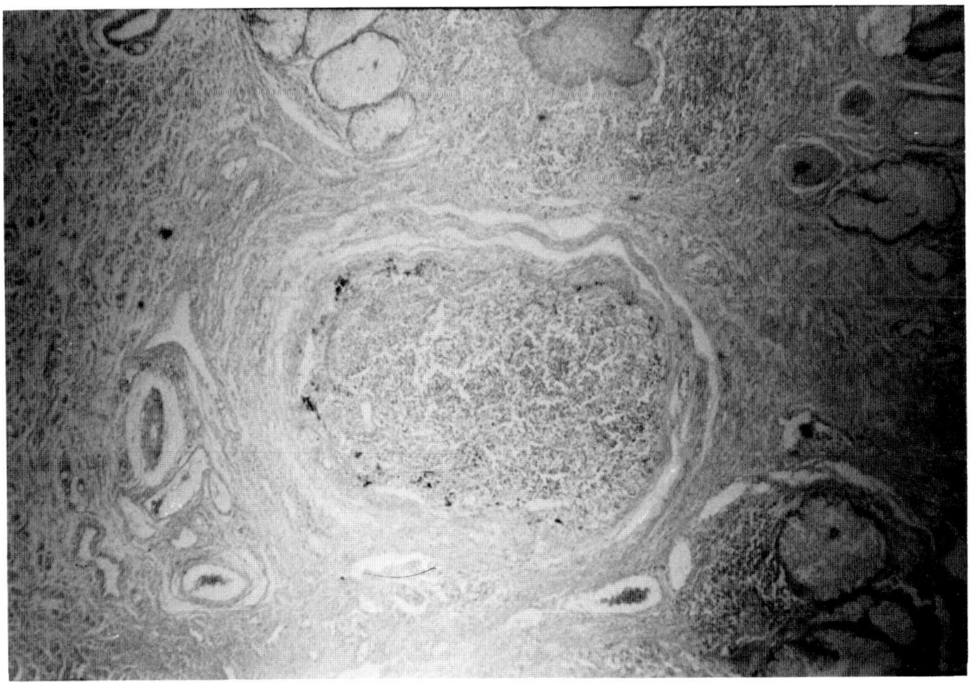

Fig. 15.28. Photomicrograph of epidermal inclusion cyst. Infective, only original wall remains identifiable. Courtesy of J. F. Yale.

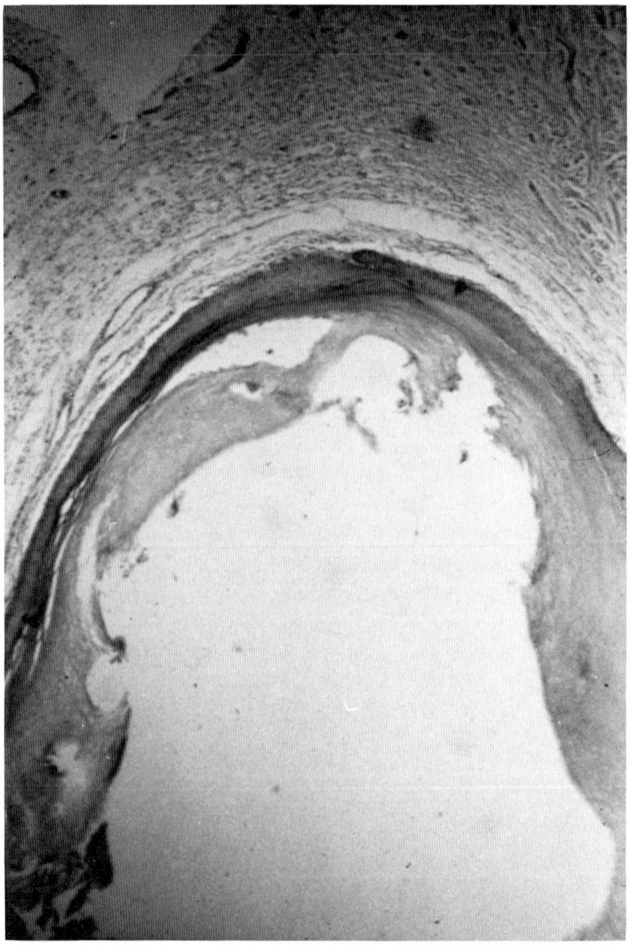

Fig. 15.29. Photomicrograph of epidermal inclusion cyst. Basement membrane is intact and the squamous elements are easily recognized and maturing in an orderly fashion. Desquamated squamous cells are noted in the center. Courtesy of J. F. Yale.

surfaces and dark red bases. Both of these lesions were elevated. Another lesion, 1.5 cm. in diameter, was elevated, red-purple in color with a smooth surface.

Treatment of Kaposi's sarcoma is complete excision of the sarcomatous masses. Removal of the lesions does not cure the condition but very often can relieve discomfort especially if the lesions have developed on the weight-bearing surfaces of the foot.

Melanoma. According to Pack (1957), about 15% of melanomas occur on the feet and about 8% occur around the nails. These tumors are usually pigmented but may be non-pigmented. Pack states that 9% occur on the soles.

Pigmented nevi should be carefully observed for evidence of growth. Davis (1955) has stated that when these lesions become cancerous they are the most dangerous of all malignancies. When deeply pigmented and on an area of friction it is wise to remove the growth to prevent metastasis since transformation of a mole into a melanoma may be very subtle. Cammack (1956) described five types of melanoma:

1) intradermal, smooth, papillary, hairy and variously pigmented, they rarely occur below the knee; 2) junctional nevus, flat, pea-sized, slightly raised, hairless and pigmented tan to black, they occur below the knee and most melanocarcinomas are thought to arise from them. 3) compound nevus, a

combination of intradermal and junctional nevi, is potentially dangerous; 4) juvenile nevus, follows a benign course; 5) blue nevus, rarely becomes malignant and appears as a blue-black, flat or hemispherical elevated asymptomatic mass.

The original growth may spread by development of nodules in an erythematous area in the periphery, surrounding the lesions. The peripheral lesions often enlarge and metastasis may take place in distant parts of the skin, to the lymph glands, the lungs, or the liver. The tumor is nodular with a broad, pedunculated base. The growth may ulcerate and be covered by serous or sero-purulent exudates.

The "melanotic whitlow" elevates the nail and is often difficult to differentiate from glomus tumors, subungual exostoses and profuse granulations. The great toe is the common site for all of these lesions. Observation of the nail plate in typical melanoma will disclose pigmentation at the periphery of the suspicious lesion. The lesion beneath the elevated nail may be a black, well-demarcated, fungating, ulcerated tumor.

Treatment of melanoma is wide radical excision with adequate closure or skin graft. Proper microscopic examination is essential in order to establish a diagnosis. Regional lymph nodes are excised or radiated. If there is evidence of an extension of the lesion or metastasis, x-ray therapy must be instituted by a radiotherapist.

Carcinoma. Primary carcinomas are uncommon on the feet. Although the lesion is commonly believed to be caused by mechanical pressure, friction and old skin lesions and scars, there is no evidence to suggest formation of carcinoma from corns or calluses.

Keratoses as precursors to carcinoma develop from sun, wind irritants and lowered resistance of the skin. Scars from burns or lupus erythematosus are etiologic. Carcinomatous lesions may develop in chronic ulcers and at sites of benign tumors that have been irritated or irradiated.

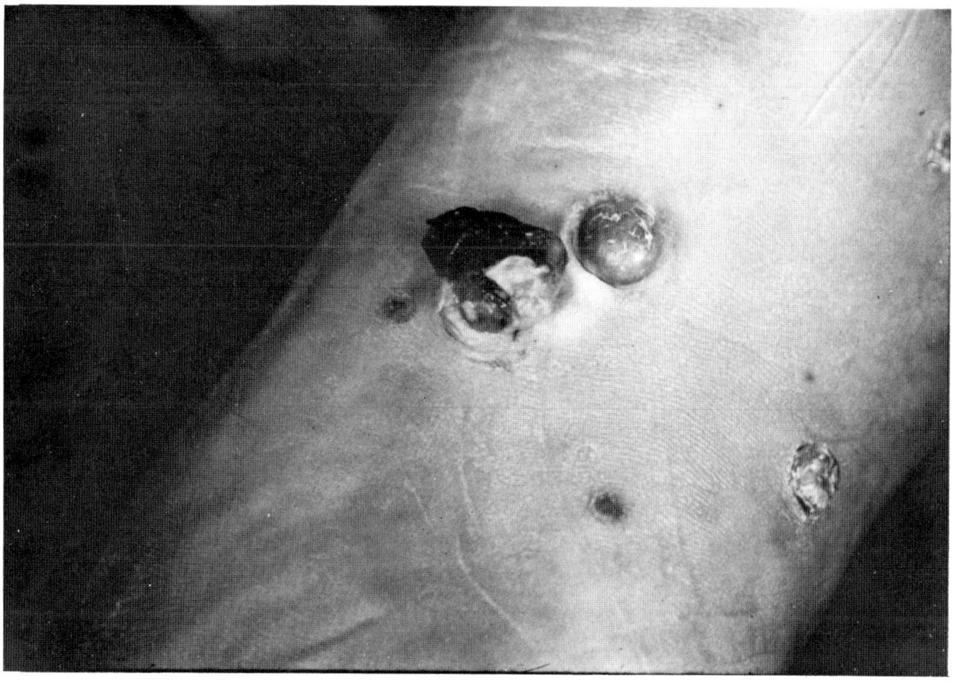

Fig. 15.30. Kaposi's sarcoma.

Early carcinomatous lesions may be indurated nodules with a dry parchment-like surface. A verrucous-like hyperkeratosis may develop slowly and ulceration can be the sequela. When untreated, the lesion may become malodorous and fungating.

Treatment. Early excision and radiotherapy of the affected site is necessary and may be lifesaving.

Squamous Cell Carcinoma--Epithelioma. These lesions may or may not ulcerate and are more prevalent in males.

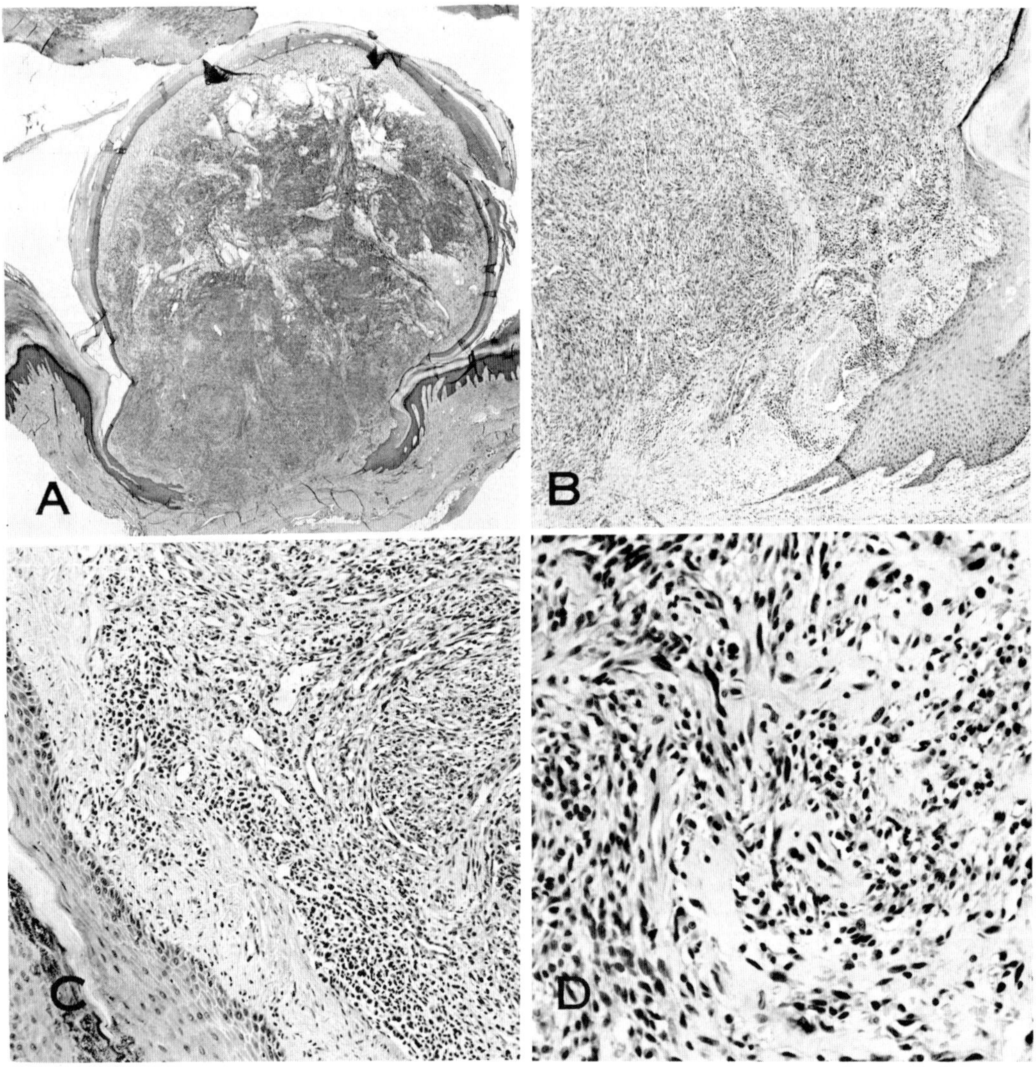

Fig. 15.31. Photomicrographs of Kaposi's sarcoma. *A*, note polypoid nature of the lesion which is unusual for Kaposi's sarcoma. Many dilated vascular spaces are present in the edematous stroma. This is usually seen secondary to trauma. Thin, pale relatively acellular stroma completely surrounding tumor and separating it from the epidermis. No tumor in epidermis. *B*, hypercellular sarcomatous pattern, *upper left*. Below this, a fibrous reaction and chronic inflammatory infiltrate. *Lower right*, hyperblastic rete pegs. *C*, note somewhat whorled pattern suggesting fibrosarcoma, *upper right*. Large vascular spaces of tumor. Chronic inflammatory infiltrate with plasma cells. Fibrous stromal reaction. *D*, fibrosarcomatous appearance, *lower left*. Capillary spaces and vascular clefts. Acellular stroma.

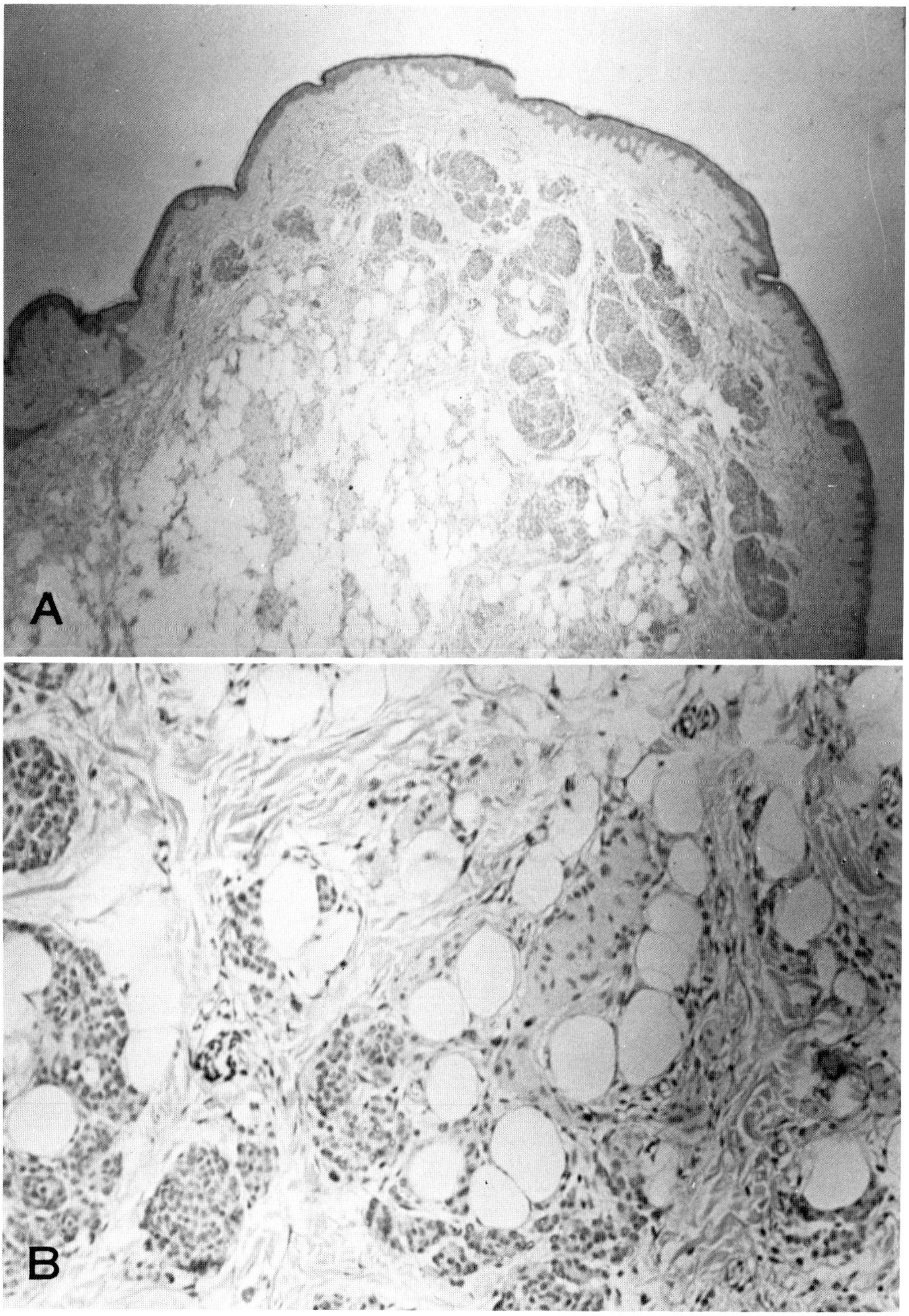

Fig. 15.32. Photomicrograph of intradermal nevus under low power *(A)* and high power *(B)*. Islands of nevus cells are scattered randomly through the soft tissues. No inflammation. Courtesy of J. F. Yale.

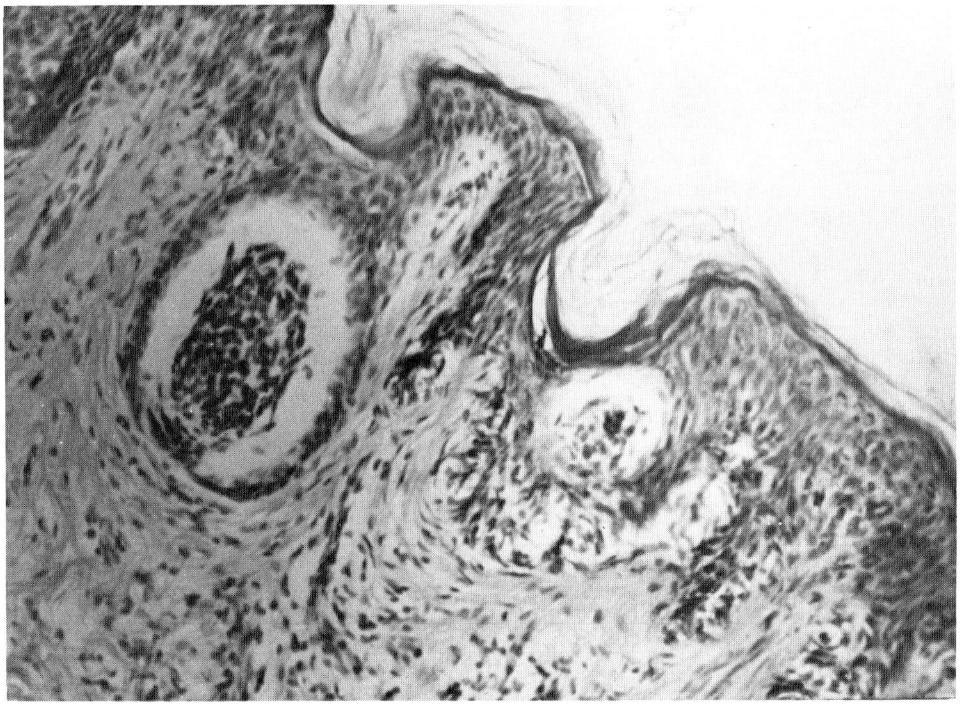

Fig. 15.33. Photomicrograph of junctional nevus. Blurring of the basement membrane by marked proliferation of nevus cells. Courtesy of J. F. Yale.

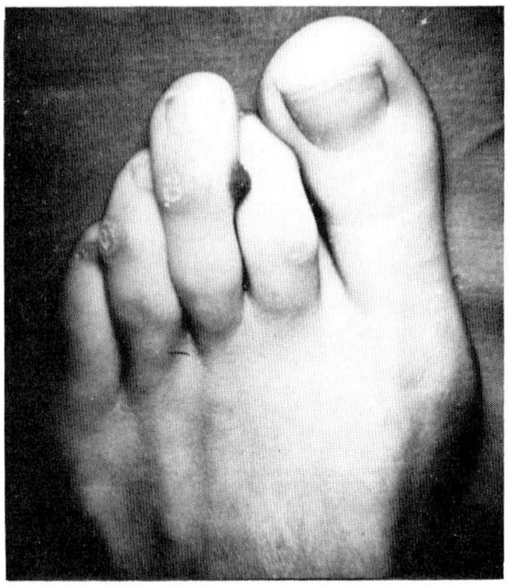

Fig. 15.34. Black elevated verrucoid lesion on the medial aspect of the third toe. Occasional bleeding suggests the need for early excision and microscopic study. Excrescences on the dorsum of the third and fourth toes due to back pressure from ill-fitting hose and an incorrect shoe.

Metastasis is rare and is usually induced by trauma. The diagnosis is confirmed by histopathologic examination. Squamous cell carcinoma are malignant but have an activity similar to benign growths. They may, however, metastasize.

Epithelial cancer of a toe originating locally from an inflamed soft corn aggravated by "corn remedies" has been reported. The malignancy diagnosed upon biopsy and subsequent surgical removal as a squamous cell epithelioma was accompanied by an extreme cellulitis of the foot. The malignant growth measured 1½ x 2½ cm.

Squamous cell carcinomas on the foot have appeared clinically as an ulceration about 0.5 cm. in diameter with surrounding induration and infiltration. The margins are elevated, hard and undercut. The base resembles poor granulating tissue and is gray in color.

Carcinoma may be caused by prolonged exposure to x-rays. The new growth has the microscopic characteristics of a squamous cell lesion. This lesion is accompanied by a numbness, roughening and fissuring of the skin. The fissures become painful and the skin may become a mottled gray to dark brown. A

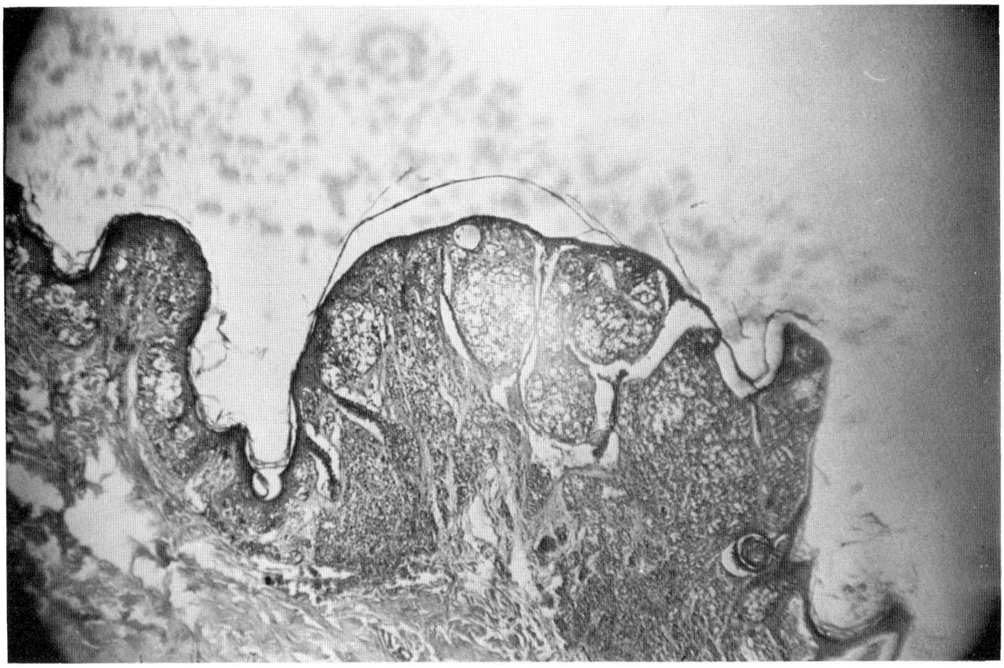

Fig. 15.35. Low-power, cross-section photomicrograph of a pigmented mole. Note typical papilloma-like enlargement of the dermal papillae and the presence of pigment in the tissue. Courtesy of A. T. Sharpe, Department of Pathology, Pennsylvania College of Podiatric Medicine.

general inflammatory infiltration and typical squamous cells are present on microscopic examination.

Treatment. Robins (1970) reported a 98% cure rate in the chemosurgical treatment of basal cell carcinoma where electrodesiccation, surgery and irradiation had failed. The treatment consists of dichloroacetic acid applications to the mass to break down the keratin in preparation for further treatment. Zinc chloride is then applied to fix the tissues. After several hours, the lesion is removed. The tissue is fixed and mapped prior to examination and the boundaries are checked for tumor tissue. The process is repeated until all boundary tissue is negative.

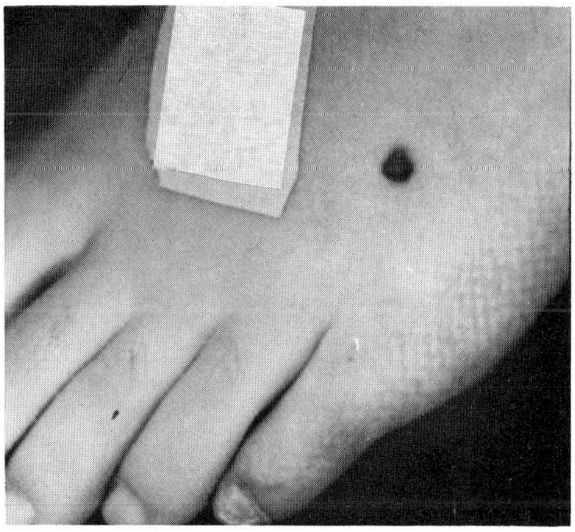

Fig. 15.36. Blue nevus.

Berger *et al.* (1966) state that "basal cell epitheliomas of the sole occur with extreme rarity."

Synovial Sarcoma. These tumors are malignant growths of connective tissue origin involving the tendon sheaths and synovial membranes. The duration of symptoms varies from several months to several years. Pain, swelling and abnormal function of the limb are the usual outstanding symptoms.

The tumor is attached to or invades the tendon, synovial membrane or joint capsule. It is usually soft, white and fleshy (depending on its vascularity) or it may be velvety, purplish appearance.

Geshicker and Copeland (1949) report a case of synovial sarcoma involving a

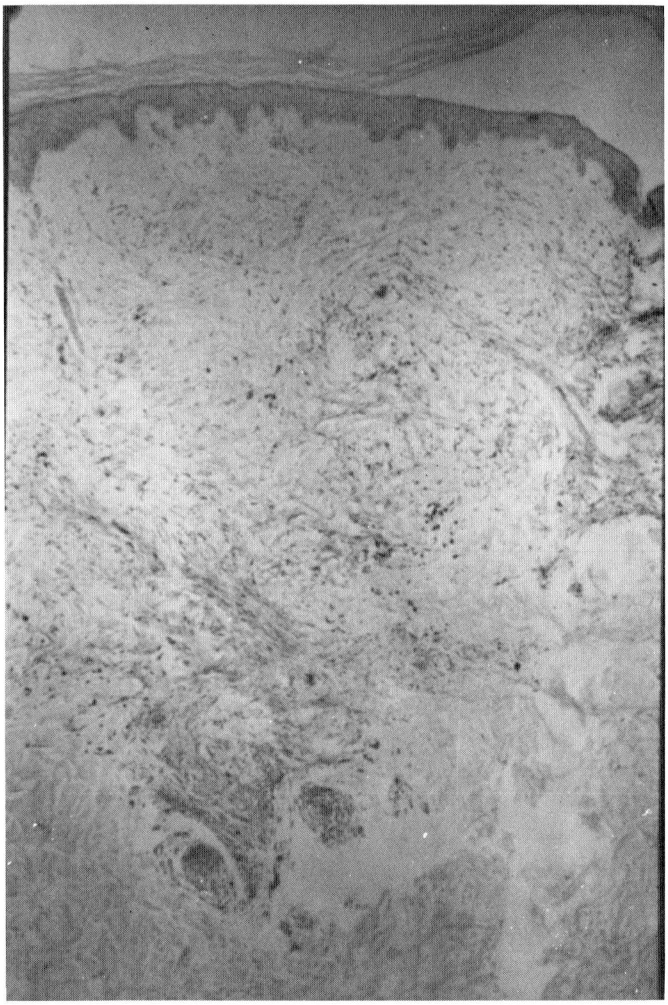

Fig. 15.37. Photomicrograph of blue nevus. Common cellular nevus deep in the subcutaneous tissues. Fibroblastic proliferation. Courtesy of J. F. Yale.

toe. The patient died with widespread metastases to the lungs and brain 5 years after resection. They also report on four cases of synovial sarcoma in the foot and two cases in the ankle. Early diagnosis and amputation may be lifesaving.

Treatment. Extensive surgical removal of the growth and adjacent glands followed by radiation therapy may be adequate treatment. Amputation is indicated where metastasis is in evidence.

Neuroma. Tumors of the nerves are not common. Neuromas may be seen at the end of amputated stumps and are excruciatingly painful. Some investigators have found a small neuroma on the digital branch of the lateral plantar nerve extending to the fourth toe in Morton's neuralgia.

Hard, indurated tumors on the tendons or in subcutaneous tissues may be neurofibromas as seen in Recklinghausen's disease. They occur in all parts of the body and are usually multiple. Occasionally a neurofibroma may prove malignant on histologic examination. The ankle joint is the usual site of a neurofibrosarcoma. Neurofibromas are often grayish-white in color.

Neurofibrosarcoma may arise from the

tendon sheaths or joint capsules. Many of the sarcomas containing spindle cells originate from connective tissue cells in or around the nerve tissue. The round cell sarcomas grow rapidly and present an irregularly outlined tumor which is pink in color and prone to metastasis.

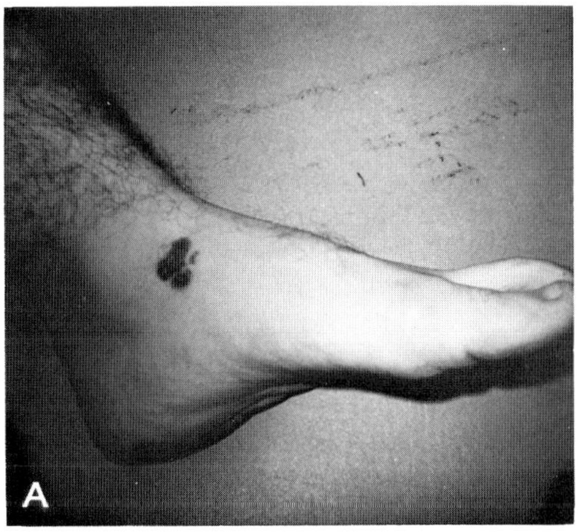

Fig. 15.38A. Melanoma.

Treatment. Total excision of the mass is the treatment of choice.

Tumor in Morton's Toe. McElvenny (1943) and Betts (1940) have expanded

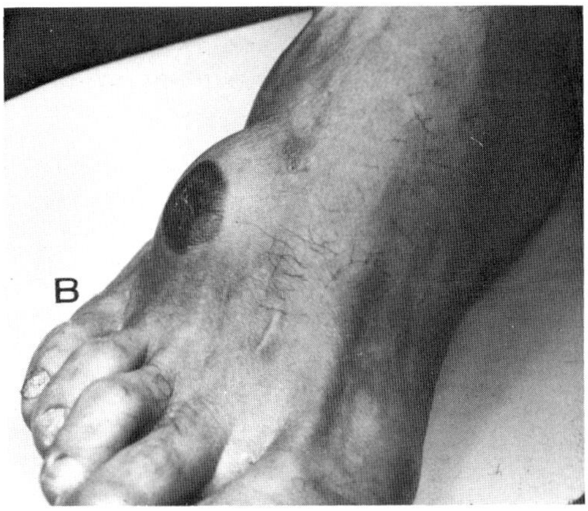

Fig. 15.38B. Melanoma. Malignancy manifest by rapid growth, indurated swelling, firm mass, adherent to underlying tissue. Skin is pigmented overlying mass with evidence of central necrosis.

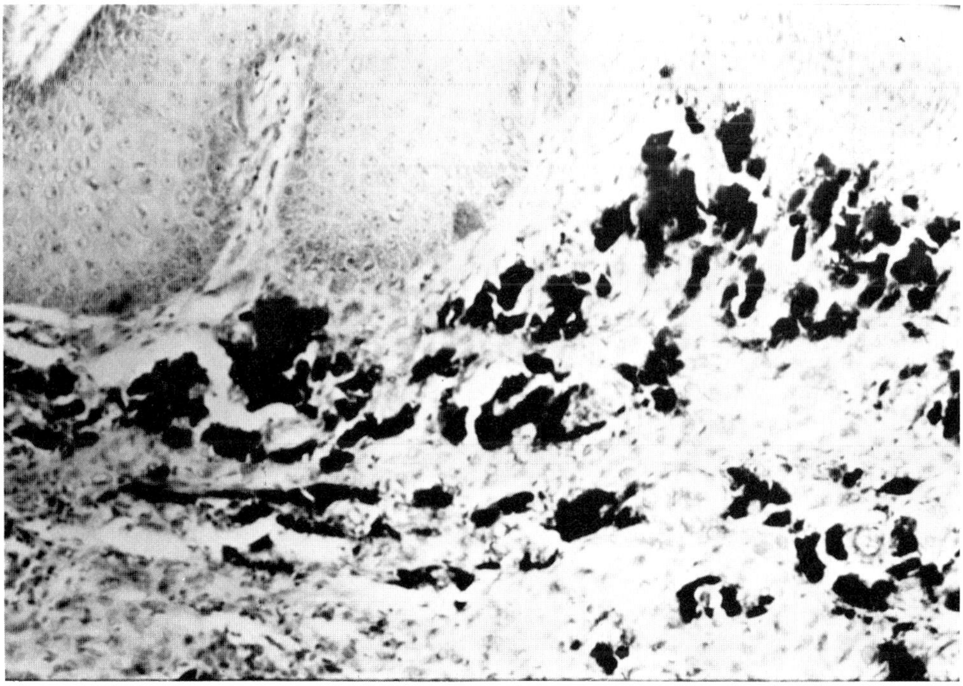

Fig. 15.39. Photomicrograph of melanoma. Note unusual heavy melanin deposit. This is seen in both benign and malignant lesions. Courtesy of J. F. Yale.

the earlier studies of Morton by surgically removing and performing gross and microscopic examinations of neurofibromas on the most lateral branch of the medial plantar nerve in the third intermetatarsal space. Grossly, the outside of the tumors are soft and contain connective tissue cells and fat cells; the central portion is dense, fibrous in texture and gray-white in color.

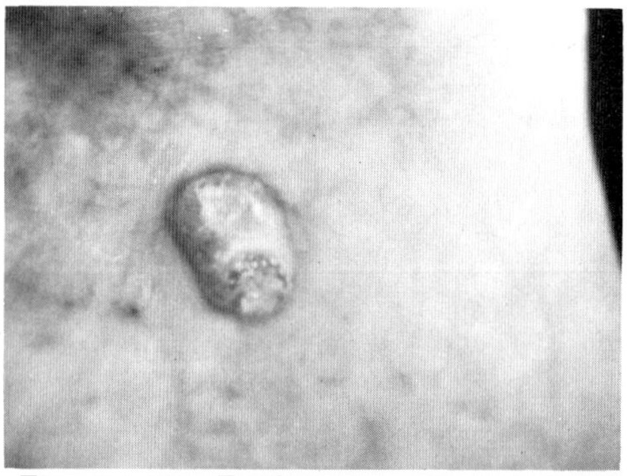

Fig. 15.40. Epithelioma. Ulcerated skin nevus.

Trauma or irritation of the nerve is thought to be etiologic. The neurofibromatous lesion is usually found between the bases of the proximal phalanges of the third and fourth toes. The nerve at this point is rather thickened due to its origin from the communicating branch of the lateral plantar nerve and the most lateral branch of the medial plantar nerve. This neurofibroma is often enveloped by a bursal sac and also has tendencies toward development of an angioneurofibroma. Multilocular ganglionic cysts have been the cause of pain. Some pathologists describe a neurinoma as the etiologic factor. This is generally the result of a thickening of the sheath of Schwann. Neurinomas can involve any of the distal nerves. Scotti (1962) states that the affected nerve becomes demyelenized; nerve fibers are lost and fibrosis with localized swelling of the nerve occurs.

Pain is dull at first with a slight burning and stinging and a peculiar feeling of discomfort involving the

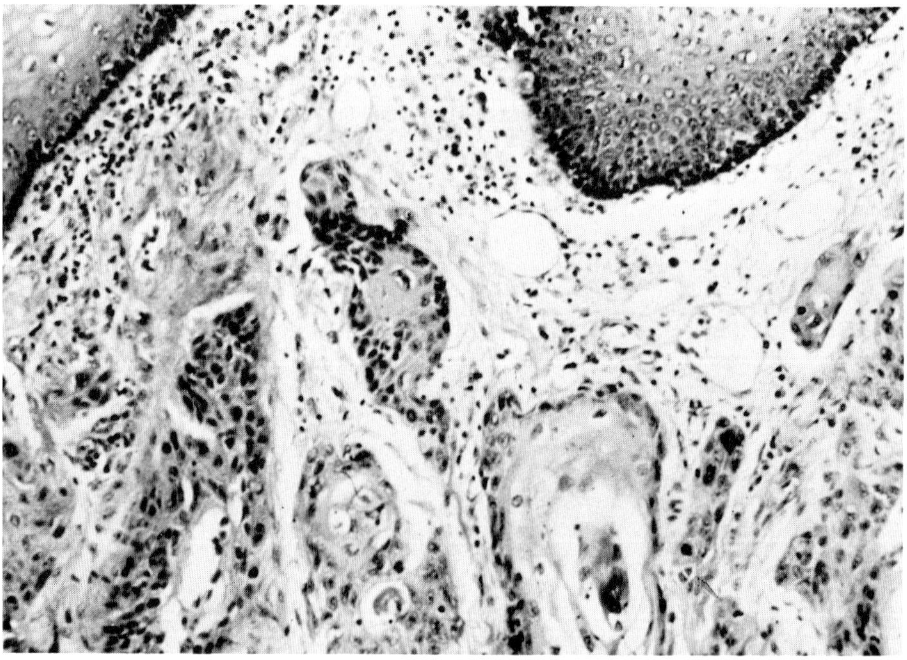

Fig. 15.41. Photomicrograph of squamous cell carcinoma—epithelioma. Islands of tumor composed of abnormal squamous cells. Several pearls are noted. Abnormal mitotic figures are present. Courtesy of J. F. Yale.

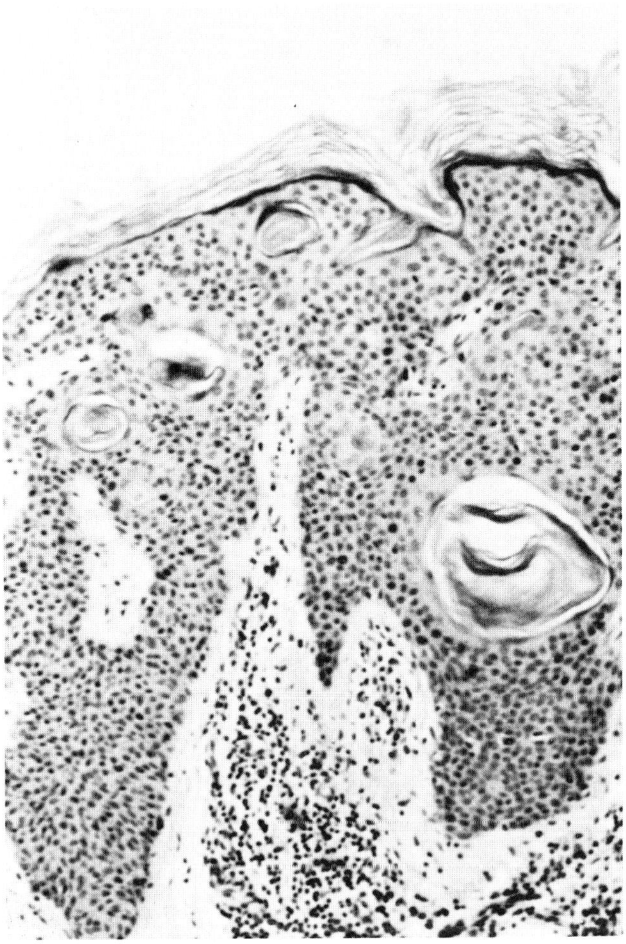

Fig. 15.42. Photomicrograph of basal cell tumor (one form). Basement membrane is distorted. Cuff of lymphocytes in the upper dermis is commonly the result of secondary irritation. Courtesy of J. F. Yale.

fourth metatarsal and fourth toe. In the second stage of this illness, the patient has severe excruciating pains spasmodically. This discomfort is real and so severe that it often radiates to the second, third, fourth and fifth toes and frequently to the posterior calf muscles. The patient is compelled to remove his shoes, flex, extend and compress the toes in an effort to gain relief.

In the later stages the slightest provocation such as alterations in the pavement, trying on shoes, a misstep or even atmospheric conditions or nervous strain will result in attacks of the characteristic pain, hysteria and nausea.

This lesion is most commonly found in women at any age and is characterized by a painful affliction of the foot that is often resistant to conservative treatment. The symptoms are produced by a tumor on the most lateral branch of the medial plantar nerve and is pinched between the third and fourth metatarsal heads or proximal phalanges.

Frost (1959), in his series of 78 plantar nervectomies on 60 patients, calls attention to unilateral multiple neurofibromas. He proposes a diagnostic nerve block to rule out the possibility of more than one lesion. Unilateral multiple neurofibromas were observed in 7 of the 60 cases. Frost was the first to recognize this possibility and he wisely advised a diagnostic test. He notes that the tumor can occur in more than one intermetatarsal space. An injection of a local anesthetic accompanied by a metatarsal raise may relieve pain.

Cozen (1958) notes that a point of

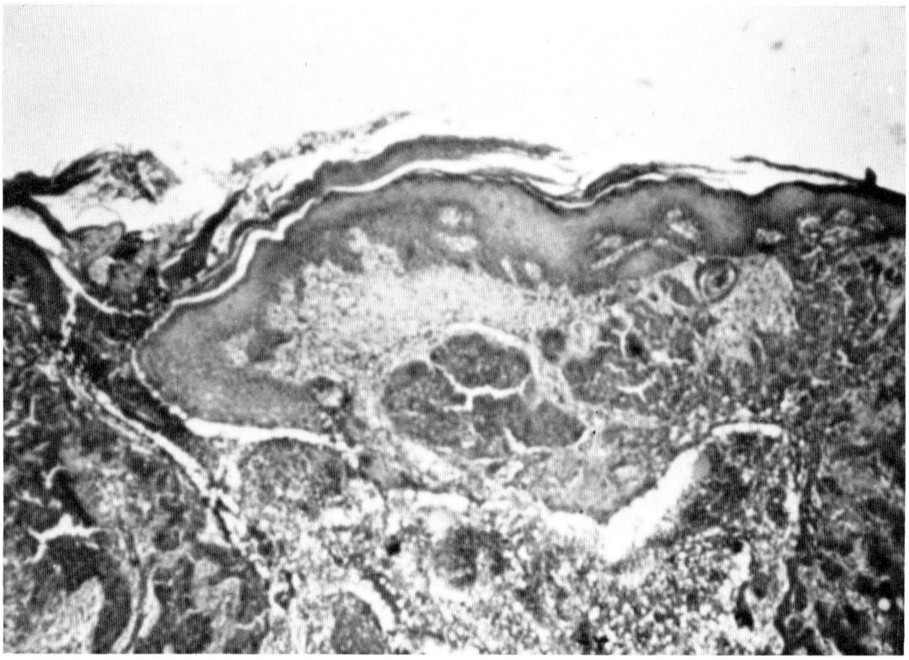

Fig. 15.43. Photomicrograph of basal cell carcinoma. Tumor in dermis. Overlying epidermis is intact. This is responsible for the rolled edge around the ulceration. Courtesy of J. F. Yale.

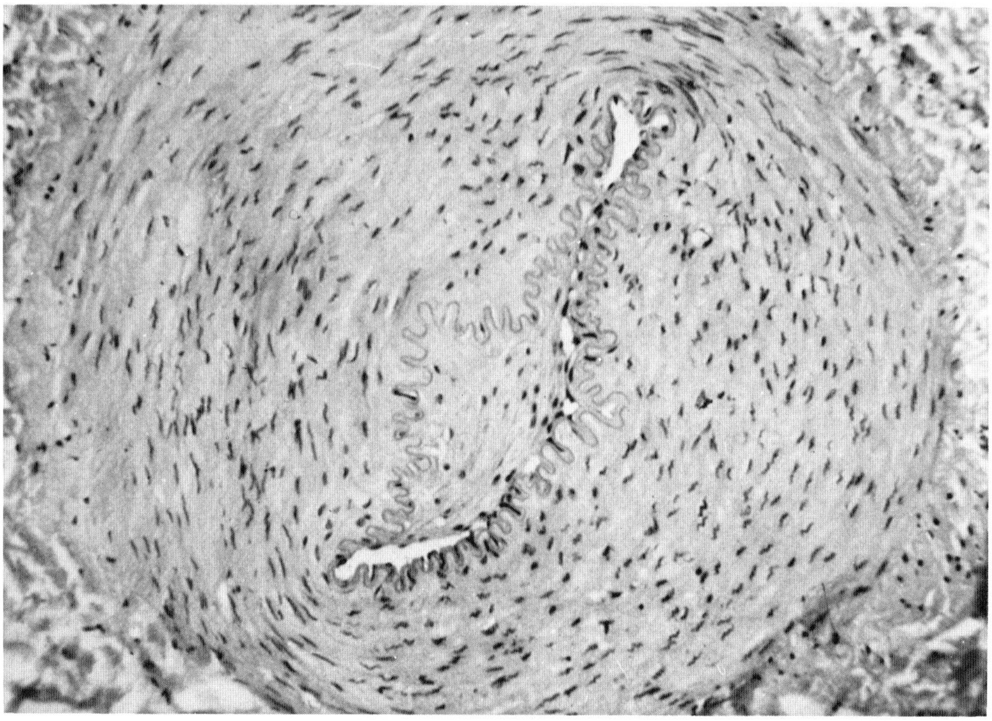

Fig. 15.44. Photomicrograph of fibrosed artery (low power). Often seen in close proximity to neuroma. Note the fibrosis. Courtesy J. F. Yale.

tenderness can be felt in the web between the toes, usually between the third and fourth, but sometimes between the fourth and fifth or second and third. A diagnostic aid is a painful click elicited when the metatarsal heads are pressed together. It is significant only if pain accompanies the click. Cozen states that injection of 0.5 ml. of hydrocortisone into the region of the neuroma affords relief and should be considered before subjecting the patient to surgery.

Treatment. There are several approaches to treatment for Morton's neuralgia or neurinoma. Conservative methods are used first followed by more radical measures when necessary. Relief of pain can be obtained in 40 to 60% of such cases by prescribing adequate footgear and constructing an appliance which lifts the fourth metatarsal bone into a different position. This is believed to relieve the compression on the digital branches of the lateral plantar nerve.

The second technique which is sometimes used along with the first mechanical procedure is to inject a local anesthetic into the third intermetatarsal space directing the needle downward and forward from the dorsum to between the heads of the metatarsals. Raise a wheal about 1/2 in. proximal to the third and fourth metatarsophalangeal joints and then direct the needle point plantarwise through the intermetatarsal area to the plantar surface of the foot just superficial to the plantar skin. Withdraw the needle approximately 1/8 in. and then deposit approximately 3 ml. of local anesthetic. This approach may give the patient complete relief for periods of from 1 day to several months. Complete alleviation of the symptoms is common.

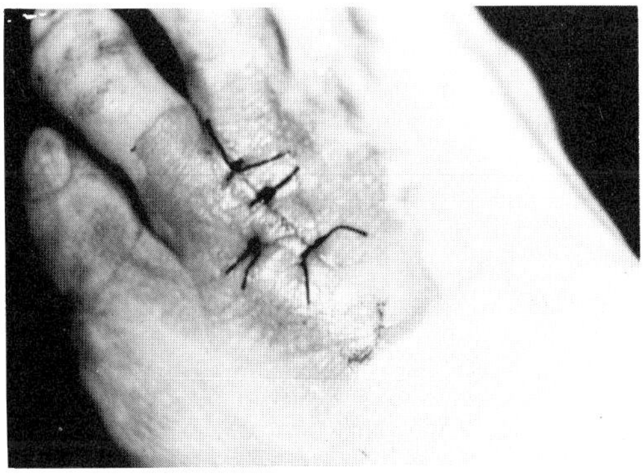

Fig. 15.45. Neuroma removed showing postoperative wound.

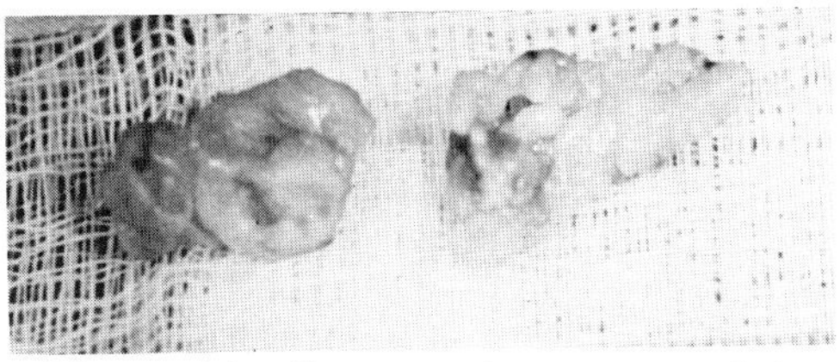

Fig. 15.46. Gross specimen removed from third interspace—neuroma-fibroma.

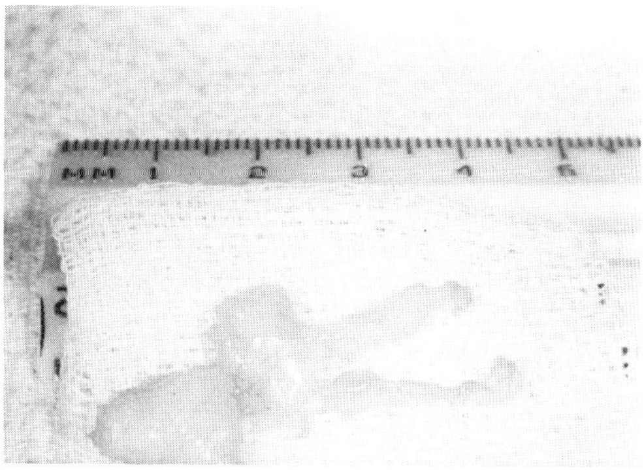

Fig. 15.47. Neuroma-fibroma at bifurcation of digital nerves.

Additional injections may be necessary. I recommend a maximum of three injections before discarding this form of therapy.

Steinberg (1955) prefers a therapeutic test with vitamin B_{12} and procaine solution. A standard 2% procaine HCl solution 1:100,000 epinephrine is mixed with a standard vitamin B_{12} solution, 100 μg. of B_{12} per ml. Equal parts of each solution to make a mixture of 3 ml. is used for injection. He suggests injecting 1½ ml. into each of the third and fourth intermetatarsal spaces. Results have been gratifying in a high percentage of cases.

Polokoff (1961) discusses a negative galvanism technique for treatment of Morton's neuralgia. Using an aseptic procedure and local infiltration of anesthesia into the third intermetatarsal space, a negative galvanic needle is inserted into the site of the digital branches of the nerve to the third and fourth toes. The indifferent electrode is attached to the sole of the same foot or any other part of the body. The current is turned up to 5 milliamperes. As the current volume is increased, the patient may feel heat at which time the current is reduced 2 to 3 milliamperes to tolerance. Pressure from the plantar will push the nerve up between the metatarsals allowing for easier contact with the needle electrode. When the tissue appears easy to penetrate with the negative current, and when resistance has been removed in about 8 to 12 min. of treatment, the machine is turned off and the needle electrode withdrawn. Warm foot soaks aid in resorption of the destroyed tissue. According to Polokoff, patients are relieved of discomfort without undue surgical risk.

In my opinion, Polokoff's technique may be too destructive to adjacent tissues not involved with the pathology. In the resistant case, I prefer the following procedure.

After administration of adequate anesthesia, a longitudinal incision is made over the third intermetatarsal space extending approximately 2.5 cm. from the web back into the space. This is deepened through the dermis and subcutaneous tissue. The tissues are retracted exposing the transverse plantar ligaments. These ligaments are incised longitudinally and the metatarsal heads are separated. Pressure is exerted from the plantar surface between the heads forcing the plantar nerve up into the operative site. The nerve is cleansed of adjacent clinging fascia and grabbed by an Allis forceps. Now the nerve is excised approximately 1.5 cm. proximal to its bifurcation and excised forward from its bifurcation at its digital extensions to the third and fourth toes. The entire mass presents itself as a gray-white tissue and is delivered through the operative wound. The wound is carefully closed in layers. Very often one will find many small nerve fibers gathered around in a fine wire-like mass at the juncture of bifurcation of the nerve. Microscopic examination is necessary for proper evaluation of the lesion.

Pincus (1962) recommended the plantar approach as being less damaging to tissue and providing better visualization.

Ganglia are not new growths but are the result of herniation of a tendon sheath or joint capsule. Very often crepitus on motion and movement of the "growth" with the function of the tendon allows for simple interpretation. Ganglia are common on the anterior of the ankle and dorsum of the foot. The extensor tendons are most commonly affected. Ganglia are circumscribed subcutaneous herniations of tendon sheaths or joint capsules and contain a clear viscid fluid which sometimes becomes jelly-like in character. The capsules are continuations of the tissue from which they develop and are firm and fibrous. The skin is smooth and freely movable over the ganglion which commonly resembles a bursa. They have a fibrous outer coat and an inner synovial layer resembling the synovial membrane of a joint. Ganglia must be differentiated from a bursa, synovioma and xanthoma.

Treatment. The treatment of a ganglion can be frustrating. Surgical intervention often results in a collapse of the lesion unless great care is taken to dissect the mass *in toto.* I advise making an incision to one side of the mass using blunt dissection to free the tissues around the ganglion. It is necessary to handle the lesion carefully while dissecting and to free the mass from its surrounding attachments. Should the ganglion be the result of a herniation of the joint capsule, it is necessary to free the mass from the surrounding tissue as it is grasped firmly with Allis forceps. Then it can be excised from its attachment. After removal of the ganglion it is essential to use adequate subcutaneous closure of the tissue layers followed by compression bandaging to close the dead space created by removal of the mass.

Many techniques have been used other than surgical excision with various results. One method used field block anesthesia followed by aspiration of the fluid within the ganglion using a 10-ml. syringe and 18-gauge needle. Irritation of the walls of the lesion is followed by compression bandages to flatten the collapsed mass. The end result is often gratifying and the irritated inner lining of the ganglion adheres to its opposite wall resulting in obliteration of the lesion. The use of corticosteroids in 0.3- to 0.5-ml. dosages injected directly into the cavity is helpful in relieving inflammatory changes. I

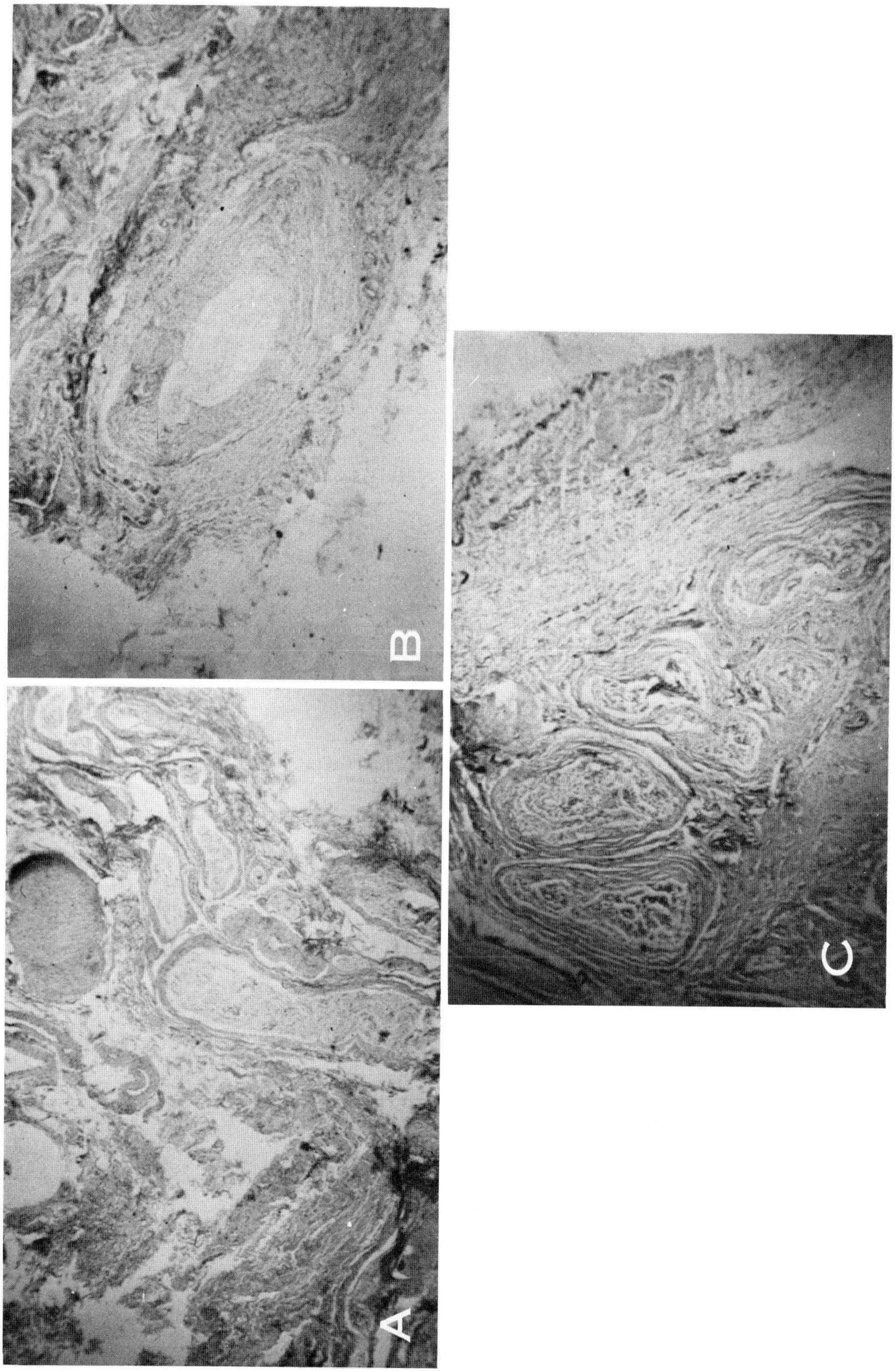

Fig. 15.48. Major microscopic components of neuroma. *A*, perineural fibrosis; *B*, fibrosed Vater-Pacini corpuscle; *C*, intrafasicular edema.

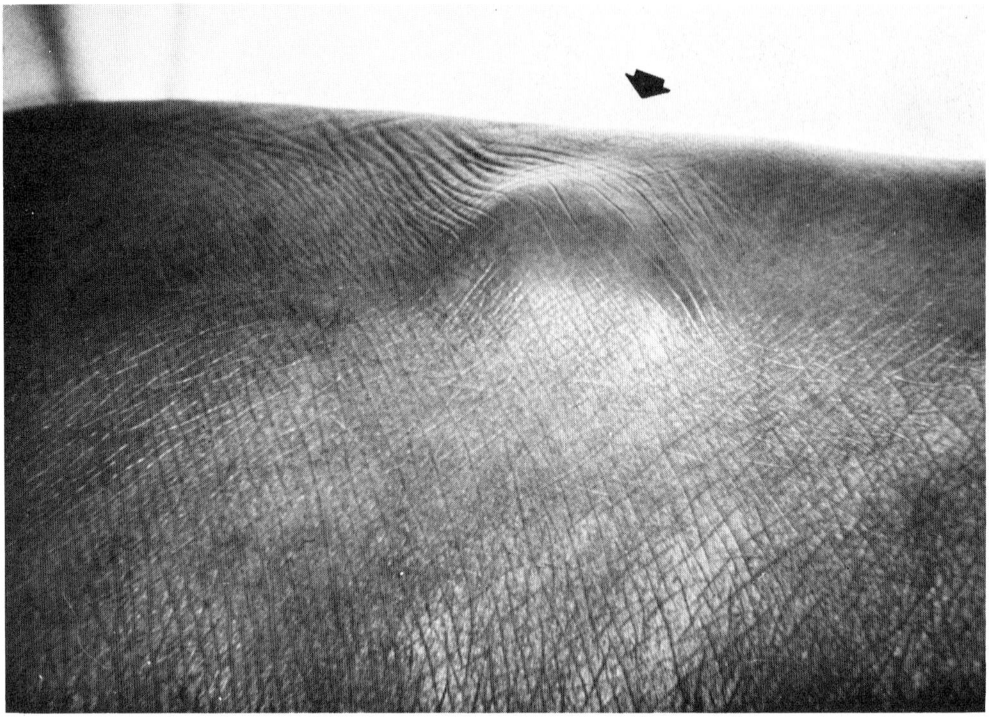

Fig. 15.49. Ganglion on dorsal surface of the foot.

do not advise the use of sclerosing agents in ganglia.

Bursitis. Trauma, infection and metabolic disorders are usually the cause of bursitis. Common sites of traumatic bursitis are at those joints which are exposed to shoe pressure. The medial aspect of the first metatarsophalangeal joint, fifth metatarsophalangeal joint at its lateral surface, the base of the fifth metatarsal laterally, the dorsum of the interphalangeal joints of the toes, the tuberosity of the navicular, the medial tubercle on the plantar surface of the calcaneus, the posterior bursa between the skin and the attachment of the tendo achillis, and the anterior achillo-bursa between the tendo achillis and the upper angle and posterior surface of the os calcis are the more common sites for bursitis. Intermetatarsal bursitis and bursitis secondary to rheumatoid arthritis and gout are not uncommon.

Occasionally inflamed bursa develop at the medial and lateral malleolus as well as the plantar surface of metatarsal heads from strain or trauma. The trauma may be acute or multiple and minimal in character. A sudden blow or kick or having the part stepped on may cause a bursitis. Exposure to extremes of temperature may be an exciting factor. Old frostbites or chilblains may predispose to bursitis.

Pathology. With trauma a local hyperemia may develop, followed by marked distention of the bursa. In swelling of the bursa the synovial fluid often breaks through the sac following the lines of least resistance.

Distended areolar tissue may occur in the intermetatarsal space or under any of the metatarsal heads from abnormal friction or pressure. The sesamoid region at the plantar surface of the first metatarsal head is commonly inflamed. Bursae may be acutely inflamed, subacute or chronic. A highly inflamed bursa must be differentiated from infectious

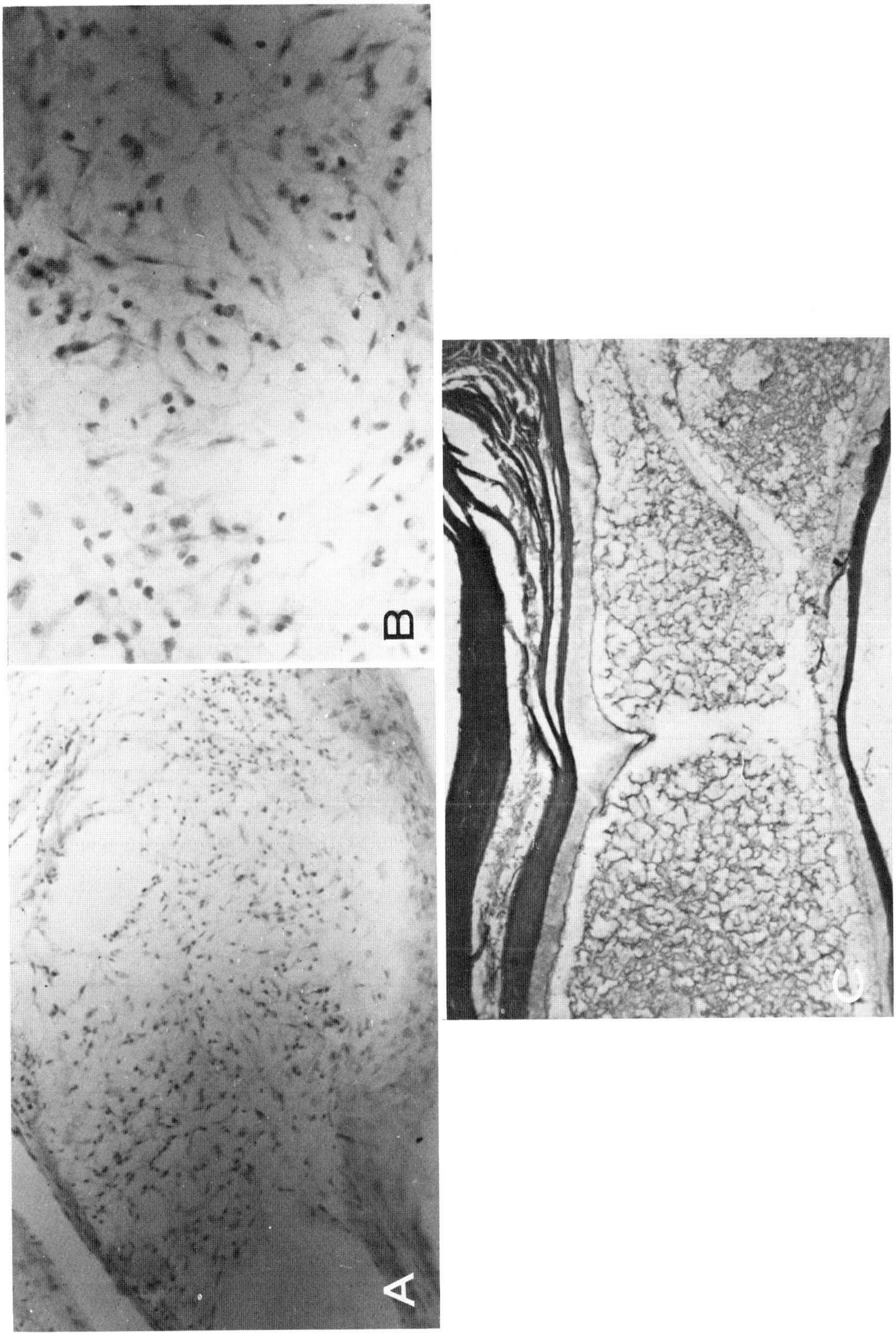

Fig. 15.50. *A*, Photomicrograph of ganglion. *B*, large spaces represent ganglion stroma. Myxomatous tissue between ganglion cyst spaces. Triangular-spaced myxomatous tissue. *C*, ganglion (low power). Well encapsulated edematous myxomatous stroma. Courtesy of J. F. Yale.

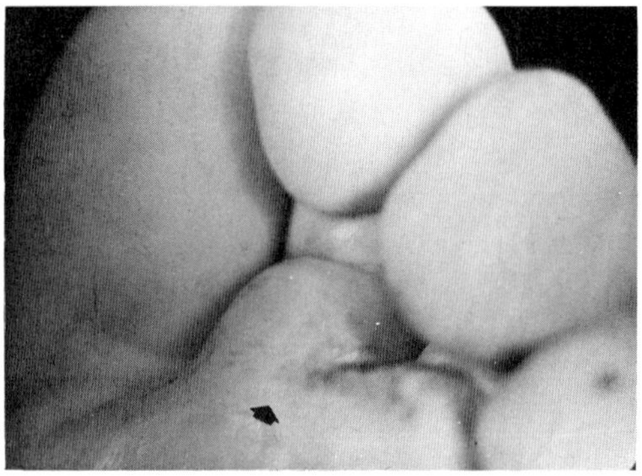

Fig. 15.51. Ganglion, plantar surface of second toe.

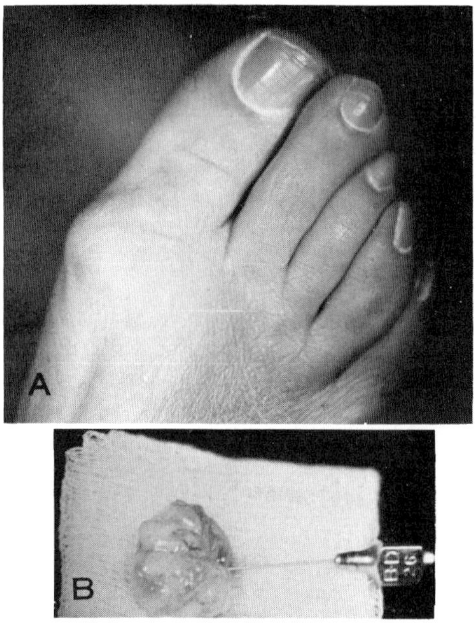

Fig. 15.52. *A*, chronic bursitis, hallux joint, gross specimen, multilobulated mass. *B*, gross specimen.

lesions, periarticular arthritis, effusions or edema of inflammation.

Occasionally bursae are infected by invasion of bacteria from an abrasion or through a small opening in the skin. The infection of callous-covered bursa through injudicious cutting or dermatitis venenata from corn remedies is common. A sinus infection, sometimes involving low grade osteomyelitis, may develop. Cellulitis and lymphangitis are often sequelae to secondarily infected bursae.

Radiographic examination of bursae may disclose multiple loose bodies within the bursa or in the adjacent articular capsule. The capsule or articular ligaments undergo fibrosis, chondrification and later calcification. Very often the bone underlying the inflamed bursa decreases in density as a result of the local hyperemia. This superficial demineralization must not be interpreted as early osteomyelitis or infectious periostitis.

Patients with rheumatoid arthritis are prone to develop inflamed bursa. In gout

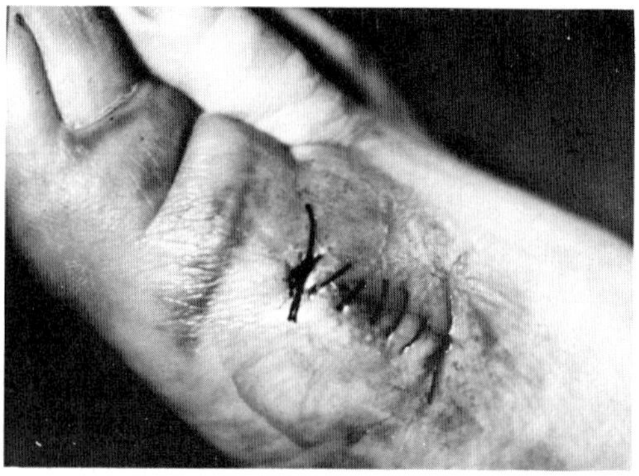

Fig. 15.53. Excision of bursa, medial aspect of hallux joint and ganglionic cyst on tendon of extensor hallucis longus.

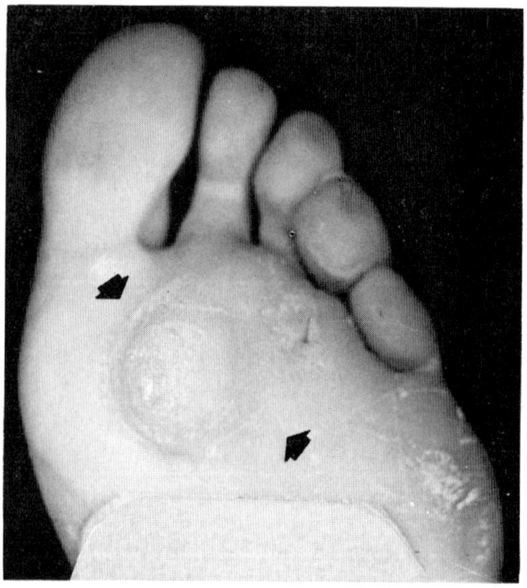

Fig. 15.54. Bursitis with overlay of callus, plantar surface of second metatarsal.

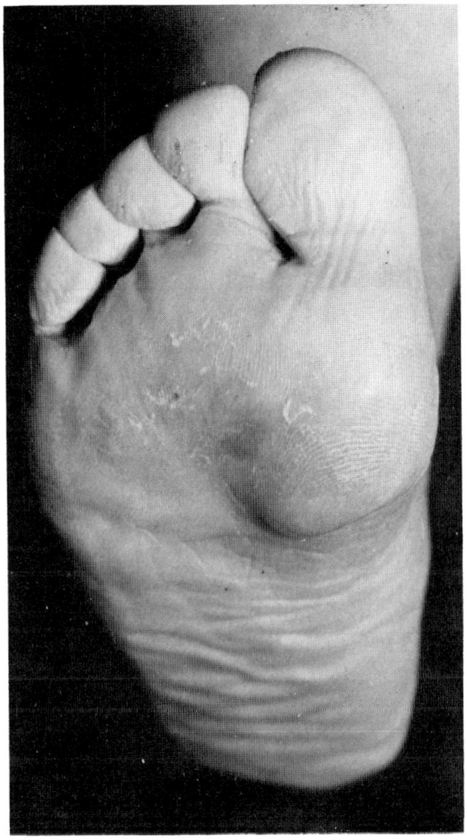

Fig. 15.55. Acute bursitis, plantar hallux joint.

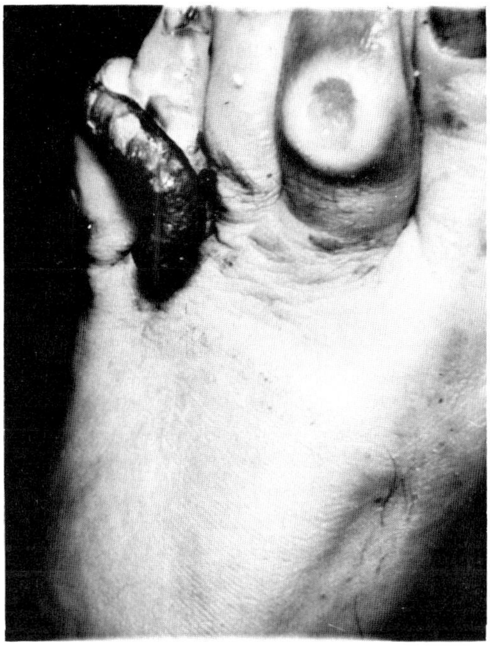

Fig. 15.56. Breakdown of infected bursa in diabetic patient, onychogryphosis, ulcer. Courtesy of J. F. Yale.

the swelling is diffuse and acute involving most of the soft tissues in the adjacent area.

Clinical Manifestations. Clinically the gross lesion is usually circumscribed, elevated and even in outline. Its surface is smooth and the tissues usually range from soft to fibrous and firm texture. The color may range from a soft, normal-colored, chronically developed hypertrophied tissue to a deep red or blue, firm, nodular mass or a bright red, tense, hot, painful mass in acute inflammation.

Occasionally a bursa may develop between the metatarsal heads or shafts. It is manifest clinically by pain on weightbearing especially while the patient is wearing a constricting shoe. Circumscribed swelling, tenderness on

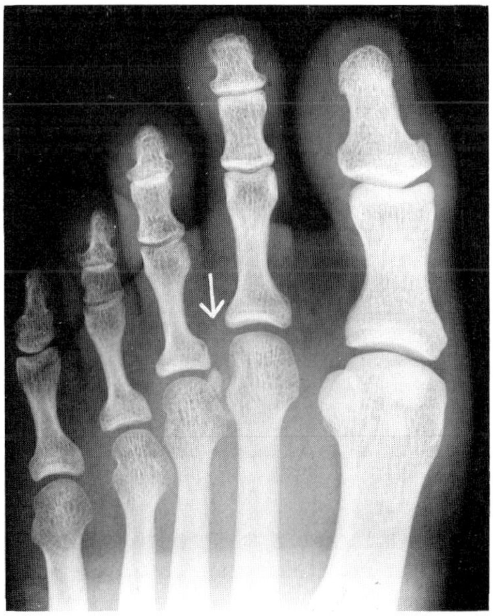

Fig. 15.57. Bursitis, intermetatarsal calcification. Courtesy of *Clinical Foot Roentgenology*, Baltimore: The Williams & Wilkins Company, 1966.

palpation, redness and heat are noted over the affected intermetatarsal space on the dorsum of the foot. Pressure exerted in opposing directions on the fifth and first metatarsals toward the midline of the foot usually elicits excruciating pain in intermetatarsal bursitis.

Bursal-like developments have been found in the third intermetatarsal space enveloping a neurofibroma or angioneurofibroma which has developed on the most lateral branch of the medial plantar nerve in Morton's neuralgia.

Treatment depends on whether the bursitis is acute, subacute or chronic. In acute bursitis, eliminate trauma, treat any infection present and provide consultation treatment by an internist for underlying systemic disorders when indicated. Occasionally, heat aggravates and cold ameliorates acute symptoms. Burrow's solution wet dressings generally reduces the swelling and inflammation.

Injections of minimal dosage of corticosteroid compounds or chymotrypsin 0.1 ml. to 1.0 ml. help to relieve acute pain and generally reduce the size of the bursa. In independent studies, Locke (1963) and Rosen (1963) noted a high percentage of good results in treating bursitis by injection of dexamethasone 21-phosphate and lidocaine in combination. White (1966) described the highly effective betamethasone injection for acute and chronic inflammatory disorders. Intra-articular and intralesional injections are relatively free of postinjection flare.

Medical ionization with magnesium sulfate shrinks the mass. Galvanism with iodine often reduces the size of the bursa and decreases pain.

Antibiotics are used in the presence of infection.

In subacute bursitis, treatment is basically the same as that for acute problems.

Aspiration and the use of ultrasound followed by protection of the affected part is helpful. Following aspiration, the intrabursal injection of 0.1 ml. to 1.0 ml. of chymotrypsin reduces the size of the bursa.

In chronic bursitis, excision of the growth *en masse* relieves pressure on underlying tissues. Provide for elimination of pressure by construction of a protective shield. Physical therapy may be needed.

Surgical excision of the mass and any degenerative calcification within the bursa by sharp and blunt dissection may be indicated.

If gout or rheumatoid arthritis is a suspected factor, diagnosis should be confirmed by laboratory studies. Systemic conditions are treated by the family physician.

Where bursae exist on the plantar surface of the weight-bearing foot, relieve the acute symptoms and maintain relief through proper shielding. Various dynamic moldable materials may be used to construct an inlay with cutouts at the site of bursal swelling.

The complications of bursitis such as cellulitis, sinus tract formation, calcifications, ulceration, or underlying bone and joint involvement can be treated according to the degree of pathology noted.

Xanthoma. In examining 150 patients with elevated blood cholesterol levels, Bloomquist (1962) noted that 22 were found to have xanthoma of the Achilles tendon. In some instances the presence of xanthoma was an indication of hypercholesteremia. Characteristic fusiform swellings were noted with some containing calcific deposits. The tendon was thickened and tender. Xanthoma cells, giant cells, cholesterol and connective tissue degeneration is noted histologically. X-ray examination shows evidence of rounded, clearly delineated masses of increased soft tissue density.

Xanthomas may occur around the ankle joint and toes and on the plantar surface of the foot. Small lesions around the toes may have to be differentiated from mucoid cysts.

Xanthoma tuberosum multiplex are

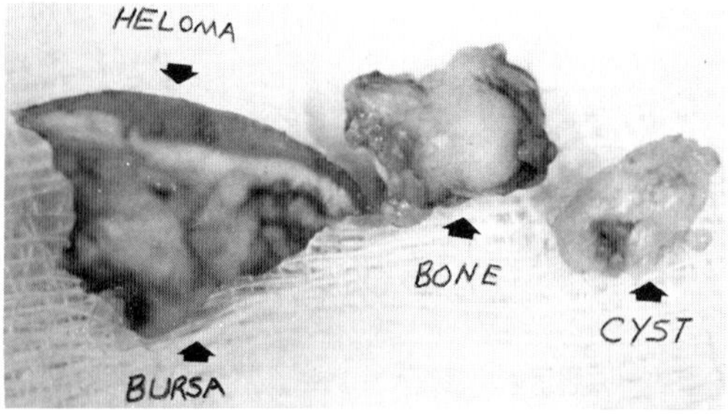

Fig. 15.58. Arthroplasty, heloma, bursa, bone, cyst. Gross specimens.

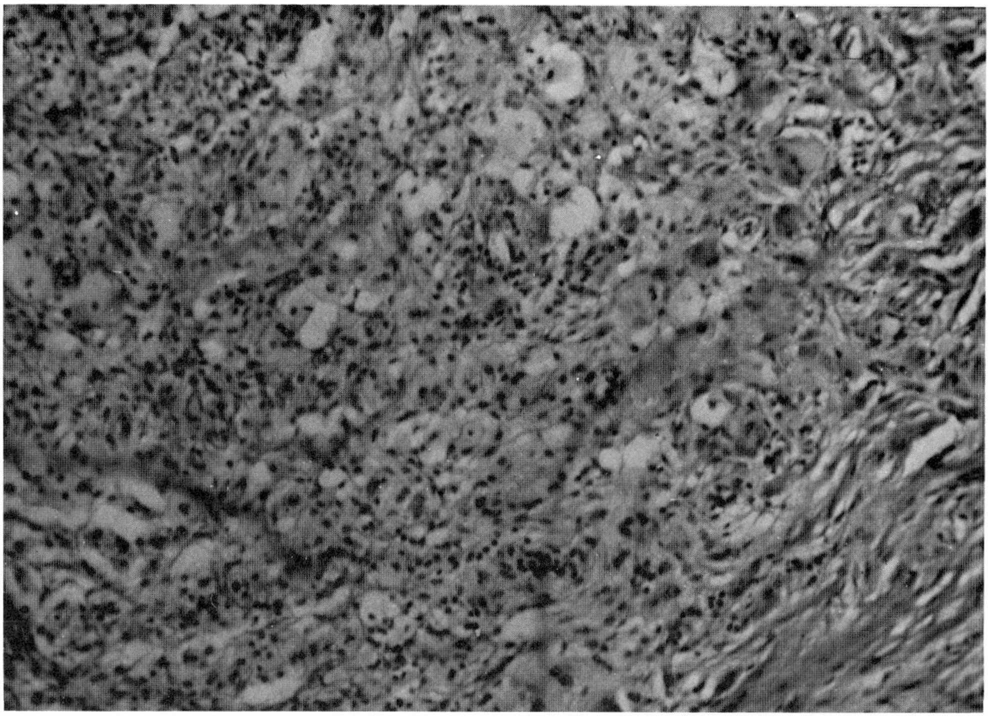

Fig. 15.59. Photomicrograph of xanthoma (low power). Note large and small giant cells in a cellular stroma with hemosiderin deposits. Courtesy of J. F. Yale.

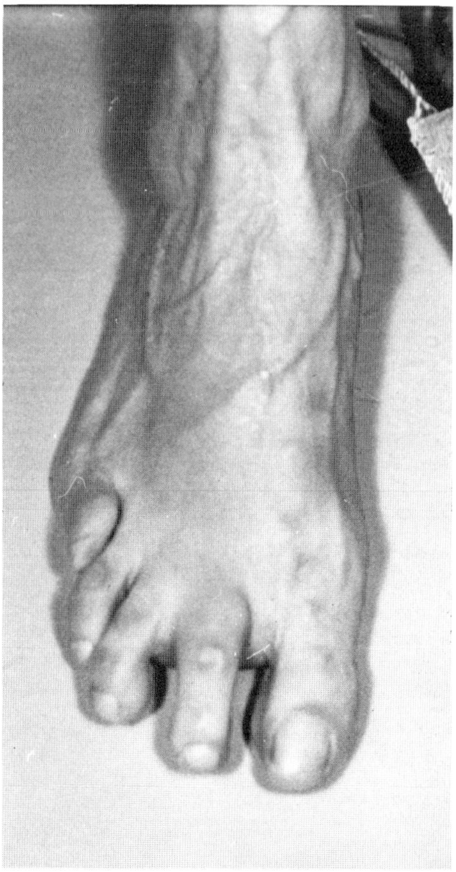

Fig. 15.60. Xanthoma forcing the toes apart.

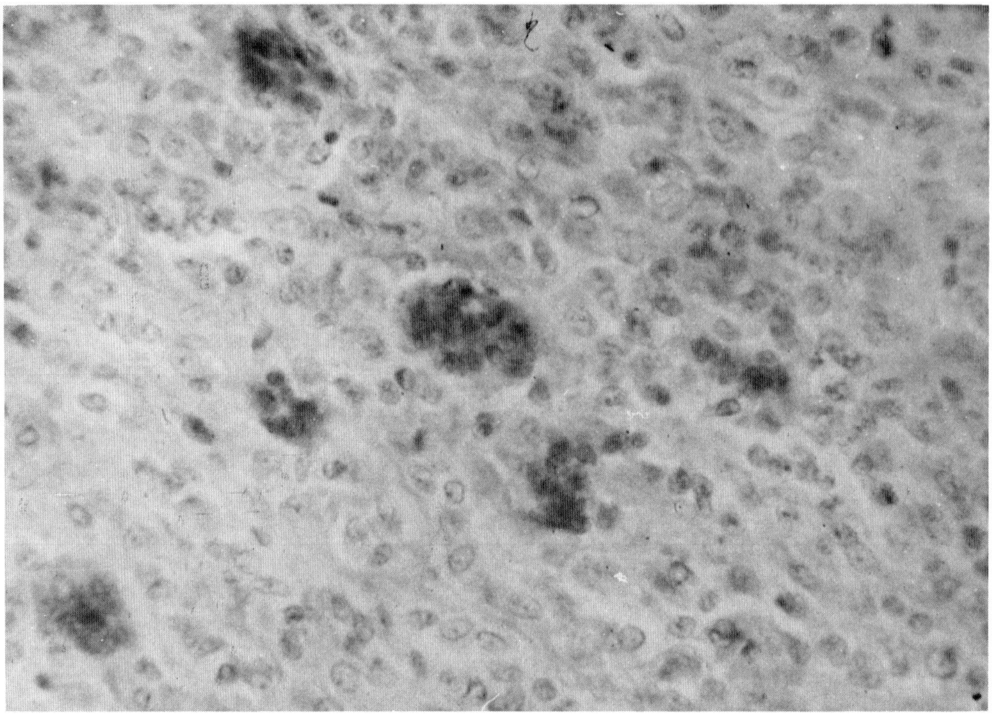

Fig. 15.61. Photomicrograph of giant cell tumor. Note large and small giant cells. Typical findings in xanthoma, tenosynovitis, bursitis.

well-defined neoplastic nodules or macules associated with jaundice and occur around the larger joints of the body. They involve the palms, soles and extensor surfaces of the extremities.

Treatment of xanthoma is based on the location and the extent of the lesion. Should these lesions affect the normal function of the foot and diminish the ability for adequate weightbearing, surgical removal is suggested. However, it is wise to limit surgical intervention since the patient with multiple lesions of this type is generally ill and requires treatment for the medical problems that exist.

16

Primary Inflammations of the Foot Structures

In discussions of the biomechanical problems affecting the foot I have been impressed by the ability of foot specialists to relate faulty foot structure and function to the complaint of pain. The science of biomechanics is undergoing revolutionary changes. A strong effort by a small group of scientists is providing fuel to the establishment of a steady flow of working propositions and definitions. Texts are standardizing diagnosis and treatment of structural and functional disorders.

In this chapter, I will discuss a variety of painful pathologic entities, most of them related to a malfunctioning foot. No attempt is made to elaborate on the biomechanical mechanisms involved. However, a study of these inflammations provides an adequate background for their diagnosis and treatment. Additional information about the x-ray findings is described in *Clinical Foot Roentgenology*. Biomechanical information is available in the new literature.

Periarthritis of the Metatarsophalangeal Joints. This is a painful enlargement of the tissues of the plantar surface of metatarsal heads. The condition may occur from dancing excessively in high-heeled, narrow-soled shoes and from multiple, minimal trauma. The underlying structures are painful to palpation and weightbearing, and the patient complains of a throbbing pain and usually a dull ache. Indurated edema is present and limitation of function typically occurs. An adventitious bursa or cyst may develop subcutaneously. Gout or rheumatoid arthritis may be an underlying factor. A stress fracture must be ruled out by radiographic examination. Marked soft tissue thickening and effusion are present. Calcifications may develop in degenerated tissue or a bursa. The joint space is widened or narrowed depending on the degree of effusion and extent of trauma.

Treatment. Oral analgesics and muscle relaxants are helpful. Shortwave, ultrasound and other physical modalities may be necessary to relieve pain.

Felt raises skived to remove weightbearing from the affected part are placed in shoes or strapped to the foot. Construction of a balanced inlay appliance to distribute weight from the affected part is generally successful.

The foot can be rehabilitated by low-voltage sinusoidal currents and active and passive exercises.

If pain persists, an injection of local anesthetic followed by injection of 0.4 ml. of an effective corticosteroid into the acutely inflamed site relieves discomfort.

Epiphysitis of the Metatarsals. In examining children prior to complete union and ossification of the epiphyses, the examiner must be cautious in interpreting forefoot symptoms.

A history of injury to the forefoot from a misstep, a jump from a height in which the patient landed on the ball of the foot, or direct trauma should lead the podiatrist to suspect epiphysitis of the metatarsals. This condition is characterized by swelling on the dorsum of the foot over the affected epiphysis. The second, third and fifth metatarsal epiphyses are usually involved. Often the styloid epiphysis of the fifth base may be displaced. This epiphysis is not constant. Pain on palpation is noted at the head of the affected metatarsal. Slight heat and bluish-red discolorations are present around the affected parts and involve the toes. The extensor tendons are usually contracted and very often inflamed with limitation of function accompanied by pain and swelling.

X-ray Examination. A soft tissue swelling follows the fascial planes. The joint may have an effusion presenting a symmetrical fusiform outline. The epiphysis may be subluxated at the metaphysis. In long-standing cases, a local demineralization may be evident anterior to the epiphyseal line. Very often a fracture involves the metaphyseal end of the bone. Fibrocartilaginous tears at the epiphyseal line may be suggested but not visible. When the injury occurs in early childhood and is of sufficient severity it is possible to note a failure in future normal longitudinal development of the bone. The epiphysis is very often displaced with trauma.

Treatment. Physical therapy such as whirlpool, ultrasound, infrared, short wave and contrast foot baths help relieve pain. Immobilization by adhesive materials, plastic dressings, Celastic, plaster and appliances are necessary to maintain a limitation of motion. Firm footgear and rigid foot orthotics coupled with shoe wedging to limit motion and protect the affected part is indicated in epiphysitis. A Jones bar on the sole of the shoe relieves excessive trauma.

Injection of corticosteroids prior to maturation and union of the epiphysis is not usually acceptable treatment since corticosteroids tend to stimulate maturation and thus inhibit normal bone growth.

Prescriptions of mild analgesics generally help bring about relief during the period of repair.

Sesamoiditis. Painful sesamoids suggest injury. Swelling, pain, discoloration and sometimes crepitus at the plantar surface of the head of the first metatarsal are the usual symptoms.

Ingersoll (1955) described this problem as a "sesamoidalgia." He refers to: enlarged sesamoids, displaced sesamoids, anomalous sesamoid bones, traumatically fragmented sesamoid bones and fusion or adhesion of one or both sesamoid bones. Clinical examination presents marked edema with redness which may involve the entire metatarsophalangeal articulation. Pain and often crepitus is felt on palpation over the affected bones. Bursitis is common.

One sesamoid may be grossly enlarged compared to the other. Occasionally a sesamoid is comminuted or presents a fracture. An interpretation of fracture must never be made unless a definite fracture line is present. Stippling or multiple hazy areas of demineralization may be visible in a sesamoid which has been painful for some time. This local demineralization usually occurs with marked hyperemia and resultant resorption of bone elements. Sesamoids may have spurs, osteophytes and lipping at their margins. Frequently a tear of the fibrocartilaginous attachment of one part of a multipartite sesamoid from the other may be noted on x-ray examination. Subluxation or dislocation of the sesamoids is a common cause of sesamoiditis.

Treatment. Reduce overlying callosities and shield or disperse pressure from the affected parts by using conventional shielding or parallel stress pads as described by Sansone (1970) or the well known dancer's pad used for many years by podiatrists.

Inject a local corticosteroid into a bursa beneath the sesamoids if necessary.

Short wave and ultrasound therapy twice weekly help relieve pain. Analgesics should be prescribed if pain persists.

Firm-soled, well-fitting footgear with anterior heels or Jones bars are helpful in relieving multiple minimal trauma.

Construction of appliances of the molded balance inlay type with a cut-out under the sesamoids may be necessary. The height of

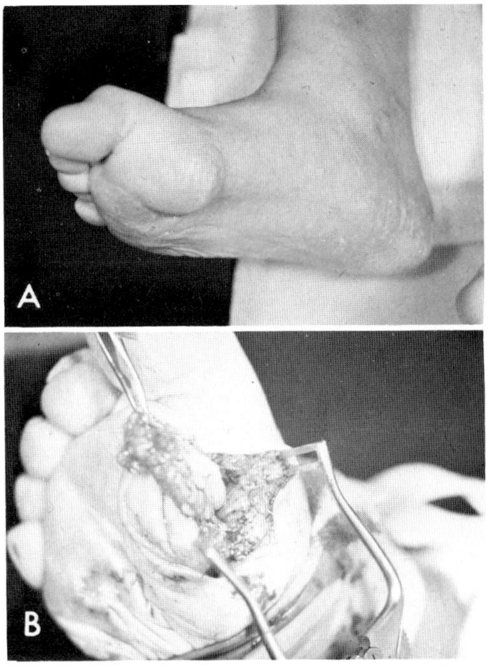

Fig. 16.1. *A*, chronic bursitis beneath enlarged seamoid. Note compensatory flexion of hallux. *B*, Surgical excision of chronic bursa and enlarged sesamoid bone.

raises is a personal podiatric judgment.

Properly posted Rohadur orthotics may correct the subtalar valgus and compensate for a first metatarsal equinus that often predisposes a patient to sesamoiditis.

Surgical removal of a chronically painful, dislocated or subluxated sesamoid may be necessary. This is accomplished by an incision at the medial plantar aspect of the metatarsal head.

Hypertrophy of the First Metatarsal Cuneiform Articulations. Thickening of the first metatarsal cuneiform joints is not common. Frequently only one aspect of the articulating surface of the affected part presents osteophytic changes at the anterior surface of the medial cuneiform or the posterior articulating surface of the first metatarsal base. Usually the dorsal and medial aspect of the articulation are involved.

On gross examination the enlargement on the dorsum of the foot looks like a tumorous mass. Careful examination may reveal an inflamed superficial tissue with overlying 1- to 3-mm.-sized helomas. A bursal sac may overlie the enlarged bone. Very often this lesion is found alone without bone pathology. X-ray examination should substantiate these findings.

The pathology in the affected part suggests enlargement and thickening of the joint capsule due to chronic irritation.

The involved bone is hypertrophied and an overlying adventitious bursa may be noted. Often the bursa is hypertrophied, inflamed and fibrotic. The sac

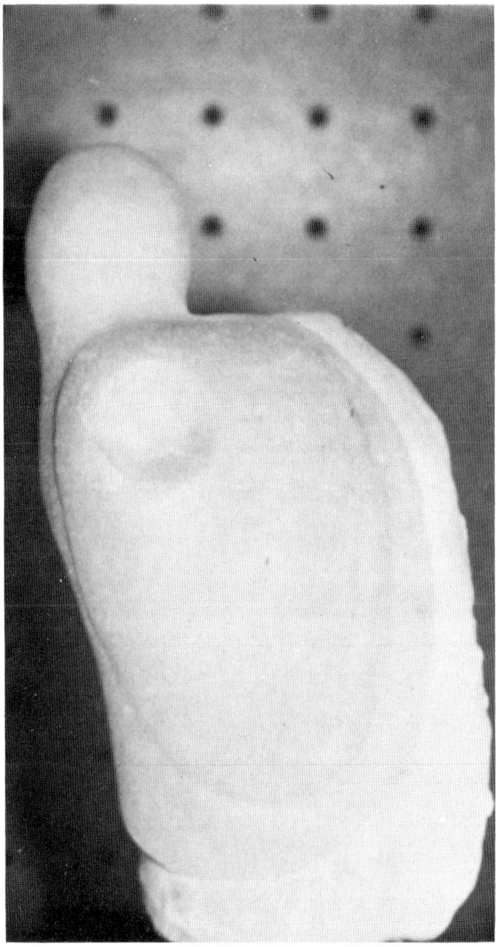

Fig. 16.2. Latex shield may be modified to protect a bursa, intractable plantar keratosis or sesamoiditis in poor surgical risks. Courtesy of Liquid Rubber Appliance Laboratory.

fluctuates in size depending on the degree of friction and irritation. The overlying skin is thickened and commonly develops helomas. Occasionally the tendon of the extensor hallucis longus becomes inflamed resulting in a tenosynovitis over the hypertrophied bone. Pressure on the medial branch of the medial dorsal cutaneous nerve may cause paresthesias along the inner side of the great toe. The medial marginal veins and an anastomotic branch overlying the hypertrophied joint may become inflamed by pressure causing a local phlebitis. Local infection may occur at the site of pressure.

X-ray examination may reveal hypertrophy of the margins of the first metatarsal cuneiform joint. The joint space narrows and the margins of the articulating surface show evidence of lipping, osteophytes, spurs or exostoses. Occasionally an accessory bone may develop over the body of the cuneiform. This must be differentiated from a calcification in the soft tissues or a degenerative calcareous tendonitis. Bursa may degenerate, become fibrous and eventually calcify leaving flaky, amorphous, calcareous deposits.

Treatment. Excise the dorsal heloma or tyloma. If a bursal sac is acutely inflamed, corticosteroid of choice may be injected.

Remove eyelets on shoes overlying the enlarged bone and shield the affected part with felt. Soothing ointment should be used.

Construct a permanent shield of latex, felt latex, plastic or silicone-gel. A foot orthotic to control pronation relieves the stress from the first metatarsal cuneiform joint.

If pain persists, local applications of ultrasound or injections of corticosteroid medications into the painful articulation is helpful.

Surgical excision of a chronic bursa and its underlying bony prominence will relieve pain and eliminate the cause.

Shortened Metatarsal Segments. With the advent of Dudley Morton's theories on the shortened first metatarsal segment, there has been much concern relative to the shortening or dystrophic involvements of one or more of the lesser metatarsal bones.

Morton felt that many of the existing foot complaints of a biomechanical nature were related, either singly or in combination, to a shortened first segment, hypermobility of the first segment or posteriorly placed pivotal sesamoids.

Podiatric observers have noted that shortening and hypermobility of the fifth metatarsal segment occur with the same frequency as the shortened first. Relief of symptoms has been accomplished through treatment of short metatarsals by affording better weight distribution.

Frequently the fourth metatarsal is short but well developed. Faulty weight distribution results with subsequent callus formation under the pivotal heads of the longer metatarsals. The toes are usually dorsiflexed, the extensor tendons are contracted and a concavity is present over the fourth head on the dorsum of the foot. Occasionally two or more metatarsals may be shortened. It is conceivable that a neurotrophic disorder or an injury to the distal epiphysis of a metatarsal could result in early union and a cessation of growth. The danger of shoe fitting fluorscopic devices producing cumulative x-ray injuries to the epiphyses is great. Reports of early union of the epiphyses from accumulation of exposures to x-rays are not uncommon. Shortening of any of the long metatarsal bones may result.

With shortening of the fifth metatarsal, the fifth toe usually falls medially against the fourth toe and very often causes a soft corn.

X-ray studies of the foot on weight-bearing give the necessary information in suspected cases of shortening and variations in the metatarsal parabola.

Sansone (1956) describes the metatarsal parabola as representing the area of weight transmission in the forefoot. It varies according to the width and length of the foot. Sansone suggested a "Rule of Forefoot Weight Distribution." "The arc of the metatarsus parabola deviates directly with any inconsistence in the

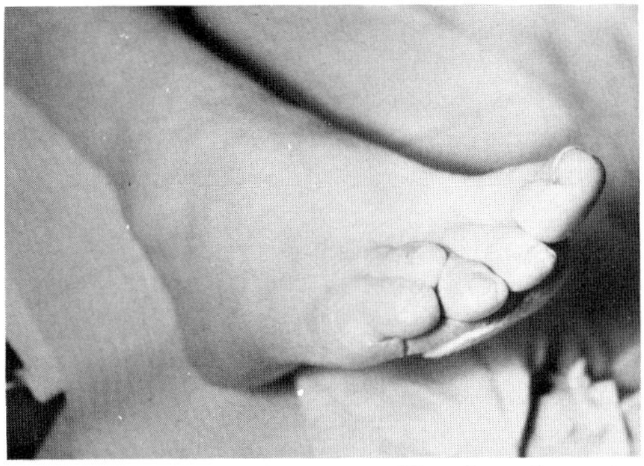

Fig. 16.3. Brachymetapodia, fourth metatarsal bone. Note short dorsiflexed fourth toe with underlapping third toe.

metatarsal lengths and the regular weight distribution pattern varies accordingly." He discussed variations in metatarsal length and the pathology they caused. Compensating pads are described to provide proper forefoot balance.

Treatment. X-ray examination establishes the presence of short or elongated metatarsal segments.

Deep excrescences occurring under longer metatarsals are reduced and shielded. The site of excrescences is marked off with skin pencil and impressions are taken for construction of an accommodative appliance. Felt-latex orthotics are constructed to accommodate the shortened bones and the deep excrescences commonly found on fulcrum serving long bones.

If feet are hypermobile, a rigid orthotic is constructed for the rearfoot with a flexible accommodating forefoot extension.

Weiner (1957) recommended a felt pad for metatarsalgia that covered a wide area of the metatarsus. It is longer and wider than the conventional metatarsal pad extending from the interdigital spaces backward to the bases of the metatarsals. It covers all the metatarsal heads with a long forward bevel to the interphalangeal joints.

Sansone (1957) described balancing of the forefoot parabola. For short metatarsal bones, extensions beyond the metatarsal heads of 1/8- to 3/16-in. pieces of felt are used to balance the foot. Cutouts are made under longer metatarsal heads while other metatarsals covered accept more of the body weight. Pads are devised to balance the forefoot when there is a long second metatarsal, Morton's syndrome, pseudoshort metatarsal, short first and second metatarsals, metatarsus proximus, or when the second and third metatarsals are long, the first and fifth are short, the first or the first and second are long, the fourth and/or the fifth are short.

Rigid orthotics are necessary to control rear foot subtalar valgus and forefoot varus or valgus incidental to this problem.

Strain at the Attachment of the Plantar Fascia and Flexor Digitorum Brevis. The plantar fascia and short plantar flexors of the toes originate at or near the medial tubercle of the plantar surface of the os calcis. The onset of pain is very often acute, yet many instances are reported wherein a dull pain, persisting for several weeks or months, had become progressively worse. Pain is noted in the region of the plantar fascial attachment and also anterior to this along the course of the painful structure. Weightbearing and digital pressure under the medial tubercle of the os calcis elicit pain. Swelling, when present, is usually slight. The condition is unilateral when caused by trauma, but if it has an infectious origin a bilateral affliction is not uncommon.

Pathologic changes or organic bone disturbances may be the result of constitutional defects such as syphilis or tuberculosis or may follow gonorrheal and rheumatic diseases.

An increase in body weight, long working hours on the feet and a vocation of standing or walking on hard inelastic surfaces cause strain. A strained plantar fascia may be caused by jumping from a height, the use of a foot pedal or a sudden change from a high to low, flat-heeled shoe which causes an excessive pull on the musculature. Prolonged rest in bed weakens the musculature. When high heels are worn for a prolonged period of time, the musculature contracts. The change on weightbearing without shoes causes strain. Strain of plantar connective tissue is usually accompanied by pain on arising after a period of rest.

Treatment. Pain is relieved by oral analgesics and inunction of rubefacients. Whirlpool, ultrasound, paraffin baths, short wave and infrared treatments are helpful. Contrast foot baths at home, b. i. d., for several days are helpful.

Adhesive immobilization by low Dye strapping shortens the distance between the origin and insertion of the plantar musculature and fascia and thus relieves strain.

In acutely inflamed plantar fascia, injections of corticosteroids at trigger points help to relieve symptoms.

Changing shoes from flexible shanks to firm rigid shanks is mandatory. Flexible shanks allow for stretching of already inflamed plantar structures.

If a structural deformity exists the problem should be corrected. Foot orthotic devices or balance inlays are helpful.

Calcaneal Spur. The calcaneal spur which causes pain on the plantar surface of the heel is defined as a bony projection extending from the tuberosity of the calcaneus, forward and downward in the direction of the plantar fascia. It may appear sharp, sclerosed, condensed or neatly demarcated with central reticulation.

The patient complains of a painful heel on arising in the morning or following periods of rest. The pain is acute with each step and in the early stages disappears after a few steps only to return after prolonged weightbearing or stress. It feels like a nail sticking into the foot or as a bruise localized to a definite area in the heel. The medial tubercle at the plantar surface is painful and an inflamed plantar fascia or acute bursitis may coexist. Pain on palpation is acute at the medial tubercle on the plantar surface. The x-ray examination is essential for diagnosis.

Treatment. Short wave and ultrasound treatments every 2 or 3 days and contrast foot baths at home t. i. d. are recommended. Analgesics by inunction and oral pain relieving medication are helpful.

Adhesive immobilization by low Dye strapping with a 1/4-in. felt raise may be used. The posterior skive is abrupt to raise the body of the calcaneus off the medial tubercle. Occasionally a donut-shaped felt or sponge pad around the painful area is helpful.

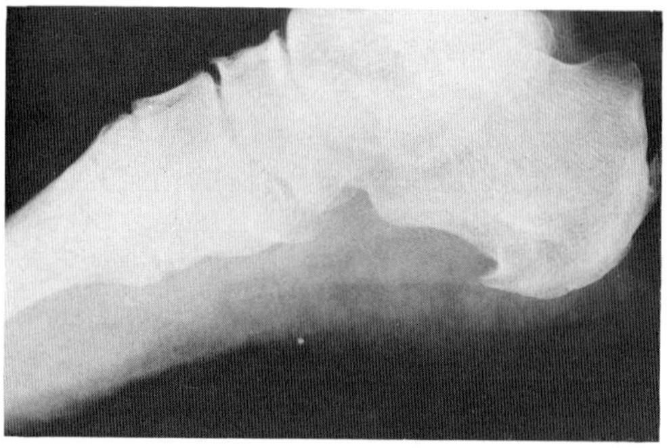

Fig. 16.4. Calcaneal spur. Note the degenerative lipping and osteophytes at the dorsal posterior and anterior articulations of the navicular.

Injections of lidocaine, procaine and/or corticosteroids into the soft tissues adjacent to the spur are indicated when pain persists. This relieves an acute bursitis which often accompanies the spur.

Construction of a foot orthotic device designed to cradle the heel with a high longitudinal raise is desirable to alter weight distribution and relieve pain. A rigid appliance is desirable if it is well fitted.

Carleton (1954) described a leather Shaffer shell designed to distribute weightbearing to the structures anterior to the calcaneus and just posterior to the metatarsal heads. The heel area is cut out and a 1/4-in. thick sponge skived at its margins is placed on top of the shell. Both top and bottom are covered.

A metal, Prenyl, Rodan or Rohadur or other firm, rigid or semi-rigid appliance may be constructed to re-align the weightbearing foot and remove pressure from the site of pain. The success of treatment depends on the skill of the foot specialist rather than the material used.

Analgesics with muscle relaxants may be prescribed for relief of pain and secondary spasm, e.g., Methacarbamol, 500 mg. (Robaxin); Chlorzoxazone (Paraflex, Parafon), 250 mg. tablets 2 q. i. d.; Paraflex 250 mg. and acetaminophen 300 mg., 2 tablets q. i. d.; Methacarbamol 400 mg. with aspirin 325 mg. (Robaxisal).

Posterior tibial nerve blocks may be necessary in the acutely painful heel. Injections of

0.5 ml. of corticosteroid directly into the painful site is also helpful in relieving acute pain. Michael (1961) reported excellent results using injections of triamcinalone acetonide 10 g./ml. (Decadron, Kenalog, Aristocort, Aristospan, Depo-Medrol are all useful injectible corticosteroids.)

Calcaneal Bursitis. A calcaneal bursitis referred to here occurs on the plantar surface of the heel, usually at the origin of the plantar aponeurosis at the medial tubercle. It manifests itself as a soreness of the heel which soon becomes moderately swollen, red and painful to touch. This must be differentiated from anterior and posterior achillobursitis. It commonly develops in the presence of a calcaneal spur and subtalar valgus.

Treatment is essentially the same as bursitis elsewhere or like that prescribed for calcaneal spur. In extremely painful bursitis, bed rest is indicated along with analgesics, corticosteroids and other anti-inflammatory oral medication.

Ritchie (1966) recommends phenylbutazone (Butazolidin) or Butazolidin Alka for short-term treatment of bursitis; 100 mg. q. i. d., for 7 consecutive days, taken after meals is an acceptable dose. Oxyphenbutazone (Tenderil), one tablet 3 to 4 times daily for 3 to 5 days is anti-inflammatory.

Intrabursal injection of anti-inflammatory medication is made easier when a posterior tibial nerve block is instituted first. Using aseptic techniques, aspiration may be instituted following local anesthesia. Leaving the 18-gauge needle in the bursa, a second syringe with 0.2 to 0.5 ml. of the corticosteroid of choice is attached to the needle and injected intrabursally.

A donut pad 1/4-in. thick may be cemented to the heel or bound down with adhesive tape.

Posterior achillobursitis is also called calcaneal bursitis and is treated in the same fashion.

Insufficient Adipose Covering. Often one sees asthenic individuals with insufficient adipose tissue around the heel. This may develop following prolonged bed rest and inactivity in the elderly and the young.

Treatment. Rubber heels on shoes and sponge in the heel seat is helpful. If the tissue is acutely inflamed, bed rest and elevation removes inflammatory exudates.

Closely fitting heel cups or appliances high enough to accept weight on the arch remove pressure from the heel. Moldable insole material serves to break the shock of weightbearing.

A high raise in the arch lifts pressure from the heel.

Periostitis of Calcaneus. Periostitis of the calcaneus manifests itself as a soreness of the heel with severe pain on weightbearing and palpation. Evidence of a soft tissue mass or subperiosteal calcific deposits may be found on x-ray examination. The most common site of tenderness is palpated at the sides of the calcaneal body. Soft tissue swelling is common.

I have seen several cases of calcaneal periostitis following infections of the teeth, nose or throat. There is generally a slight elevation in skin temperature overlying the area of inflammation. Tenderness and swelling of the heel has been observed following the use of penicillin for an infection far removed from the foot. Stress fractures of the calcaneus must be ruled out.

Treatment. If stress is caused by overweight, weight reduction under an internist's supervision is indicated. Plastic heel cups protect the heel from trauma. Fiberglass, metal, Rohadur or Rodan orthotics to relieve weightbearing from the affected heel may be necessary. A plaster cast, flexible casting or Celastic immobilization of the heel may be used in acute states.

Isolation of the infecting organism of some periostitic involvements is necessary to establish the etiology and prescribe the proper antibiotics. An internist should be consulted if a systemic disease is suspected.

Osteochondrosis of Calcaneus. (Synonyms include apophysitis of the calcaneus, avascular necrosis of the calcaneal apophysis, osteochondritis of the calcaneus, calcaneal osteosis.) Gamble and Yale (1966) define an apophysis as any outgrowth, swelling or process, especially a bony process which had never been entirely separated from the bone of which it forms a part, and which does not enter into the formation of a joint and is not covered by cartilage. Apophysitis, an inflammation of the posterior epiphysis of the calcaneus, is most common in boys between the ages of 8 and 12. Direct trauma or multiple minimum injury to the apophysis may be etiologic. Muscular stress on the tendo achillis may cause a tenderness along the cartilage line. Infections and circulatory changes in the epiphyseal cartilage may cause discomfort in the apophysis. This condition is usually unilateral. Krantz (1965) felt that calcaneal apophysitis is probably caused by microtrauma.

The apophysis is placed at a distinct disadvantage by virtue of the attachment on its posterior surface of the tendo achillis. When the osteochondrotic changes become severe, osteitis and destructive lesions may occur, and, in some cases, periostitis may be evident. The apophysis may fail to develop properly if untreated, possibly resulting in a faulty ossification. Krantz (1965) found that children with medium to high arches and limited flexion seem to be subject to this problem.

At first the pain is described as a dull ache over the mid-portion of the posterior surface of the apophysis. The pain may become more severe extending to either side of the posterior of the heel. The slight pain in the back of the heel becomes severe when climbing stairs, jumping or running. Pain and difficulty in walking is most severe after a period of rest. This is post-static dyskinesia. Pain on palpation is noted at the posterior plantar angle of the heel. A thickening of the tissues may be felt laterally and on the plantar of the apophysis. Dorsiflexion of the foot may cause pain at the apophysis. Pain is less marked when a ¼-in. felt pad is placed in the heel seat to relieve the pull of the Achilles tendon. Pressure of the shoe counter causes pain. Swelling may be present, and very often the patient walks with a limp, as in an equinus gait. This is especially true in the morning with the first steps. The pain dissappears with motion only to return when the patient gets tired.

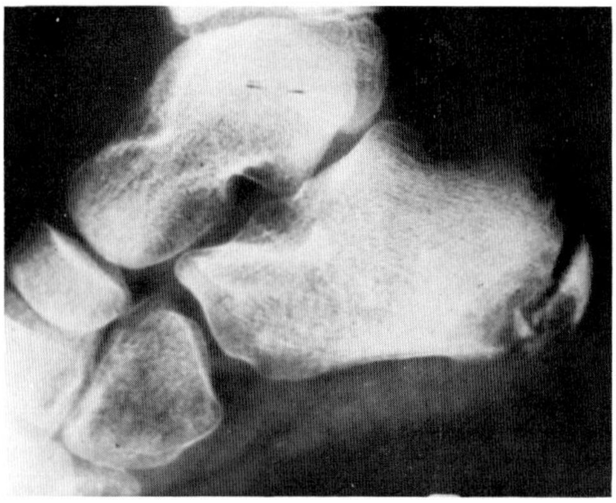

Fig. 16.5. Traumatic apophysitis with fracture of the apophysis. Courtesy of *Clinical Foot Roentgenology*, The Williams & Wilkins Co., Baltimore, 1966.

Treatment. Prescribe oxford tie shoes with rigid shanks, extended counter, rubber heels, leather soles and a snug fit in heel and arch. The patient should refrain from wearing soft soles, flexible shanked shoes or sneakers.

It is wise to limit the use of short wave and ultrasound currents to the developing apophysis as they cause alterations in the cartilage growth.

Rheumatic fever should be ruled out. A CBC, sedimentation rate, heterophile and latex fixation examination are also necessary for diagnosis.

Relieve strain on the tendo achillis and plantar musculature by strapping and padding the arch of the affected foot in a rested position. Use heel cups and appliances to correct biomechanical problems and weak feet. Protection from repeated trauma can be assured by decreasing physical activities and using a sponge heel seat.

In severe cases, a plaster cast to limit a child's activity may be necessary for a few weeks to relieve inflammation.

Use of corticosteroids in young patients is discouraged. Analgesics are helpful in relieving pain. Salicylates, 10 grains taken every 4 to 6 hr. as needed are usually adequate.

Achillobursitis Anterior. (Synonyms include Albert's disease, achillodynia, retrocalcaneal bursitis.) Achillobursitis anterior is an inflammation occurring in the bursal sac lying between the tendo achillis and the upper portion of the posterior surface of the calcaneus.

This inflammation may result from weak feet with a positive Helbing's sign, trauma or, more rarely, gout, rheumatism, tuberculosis and gonorrhea. When inflammation is the result of disease, the onset is slow, but in trauma the symptoms appear rapidly. A severe twist of the foot, especially in a high-heeled pump, may produce this condition. Sudden jumps, constant strain on the Achilles tendon, stiff shoe counters or a kick or blow to the heel may cause this inflammation. Haglund's deformity may be etiologic.

Pain is localized over and around the sides of the tendon most proximal to its insertion. Use of the foot and digital pressure may cause pain. Swelling and inflammatory changes may be evident on either side of the tendo achillis. The foot is usually everted to avoid dorsi flexion.

Treatment. Sources of trauma should be eliminated. The heel should be elevated with a ¼-in. raise in the heel seat. Salicylates, indomethacin (Indocin), propoxyphene hydrochloride (Darvon), acetaminophen (Tylenol; Valadol), 325-mg. tablets, are helpful in controlling pain. Injection of corticosteroids or other anti-inflammatory agents in less than 0.4-ml. amounts directly into the bursa affords relief. Ultrasound every other day is also helpful.

In severe cases, the heel should be immobilized by adhesive tape or plaster cast and oral analgesics may be prescribed.

If systemic disease is the underlying cause of the condition, the patient should be referred to an internist.

Achillobursitis posterior is an inflammation of an adventitious bursa occurring between the skin and the tendo achillis just above its insertion into the os calcis. It may be caused by friction and pressure from shoes that do not fit properly such as those with stiff counters, tight shoes, high-heeled pumps, sling backs and poorly shaped shoes. Rheumatoid arthritis, chilblains and frostbite affecting the heel often cause this condition which is more common in females. Haglund's deformity and pes valgus are predisposing factors.

Pain is caused by friction and pressure of the shoes. Bullae may develop. The bursal sac forms at the margin of the counter, often becoming red, hot and swollen. Sometimes fissures develop in the skin. The bursa may become chronic and cause pain at the slightest provocation. The skin over the bursa may ulcerate.

X-ray findings show a large, soft tissue mass of increased density just above the attachment of the tendo achillis. Occasionally, the bursal sac degenerates and calcification takes place. Exostosis may be present at the attachment of the tendon. The posterior superior angle of the heel may protrude as in Haglund's disorder.

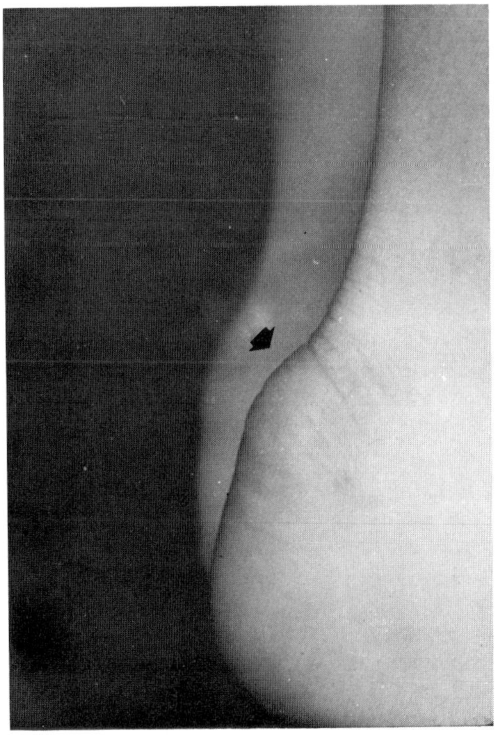

Fig. 16.6. Posterior achillobursitis. X-ray examination may reveal an underlying Haglund's deformity requiring surgical correction.

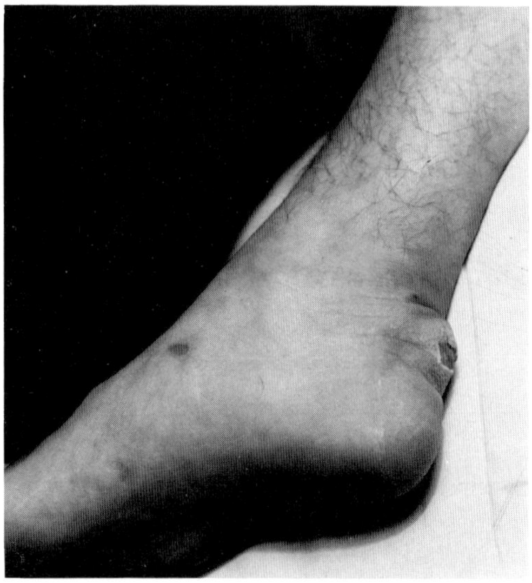

Fig. 16.7. Ulceration over posterior achillobursitis. Courtesy of Douglas Mowbray.

Treatment. Frostbite and chilblains should be treated. Vasodilators are helpful and protection is necessary. Remove pressure of the shoe by elevating the heel seat. A felt or foam donut pad over the inflamed part to relieve pressure is helpful. Injections of an acetylated corticosteroid into the bursa relieves pain. Ultrasound, hot pacs and topical analgesic ointments are also used.

Construct a permanent shield from a cast or directly over the part. Latex or liquid plastic are materials of choice. PodoSil, a new silicone gel, has simplified the technique of pad construction.

Surgical excision of a chronic bursa is indicated in intractable cases.

Causative systemic diseases should be treated by an internist.

Haglund's Deformity. In Haglund's deformity, the posterosuperior angle of the oscalcis extends upward and backward. The pressure of the tendo achillis against this bony prominence results in severe pain. An x-ray of the part establishes the diagnosis of Haglund's deformity.

Over a period of years, the prominent bone may undergo degenerative changes. Irregularity of the cortex with loss of substance and subcortical demineralization are often found with this disorder. Subacute or chronic bursitis is often the painful problem requiring relief.

Treatment. Permanent shields may relieve pressure from the bony prominence. Raising the heel seat ¼ in. lifts the bone away from the pressure of the counter.

Local physical therapy and oral analgesics are indicated for relief of pain in acute inflammations.

Surgical excision of the bony prominence is necessary for complete relief. A chronic bursa may be excised.

Traumatic tenosynovitis is an inflammation of the tendon and its sheath due to excessive use of the tendon in its sheath. The inflammatory symptoms may result from slow, prolonged friction over a tendon, such as may occur in ice skating, long hikes, multiple twists of the ankle, strap shoes and pressure on the extensor hallucis longus tendon from pumps. Sudden direct injury, such as dropping an article on the foot, may cause tenosynovitis.

Tenosynovitis is most common around the ankles. As the tendons pull at an angle they are subjected to great friction in normal use of the foot. Usually there is pain on motion and crepitus within the inflamed sheath, but on direct pressure pain is slight. The tendon sheath becomes hot, swollen, painful and tender, and in the slow, prolonged cases, marked fibrosis takes place. Over the tendo achillis the multiple minimal frictions from the counter of the shoe may cause fibrosis, especially in women. The overlying tissues may or may not show evidence of inflammatory changes. The extensor hallucis longus and the anterior tibial tendons are most commonly affected.

Treatment. Rest and removal of the causative agent are necessary. Ultrasound and immobilization help relieve pain and inflammation. Local injections of corticosteroids may be used in conjunction with aspirin, 10 grains q. 4 to 6 h., p. r. n. for pain. Oral enzymes reduce swelling and relieve pain.

Pyogenic tenosynovitis is usually

caused by the introduction of bacteria through a wound over a tendon sheath or by the extension of infection from the surrounding area through a puncture wound or laceration.

Objectively, the lesion presents all signs of acute inflammation accompanied by a marked degree of impaired function. Fluctuation is noted after organization of the pus. The severity of the condition is manifested by increased temperature and leukocytosis. The offending organisms may be either staphylococcus or streptococcus. *Neisseria gonorrhoeae* often attacks the tendon sheath of the ankle and the foot. Lymphangitis and adenopathy may result in the acute stages.

Treatment. Culture and sensitivity tests performed after incision and drainage identify the infecting organism and the antibiotic(s) of choice.

A hot magnesium sulfate poultice over the acutely infected tendon is helpful. Remove all pressure and apply moist heat with rest and elevation of the afflicted part.

Penicillin or a broad-spectrum antibiotic may be necessary where secondary infection and lymphadenopathy are present.

Systemic diseases are treated and controlled by an internist.

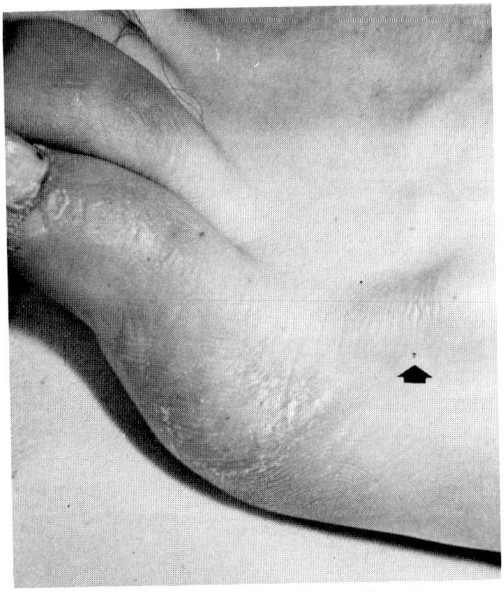

Fig. 16.8. Tenosynovitis. Note discoloration and distention of extensor tendon sheathe.

Tuberculous Tenosynovitis. The tendon sheath may be invaded by tubercle bacillus. This is characterized by a slow, progressive, mildly painful swelling over the involved sheath. Early diagnosis is difficult but it is essential to the patient's general health and comfort. The patient is referred to an internist for further examination and treatment. Rest and elevation of the part and systemic antibiotic therapy are necessary for relief while the active focus of the disease is located.

Tumors of the Tendon Sheath. Fibromas are by far the most common tumors affecting the tendon sheaths. The extensor tendons are usually affected. These connective tissue growths are characterized by slight pain, circumscribed and local development and adherence to the tendon sheath from which they develop. No inflammatory changes are noted unless precipitated by pressure over the tumor from ill-fitting shoes or trauma from other sources.

Treatment. Excision of the tumor is mandatory. Care must be taken to preserve the integrity of the tendon. The specimen should be submitted for microscopic study.

Institute postoperative treatment early to maintain good tendon function. This may consist of active and passive exercises, short wave, ultrasound and use of low voltage currents.

Chondromas may affect the tendon proper and are seen on radiographs as spotty and flaky areas of calcification lying within a localized and fairly well-outlined increase in soft tissue density.

Rupture of the Plantaris Tendon. This traumatic condition characteristically affects tennis players and is known as "tennis leg." The patient feels a sudden, sharp pain in the calf of the leg when landing on his foot after a high jump. He describes the pain as a snap or "whiplash" type of trauma. Discomfort is great on dorsiflexion of the foot. The patient walks on his toes and is relieved by elevation of the heel by mechanical means.

This condition may be seen in people of all ages, especially middle-aged females. Direct or indirect trauma may be etiologic. After a marked, sudden pull of the calf muscles symptoms may become evident. Objectively, the middle of the calf may become discolored as if contused and slight edema may be seen. Pain on palpation is evident. Predisposing factors are senility, pathologic changes, physiologic predisposition, occupation, fatigue or trauma. The podiatrist must rule out rupture of the fibers of the tendo achillis or specific damage to the gastrocnemius and soleus muscles.

Treatment. Early treatment is rest and application of ice bags to the painful site.

Oral enzymes should be used to reduce swelling and to dissipate hemorrhage. Muscle relaxants relieve spasms.

Elevate the heel with a ¼-in. heel pad in the shoe and immobilize it by strapping the foot in the extended position or by applying a plaster cast to immobilize calf muscles. A gelatin cast is helpful in mild cases. The patient may have to use a cane or crutches in walking since the foot is placed in an extended position.

Analgesics to relieve pain and facilitate early function will help bring about a rapid recovery in 3 to 5 weeks.

Strain of the Tendo Achillis. Football players and runners are subjected to the discomfort of strain of the tendo achillis. It is seen also in women who suddenly change from wearing a high- to a low-heeled or flat shoe. The tendo achillis can produce pain anywhere from its insertion in the midportion of the posterior of the os calcis upward to the triceps surae. The tendon and its surrounding areolar tissue is edematous and painful to the touch. The tissues may be red and hot along the course of the tendon. Crepitus is noted on flexion and extension of the foot on the ankle.

Treatment. Correct faulty foot function and raise the heel seat of the shoe.

Physical therapy by hot pacs, ultrasound and short wave is helpful. Rest and elevation of the part is necessary in early stages. Analgesics and muscle relaxants are used to relieve pain.

Rupture of the Tendo Achillis. This serious injury generally occurs in active men under 40 years of age and may occur during a period of inactivity. Arner *et al.* (1958) suggest that degenerative changes occurring prior to the rupture are due to circulatory changes in the tendon. Lindholm and Lindvall (1958) point out that the curvature of the tendon is turned away from the upper border of the calcaneus and its attachment. This curving away from the calcaneus, which seems to be pathognomonic of this rupture, is combined with an unimpaired forward deviation of the tendon contour proximal to the calcaneus. A limited segment about 2 to 6 cm. above its insertion on the calcaneus is ruptured.

Thompson (1962) confirmed in 22 patients that squeezing the calf of a normal leg causes a strong plantar flexion of the foot, whereas squeezing the calf of a leg with a ruptured heel cord produces no motion in the foot. In my experience this may give a false positive result when the deep muscle reflex arc is intact.

Treatment. Greenblatt and Diehm (1967) used chlorphenesin carbamate (Maolate) for musculoskeletal injuries with good results. All the conditions were acute and relieved by Maolate 400 mg., q. i. d., for 1 week. I have used this treatment successfully for several years as an adjunct to physical therapy and early rehabilitation following trauma and inflammation of the musculature.

Exploratory surgery is advised to correct the rupture and any other pathology.

Plantar Fasciatis. The plantar aponeurosis is easily strained with severe stress on weakened feet. The posterior attachment at the medial tubercle of the plantar surface of the os calcis is very often inflamed from the continued pull or trauma at its attachment.

A condition has been described which resembles strain of the plantar fascia but presents few of the predisposing causes and symptoms.

Although the onset is acute and pain is localized in the ankles, subtalar joints, plantar surfaces of the heels and the origin of the plantar fascia, the symptoms present a definite entity. They must be differentiated from infectious and rheumatoid arthritis.

The symptoms are severe with acute onset affecting the parts mentioned above. Increased temperature and swelling of the affected area is noted. Sedimentation rate is always high. Both males and females, usually between the ages of 3 and 30 may be affected.

Careful history-taking discloses a recent febrile disease about 3 to 6 weeks before onset. The disease runs its course in from 10 days to 3 weeks. Penicillin reactions have resulted in a similiar acute plantar fasciatis.

X-ray findings are reported to be indefinite and of little diagnostic value.

Plantar fibromatoses may develop following acute inflammation. They are rarely painful.

Nodular fasciatis or infiltrative fasciatis is a tumor-like fibroblastic proliferation which resembles a sarcoma but is clinically benign. Rosenberg (1969) describes the lesion as usually occurring in adults, possibly as a virus-induced inflammatory process. The overlying skin may be raised with slight brownish discoloration. It appears suddenly and is characterized by rapid growth. It may be a single lesion measuring 4 mm. to about 4 cm. in diameter.

Total excision of the mass is indicated. It is comparatively rare on the foot.

Treatment. Heat, rest and elevation of the part and use of analgesics and necessary antibiotics are the usual treatment. Carisoprodol (Soma) and methocarbamol (Robaxin) may be used successfully in the treatment of pain and spasm. Soma is prescribed as a 350-mg. tablet and a 250-mg. capsule. The usual adult dose is 1 350-mg. tablet t. i. d. and h. s.

Adhesive immobilization to reduce strain is indicated.

Blood studies are necessary to differentiate infections and rheumatic disorders of systemic origin. Sytemic diseases should be treated by an internist.

Cutaneous Herniations. Galinsky (1970) describes cutaneous herniations as "fatty subcutaneous tissue passing through a defect of the connective tissue into the fascial layer of the dermis." Cutaneous hernia is rare. Galinsky describes a unilateral case in a patient, age 27. I have seen a 6-year-old patient with bilateral cutaneous herniations around the heels as described by Galinsky. The multiple herniations on the medial, lateral and posterior of the heels measured 0.3 to 1.0 cm. in diameter on weight bearing and disappeared at rest. The lesions were painless and easily compressed.

Treatment. The treatment of this problem is compression of the heel by a shoe with firm counter, the use of a heel cup and, if Helbing's sign is positive, a heel stabilizer.

Myalgia is a symptom affecting single muscles or groups of muscles and is characterized by varying degrees of pain, stiffness and disability. The pain of myalgia is increased with movement of the muscle. The affected muscle is held in a certain position of immobilization in order to avoid motion. The pain is in some cases caused by a slight neuritis affecting the intramuscular sensory nerve ending and may also be due to inflammations and abnormal movement of the muscles themselves.

Strains or overuse of the muscles may cause myalgia. Acute infections often result in acute myalgic states.

The cause of chronic myalgia may be chronic intoxication with alcohol, lead poisoning, diabetes or gout. Chronic infections such as syphilis, tuberculosis and septic infections and unusual strain from lack of proper muscular balance and postural instability may cause chronic myalgia. It may also be caused by lesions involving joints or bones.

Acute cases may last from a few days to a week while chronic cases continue with remissions and intermissions for months or years.

The plantar flexors and plantar fascia are very often affected by this involvement. Although the central portion of the plantar fascia in the sole of the foot is most tender and painful, usually the localization of pain is at the medial tubercle of the os calcis at the origin of the short flexors or the toes. The peroneal and anterior tibial muscles are readily affected. The calf muscles, when painful, should be thoroughly checked in order to differentiate myalgia from other lesions before a definite diagnosis is made. Myalgias must be differentiated from myositis, dermatomyositis, myositis ossificans and trichinosis.

Treatment. Analgesics and oral muscle relaxants help to relieve pain. Pentazocine hydrochloride (Talwin) 50 mg. q. 3 to 4 h. may relieve the pain when the usual analgesics have failed.

Chronic intoxications must be corrected. Disease and infections should be controlled by proper medication.

Muscle and joint disorders are corrected to relieve strain.

Physical medicine using hot pacs, ultrasound, short wave and other heat-producing modalities are good adjunct treatment.

Steinberg (1957) discusses treatment for the short muscles of the foot. He cites the technique of Dr. M. F. Good who uses a spot injection of a solution of procaine hydrochloride, chlorobutanol and saline. Results were good with reduction of pain and restoration of functions. Rarely were more than 2 or 3 injections given into the myalgic "spot."

Myofascial Foot Pain. Cinzio (1963) concludes that myofascial disorders include myositis, fibrositis, fibromyositis, tendonitis, muscular strains and contusions. The pain may not coincide with dermatomal patterns. Muscle metabolism and oxidation processes are disturbed resulting in a diminution of oxygen, enzymes and other substances. The pain may be triggered by a reflex muscle spasm, organic or vasospastic circulatory diseases, vitamin deficiencies, allergies, contusions, strain and infection by bacterial or viral agents.

Symptoms may vary from a slight stiffness in the foot or leg musculature to excruciating pain with crepitus and immobility.

Treatment. Pain is relieved by physical therapy suitable for the complaint, correction of the etiology, analgesics applied topically, orally or parenterally, and with stretching exercises and injections of local anesthetics and/or corticosteroids into the trigger points of pain.

"Spot" injections of lidocaine 1% plain, and a corticosteroid into trigger points or at site of pain and stiffness relieve pain.

Carisoprodol (Soma) 350 mg., after each meal and 2 at bedtime for periods of 1 day to 3 months helps relieve pain and spasm. Muscle relaxants and combinations with analgesics are also effective in relieving pain. Banninga (1960) demonstrated a 48% improvement in a variety of musculoskeletal disorders using this therapeutic regimen.

Physical therapy, ultrasound, whirlpool, deep heat, wet hot pacs and a variety of analgesics with anti-inflammatory agents are helpful.

17

Congenital and Acquired Deformities of the Foot: Biomechanical Relationships

Podiatric medicine considers the deformities of the foot in light of their relationship to discomfort and pain. Time and space do not permit a thorough study of biomechanical relationships and treatment of foot deformities. Likewise, it is not within the province of this text to interpret the various arthritic involvements as they relate to foot structure and function. In this chapter we consider the biomechanical implications of congenital and acquired abnormalities in the foot.

The feet are subject to many anomalies of congenital and hereditary origin. These may vary from mild genetically predetermined deformities to severe deforming states requiring surgical correction to enable the pedal extremities to perform useful biomechanical functions.

Pigeon Toe. This defect generally escapes detection until the infant starts to walk. Several complicated problems are noted at birth. The common clinical deformity involves a hypermobile musculature, especially at the hip, resulting in inward rotation at the acetabulum in gait. Examination of all the body joints may reveal lax articular ligaments with hyperextensibility of the muscles with active or passive function. The joints are flaccid in the hip, knee, ankles and feet. A true pigeon toe, however, is a metatarsus varus, a varus located in the forefoot only, with a normal or somewhat everted rearfoot. Metatarsus varus is usually apparent at birth or by the third or fourth month. This type of pigeon toe is observed early enough for definitive treatment.

Frequently, the pigeon-toed patient presents a severe weak foot with inward rotation of the os calcis on its long axis, a prominent tuberosity of the navicular or subluxated talar head and poor muscular function. Careful examination may disclose that the pigeon toe gait is often a compensatory reaction to the great strain on the leg muscles from improper foot function and faulty weight distribution. The external rotators of the hip are often weak. Contractures of the internal rotators may be a factor. Pigeon toe may result as a compensatory change from myositis or dystrophic and neurogenic factors.

Where structural deformity exists in a marked varus, the patient generally has equinus and the condition must then be considered a clubfoot.

Treatment is based on the appearance of the foot at rest and its ability to perform in stance and in gait. An evaluation of the relative strength of the various muscle groups is most important in deciding on proper therapy. The extremities should be placed through various passive ranges of motion, and the podiatrist must decide whether there are restrictions to both active and passive motion at the hip or knee or in the foot. A limitation of active or passive external rotation of the limb at the acetabular articulation may be the result of a tightness of the ligaments and internal rotators at the hip. The gluteal and

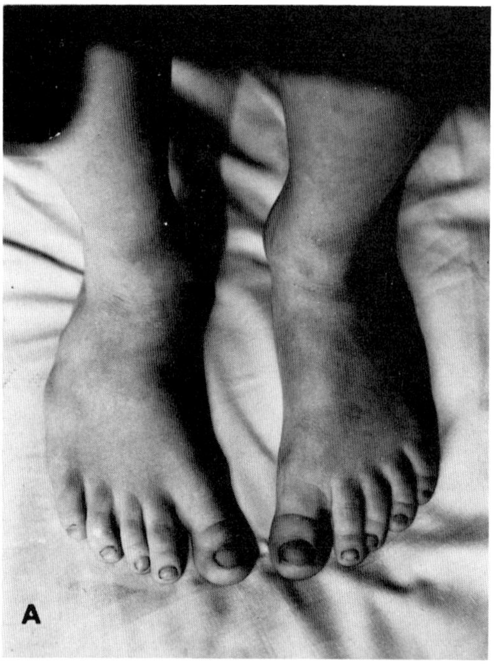

Fig. 17.1*A*. Pigeon toe—metatarsus varus.

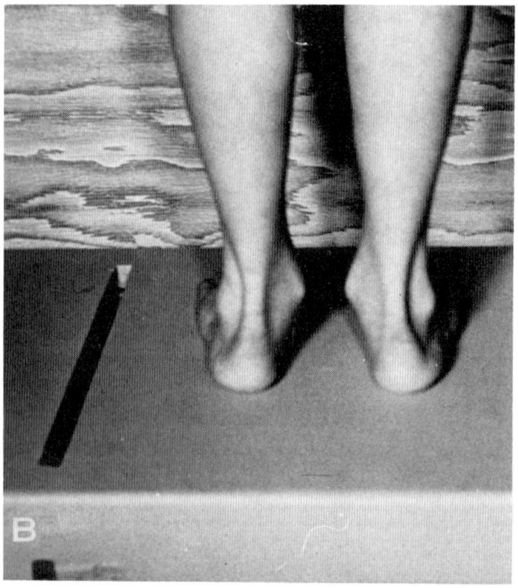

Fig. 17.1*B*. A compensating intoeing gait may develop in this pronated foot problem.

inguinal folds should be equal and bilaterally symmetrical. The knee joint flexes and extends both actively and passively. The ankle joint should perform its functions within a normal range. Abduction, inversion, eversion and adduction must be tested both actively and passively to detect restrictions which could create the pigeon toe. The gross appearance of the foot in gait and stance must be properly appreciated at this time. Deep and superficial reflexes should be evaluated and measurements in limb length and girth considered to rule out neurologic disorders and deformities of the extremities.

If, following the takeoff, the patient brings the leg and foot into internal rotation and adduction prior to heel strike, one can assume that the problem is not a foot deformity but a compensatory change due to muscular contraction. This performance may be necessary for the relief of some discomfort or restriction elsewhere in the extremities. Conversely, if, on complete weightbearing of the foot the knees appear knocked, the pigeontoe may be a compensatory change due to severe subtalar valgus and compensatory forefoot varus.

Treatment. Early treatment in infancy is accomplished by plaster casting the deformed foot in an overcorrected position. Periodic cast changes may correct the problem. The use of the Brachman Skate, Irving Yale Club Foot Splint, the Ganley Splint, Fillaur Splint, Dennis Brown Splint and Friedman Shoe correction may assist in the reversal of the deformity.

Scheimer (1957) states that the use of plaster of Paris casts is by far the best treatment for metatarsus varus.

Active and passive exercises, stretching and physical therapeutic massage and manipulation are indicated. Gait training is imperative.

When the patient starts walking, straight last shoes or varus and pigeon-toed shoes will help. Care should be taken to assure that the corrective procedures do not permanently deform the foot in a valgus state. Shoe corrections such as lateral wedges, to force the feet out should never be used without compensatory longitudinal support and a Thomas heel.

In most cases of intoeing I prescribe a straight last shoe, external rotation gait exercises and a Celastic Whitman build-up in the shoes with a lateral extension under the fifth segment. Metal, Rodan, Rohadur or fiberglass Whitman or Roberts Plate may be necessary.

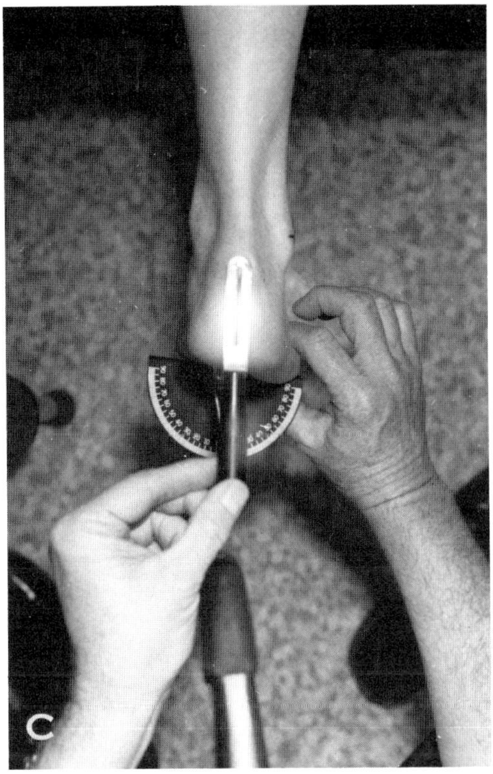

Fig. 17.1*C*. Use of the forefoot varus meter. Position the foot with the subtalar joint at its neutral position and the midtarsal joint maximumly pronated, place the slotted portion of the forefoot varus meter on the neutral calcaneous line, extend the instrument so its base is under the fifth metatarsal head, and, grasping with the thumb and forefinger, let the base plate rest lightly across the metatarsal heads. Read the dial for the forefoot aberration, be it varus or valgus. Courtesy Burns Podiatric Laboratory.

The patient wears a toe cutout shoe at night with a strap extending from one shoe to the other to externally rotate the limbs. This is the treatment of choice except when contractures require the use of a Brachman Skate, Dennis Brown or other bar splint. Surgical correction is rarely necessary. Active and passive stretching helps. Less damage to the structure of the foot is noted when tendo achillis lengthening is performed where indicated.

Counter correctors or similar straps attached to the shoes may be used as night and sleep retainers.

Hip and knee pathology should be handled by an orthopedic surgeon.

Congenital Hallux Varus. The classical clinical appearance presents the great toe widely separated from the second toe. The abductor of the great toe exerts considerable pull causing this deformity. Congenital hallux varus is rare. When it is found early before the bony transformations take place, the joint may be corrected by orthodigital treatment.

Regardless of the therapy selected, the end result will depend on judicious use of orthotics, exercises and corrective forces of an active and passive nature. One word of caution at this point should be made about the over-treatment of infants and children: the podiatrist must be constantly aware not only of the need for corrective forces and their application but also of the damage that may accrue in epiphyseal cartilage from their injudicious use.

Treatment of congenital hallux varus depends on whether the deformity is localized to the hallux or a part of a varus of the first metatarsal segment. In the event treatment is started early, it is wise to have the child wear a varus shoe or the opposite shoe on the affected foot. A plaster cast may be necessary to correct this deformity.

If therapy is instituted rather late, it may be necessary to construct an orthodigital appliance to bring about correction. An orthodigital appliance can be constructed out of felt and latex or latex and other materials such as tubegauze or plain bandage impregnated with

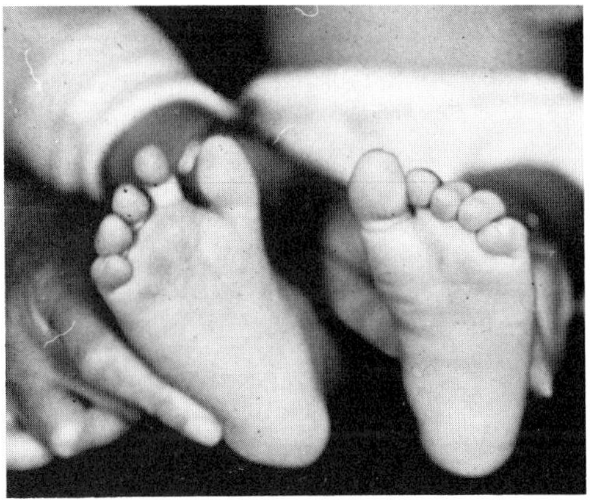

Fig. 17.2. Hallux varus—short first metatarsal. Note cleft in first interdigital space.

latex or silicone gel. The application of a ring around the hallux coming over the dorsum of the foot connected to one or more of the lesser toes or encompassing the entire forefoot, may produce an adequate force to bring about correction. This appliance pulls the hallux closer to the foot in line with the lesser toes. More sophisticated treatment may embody surgical syndactyly of the hallux to the second toe. Occasionally the treatment of choice is a surgical shortening of the adductor hallucis oblique and transverse tendon at its attachment. Lengthening the abductor tendon and incision of the medial joint capsule is also helpful. Syndactylizing the hallux to the second toe may be necessary to realign the hallux.

Overlapping and Underriding Toes. These deformities commonly involve the lesser toes. I have seen many cases of underriding hallux; usually a hallux valgus co-exists with the deformity. The great toe may extend under the second toe and sometimes under the third toe. The hallux nail, receiving the brunt of weightbearing by the dorsiflexed second toe, becomes atrophic, grayish, yellow or brown in color. The hallux may also override the second toe with severe contractures of the adductor hallucis, joint capsule and articular ligaments. Very often the extensor hallucis longus appears as a bow string due to its great longitudinal pull.

Observation of the feet of many children and adults reveals a characteristic hypermobile deformity of the lesser toes. I have seen the second toes of many individuals—often of Italian extraction—contracted through pull by extensor muscles and articular ligaments to the point of dislocation. Along with this contracture are flexions of the distal phalanges on their long axis either medially or laterally resulting in severe deformity. The third toe is similarly involved but more often presents an underlapping to the second toe which is contracted. The fourth toe is usually rotated on its long axis and underlapping the third. Many of the deformities take place at the interphalangeal joints with normal metatarsophalangeal joints. The fifth toe may overlap the fourth with contractures of the skin and joint capsule as well as the extensor tendon.

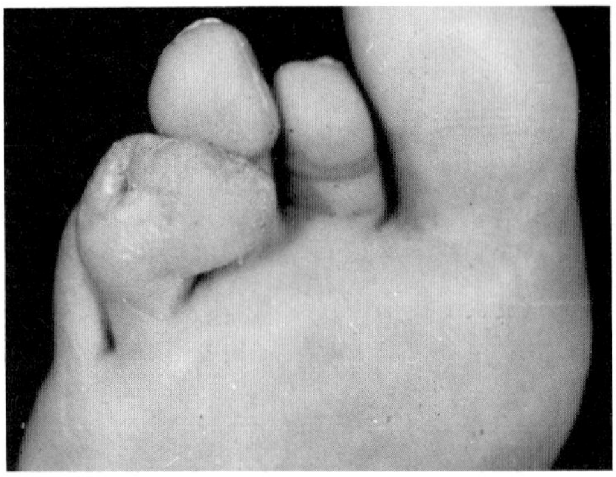

Fig. 17.3. Underlapping fourth toe. Ulceration and sinus tract.

These patients develop soft corns from abnormal friction and many patients develop hypertrophied nails from trauma. They also have difficulty in buying shoes that fit well.

Treatment. Treatment depends on the degree of deformity, the age of the patient and the extent of deformity as it relates to disturbances of the biomechanics of the foot. The usual physiologic functions of the foot may not be affected by the minor deformities of the toes. However, the presence of underlapping or overlapping toes may alter foot function creating postural disturbances a distance from the site of a local deformity. Conversely, tight flexor muscles may pull toes down to a deformed state where the feet are weak. The treatment may be divided into a conservative and radical treatment.

The conservative treatment of these deformities depends on the use of adequate footgear to provide sufficient room for function of the deformed toes. Also, it is essential that the toes be placed on a plane that will allow for maximum function within the limitations of the deformity. This can be done by judicious use of orthodigital corrective forces as prescribed by Budin, Polokoff, Whitney, McGlamry, Rosoff, and others. Roven (1959) demonstrates a simple rubber sling for correction of overlapping fifth toe. This was a modification of Budin's (1941) elastic traction loop sling. The use of orthodigital corrective or

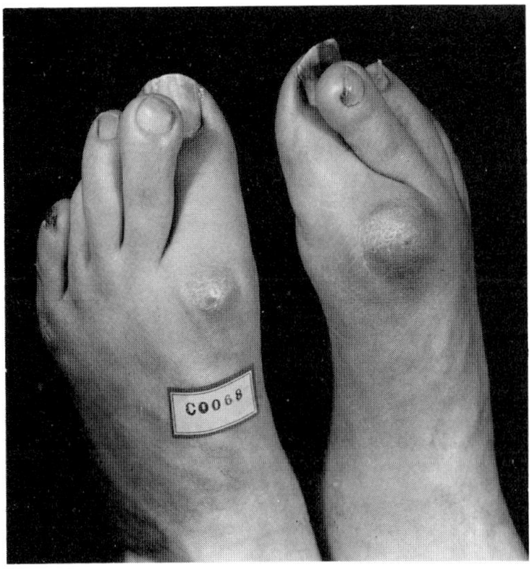

Fig. 17.4. Overlapping second toes. Hallux limitus, dorsal bunion.

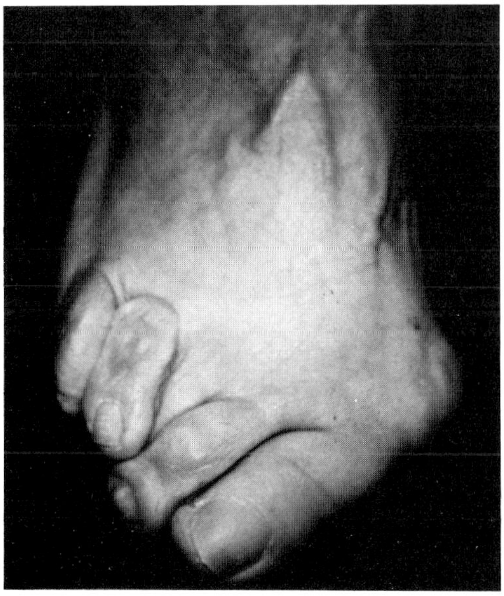

Fig. 17.5. Overlapping toes. Second and fourth toes over third.

accommodative devices to increase the efficiency of the affected parts is indicated where surgical intervention is a risk. They consist of functional splints, removable crests, and crests located on functional insoles and appliances.

The radical treatment of these disturbances may consist of a combination of surgical intervention and corrective forces and splinting in order to maintain the correction. Here the podiatrist may use the techniques of "Z" plasty, tenectomy, tenotomy, tendon lengthening, capsulotomy, syndactyly, arthroplasty, removal of an exostosis, and resecting portions of capsular tissues to tighten up the articulation with suturing. Often it is essential to use two or more of the above techniques for correction. I correct these deformities with a middle phalangectomy to bring about a more even balance between the flexor and extensors of the toes. Recent surgical approaches, described by Roven as "phalangeal set," necessitating transverse incision of digital tendons and joint capsules without bone removal have proved beneficial in correcting minor digital deformities.

Fusion Deformities. Cases are reported of congenital synostosis in several articu-

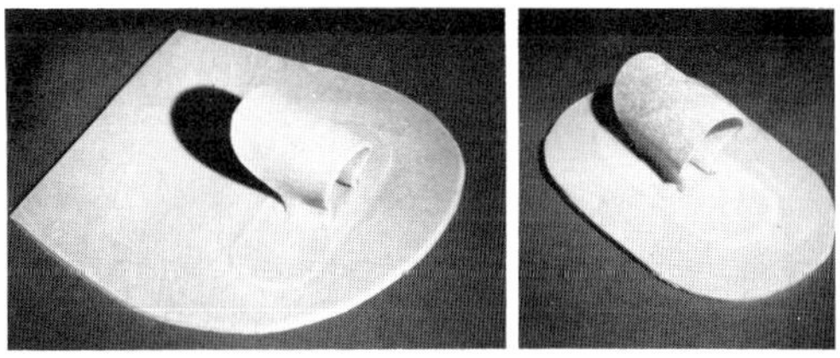

Fig. 17.6. Budin splint. Transverse for overlapping toes (left).

Fig. 17.7. Budin splint. Longitudinal for hammertoes (right).

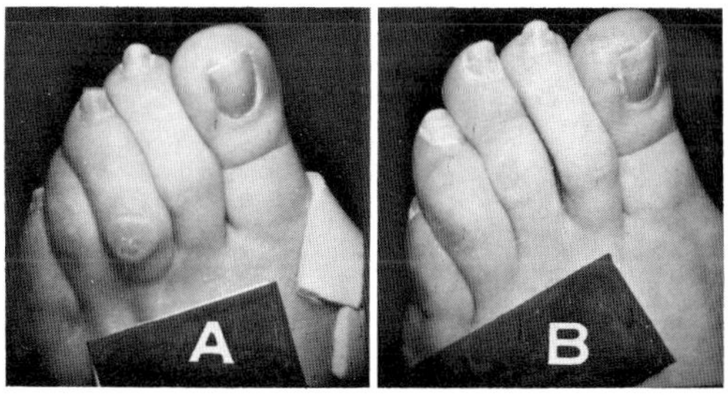

Fig. 17.8*A* and *B*. Correction of hallux and lesser toes.

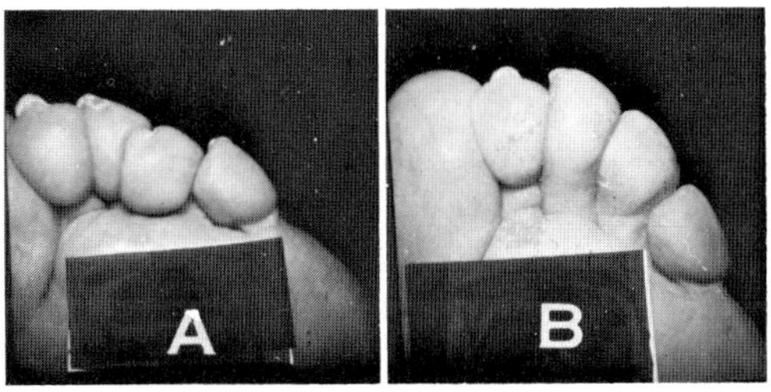

Fig. 17.9*A* and *B*. Phalangeal-set and osteotripsy. Courtesy of M. Roven.

lating bones. With congenital absence of articular cartilage, the apposing bone surfaces may unite and form a complete fusion. Bilateral fusion of the calcaneocuboid articulations has been reported. The bases of metatarsals and the tarsal bones are often fused without pathologic findings and therefore must be construed to be of genetic origin. Syndactylism is a fusion deformity involving the soft tissue of the toes. Occasionally, the phalanges are fused resulting in claw foot.

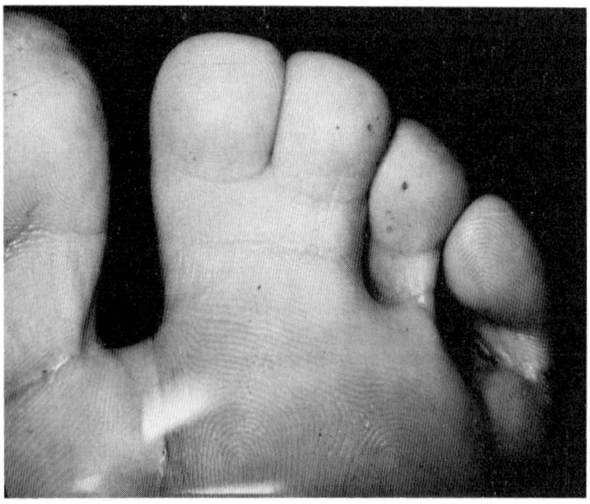

Fig. 17.10. Syndactylism.

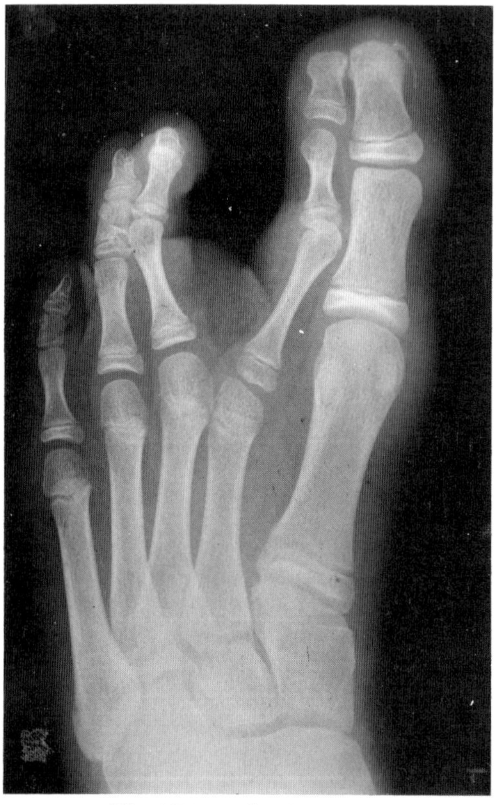

Fig. 17.11. Syndactylism.

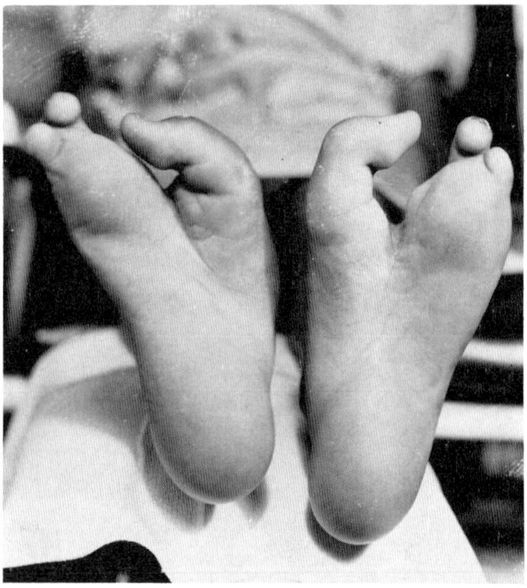

Fig. 17.12. Claw foot.

Fusion deformities may also be the basis by which the various bars develop between two or more tarsal and metatarsal bones. In this classification we would find the talocalcaneal-cuboid or the talonavicular-calcaneal synostosis. The treatment for these fusion deformities depends upon the extent of the deformity or the patient's ability to pursue normal activities with the affected foot. The proper application of a rigid orthotic appliance often alleviates the discomfort that commonly develops where a mechanical dysfunction exists due to synostosis. The orthotic is constructed to a cast of the foot. Under no circumstance should the patient with fusion deformities wear flexible-soled or shanked shoes. The motion produced by gravitational pressure against a flexible weightbearing surface increases the stress on the bony bars. Fracture of the bar is capable of causing a disabling deformity of a foot. Treatment and further discussion is beyond the scope of this text.

Polydactylism (polyphalangia, supernumerary toes). The fifth toe, as well as all other toes, may have a rudimentary center for development of an extra toe. Often the toe may have its own corresponding metatarsal or it may arise from the base of the proximal or distal phalanges, the heads of the metatarsals or form an accessory metatarsal shaft.

The treatment of polydactylism is based on the physiologic factors entering into the case and the ability of a patient to wear conventional footgear. The proper approach to treatment is surgical intervention as early as possible to eliminate the extra toe. Where additional metatarsals exist, plastic surgery to remove the extra toes and their articulating metatarsal bones is necessary. Another important reason for surgical intervention in this deformity is to remove emotional stress in patients who are often overly sensitive about the condition.

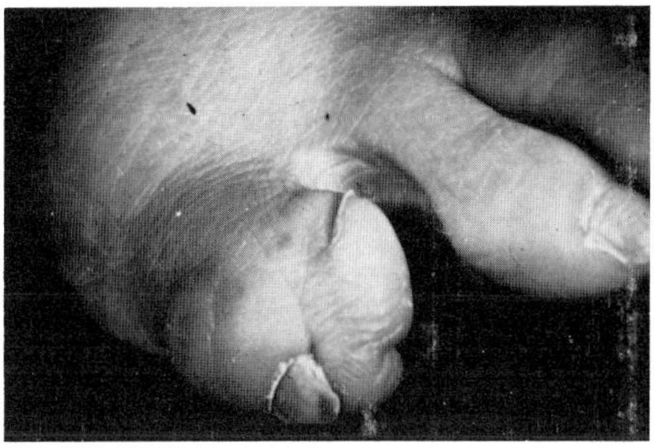

Fig. 17.13. Synpolydactylism

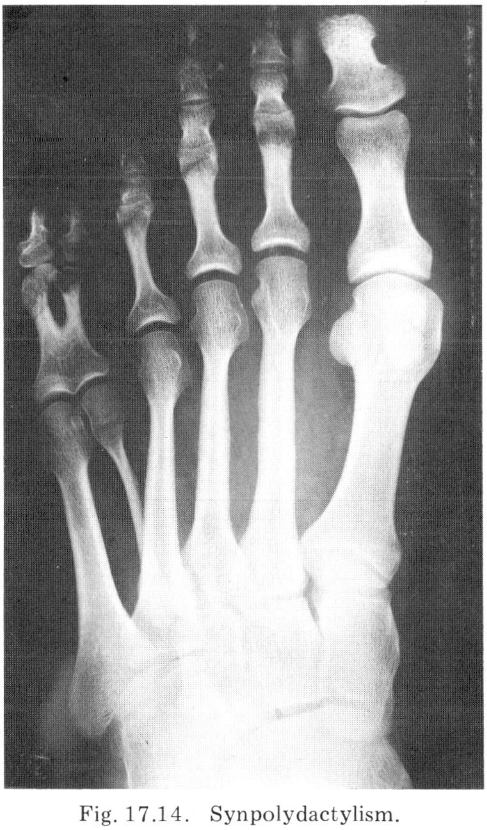

Fig. 17.14. Synpolydactylism.

Agenesis. This condition should be differentiated from intrauterine amputations of skeletal parts. In agenesis there is sudden cessation of further bony growth and the skin and subcutaneous tissue extend beyond the abruptly completed skeletal parts. The soft tissues may look like the absent skeletal part through their shape, although bony support is absent. The defect is in the skeleton and the parts show no evidence of ever having been present.

True skeletal intrauterine amputations may be differentiated where there is involvement of more than one extremity. There may be clinical and radiographic evidence of sloughing off. The soft tissues have multiple creases to differentiate them from true agenesis as previously described.

Treatment of this involvement is cosmetic unless the extent of agenesis results in faulty function and gait. I advise the early use of cosmetic devices to maintain emotional stability as well as to maintain adequate foot function and good foot posture.

Agenesis of a toe or entire forefoot may be accommodated in a shoe by a prosthetic device with shaped fillers. The prosthesis can be molded over a cast to fit the foot. An impression of the forepart of the shoe can be constructed with the foot in the shoe by stuffing wet *papier mâché* into the toe section. Other materials like rubber butter, silicone gel, or felt impregnated with latex may be used for molding. The podiatric device is ultimately a well-fitting, comfortable prosthesis. Ground smooth, covered with soft leather and fit into a shoe, the prosthesis enables the patient with agenesis to be a normally functioning individual with a minimum of physical or emotional instability.

A prosthetic device with simulated toes can be fit over the stump. In many instances it may be a necessary device for cosmetic purposes. The device can accommodate certain pressure points that exist with agenesis. Cutouts, build-ups, wedging and depressions allow for accommodation and relief of pressure pain.

Brachymetopodia is generally seen in hypoplastic malformation of the metatarsal bones. I have seen several cases of unilateral shortening of the fourth metatarsal bone. This bone is usually well formed but prematurely developed and ossified at the epiphyses. Cases of bilateral shortening of the fourth metatarsal bones and bilaterally shortened third and fourth bones are in our files. This development is considered to be either congenital or acquired. Cases of unilateral shortening have been observed presenting symptoms of a neurologic disorder unnoticed in childhood. Trauma to an epiphysis may result in premature closure and cessation of bony growth.

Treatment for brachymetopodia is based upon maintenance of good foot function. The construction of a prosthetic device to maintain proper foot balance is indicated. This obviously depends on the extent and degree of deformity and the ability of the part to function without pain.

Shortened metatarsal bones create faulty weight distribution. Adjacent longer metatarsal bones must accept a greater share of weight-bearing. Construction of a prosthesis is aimed at developing a broad distribution of body weight. Extensions of weight-distributing material beneath the short bone allow it to assume its responsibility in maintaining good stance and gait.

Absence of Toes. The fifth toe often develops with two phalanges. The proximal phalanx appears unusually long with a normal-sized distal phalanx. Absence of toes is common and is often seen with absence of other bones in the extremities. Cases of congenital absence of one or both sesamoids have been reported. Very often the distal phalanx appears fused to the middle giving a double phalanx appearance where only a single phalanx exists. These are rarely of clinical significance. However, a prominent base of the distal phalanx may be the underlying etiology for a heloma.

Treatment. Correction of foot deformities and faulty foot function due to absence of toes or bones of the feet must be considered early. Artificial toes may be constructed using silicone rubber. These may be incorporated into a latex forefoot prosthesis. Surgical excision of deformed bones may be indicated. Accommodative orthotic devices may be necessary.

Deformities of the Accessory Bones of the Foot. The accessory bones of the foot are often referred to as sesamoid bones. The only constant sesamoid bones are those that occur beneath the first metatarsal head. They develop by separate centers of ossification within the tendons of the flexor hallucis brevis. These bones may be seen on the radiograph as multipartite. The tibial or medial sesamoid is often seen as a bipartite bone. It is not unusual to find the tibial sesamoid in many parts. Each part is attached to its adjacent member by fibrocartilaginous tissue and is developed from a separate center of ossification.

All accessory bones may show evidence of trauma or pathology. The sesamoid bones beneath the first metatarsal head are subject to fracture and dislocation.

Sesamoids beneath lesser metatarsals are not uncommon. They are often multiple when present under the metatarsal heads and present a complete cortex and central ossific pattern. These sesamoids or ossicles are also commonly seen at the plantar surface of the interphalangeal joint of the great toe and must not be confused with calcium deposits.

The os trigonum, located at the lateral portion of the posterior surface of the talus, often is attached to and forms a part of the talus. A twist of the ankle or a sudden severe trauma may result in a fracture of this posterior process or a tear of its fibrocartilaginous attachment.

The os tibiale externum is posterior medial and slightly plantar to the tuberosity of the navicular. It is not necessarily bilateral as many observers have stated. This accessory ossicle may be attached by cartilage to the tuberosity of the navicular and become a part of it or it may become displaced from its articulation with the body of the bone and develop degenerative arthritis. Often it is inflamed from pressure of pes valgus when prominent on the medial aspect. A prominent tuberosity of the navicular may fracture with severe trauma resulting in a simulated os tibialis with a pseudo-articulation from nonunion. An acute adventitious bursitis may develop over the prominent bone.

The os vesalanium, os cambelli, os intermetatarseum, os cuneiforme intermedium, secondary os calcis, accessory os cuboideum, piries bone, os fibulare and os tibiale are shown in Figure 17.15. These bones must be differentiated from fracture fragments or calcifications of the soft tissues; when overlapped by bone they are often mistaken for nonreticulated areas, compact islands or innocuous bone nodules.

The presence of an os vesalanium sometimes results in a prominence at the fifth metatarsal base with an overlying callus. Acute bursitis may develop between the calloused skin and the prominence of bone.

The os fibulare at the distal end of the fibula malleolus must be differentiated from fractures of the lateral malleolus or displacement of the distal epiphyses. A cortical tear may result from a twisted ankle and rupture of ligaments. The torn cortex may simulate an accessory ossicle.

The os tibiale at the distal end of the medial malleolus must also be differentiated from fracture or epiphyses. Often a tear of the accessory bone from its fibrocartilaginous attachment simulates a fracture. Remember that the accessory ossicle has a smooth cortical outline.

There is a 2-year lag between ossification of the sesamoids in males and

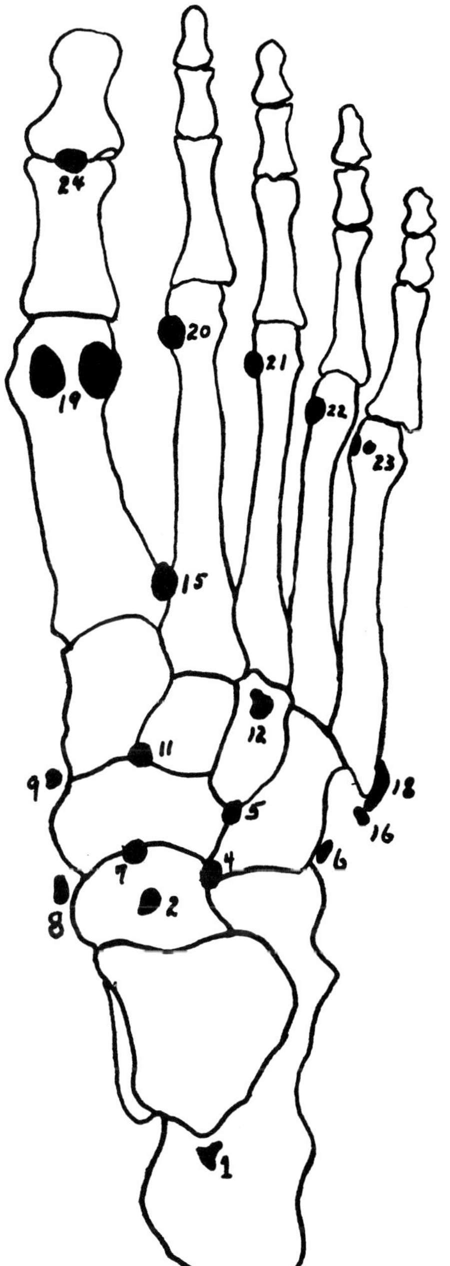

Fig. 17.15. Accessory bones of the foot.

ossification of the sesamoids in females, but there is negligible difference in the sex distribution of accessory bones.

Calcifications are amorphous with no evidence of cortex or internal architecture on the radiograph. They must not be confused with ossifications as seen in accessory bones.

Treatment of the accessory bones of the foot depends upon the status of the bone in function and structure. A sesamoid bone beneath the lesser metatarsals may be innocuous unless it has been crushed, subluxated or torn from its adjacent tissues. Resting the part with the use of felt and adhesive tape for a period of time is necessary to allow for complete repair and relief of pain. An appliance properly constructed to take pressure off the affected part may be indicated. Subluxation of sesamoids beneath the interphalangeal joints of the toes—most frequently the great toe—may be treated by immobilization, traction or both.

Damage done to the os trigonum is easily relieved with local injection of an anesthetic and steroid followed by immobilization with adhesive tape in the usual manner. A fracture of the posterior process of the talus is treated by immobilization with rigid or flexible castings to allow for repair of the fractured part. After the fracture has healed, physiotherapeutic measures may be used to hasten relief of pain and increase mobility.

Treatment of a painful os tibiale externum may be either conservative or radical. When constructing an orthotic device to compensate for some of the mechanical defects in a foot, it is essential that the podiatrist consider that a very high medial flange may result in great pressure over the os tibiale externum. It is not uncommon for a bursitis to develop over an os tibiale externum where a rigid orthotic appliance with a high flange presses on the bony prominence. I suggest that the flange be kept low and below the prominence of bone or that a pocket for the bony prominence be provided in the appliance. Where a degenerative joint disease has developed between the tuberosity of the navicular and the os tibiale externum, it may be necessary to excise the os tibiale externum if it is too large and interferes with the functioning of the foot. A semi-elliptical incision is made over the affected part, the attachment of the tibialis posterior is exposed, the os tibiale externum is dissected free from its attachments and closure is instituted in such a way as to maintain the integrity of the tibialis posterior muscle.

Hammertoe. The common digiti flexus or hammertoe deformity causes untold misery in this world. This deformity usually affects the second and fifth toe but may occur in any toe. The proximal phalanx is dorsiflexed on the metatarsal head, the middle phalanx is plantarflexed, and the distal phalanx is flexed or extended.

Hammertoes may be congenital, hereditary or acquired by trauma or disease and are usually bilateral. The second toe, because it is the longest toe, is easily traumatized by short stockings or by short or extremely pointed shoes. Hallux abducto valgus deformities are common with extreme deformities of the second toes. Rheumatoid and osteoarthritis may be etiologic.

The proximal interphalangeal joint is the highest point dorsally and is readily traumatized by shoes. Helomas, tylomas and bursae are the result of friction and pressure. The tip of the distal phalanx is very often flattened out, broadened and covered by a heloma or tyloma. The above excrescences break down in circu-

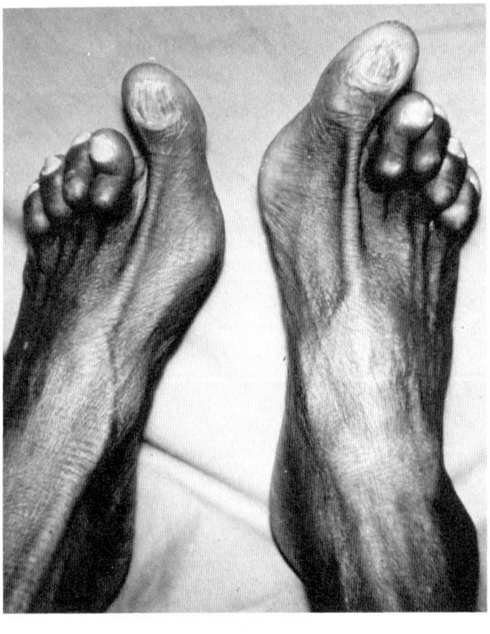

Fig. 17.16. Severe rheumatoid arthritis. Hammertoes. Note contraction of extensor tendons, prominent proximal interphalangeal joints with flexion of middle phalanx and extension of distal phalanx.

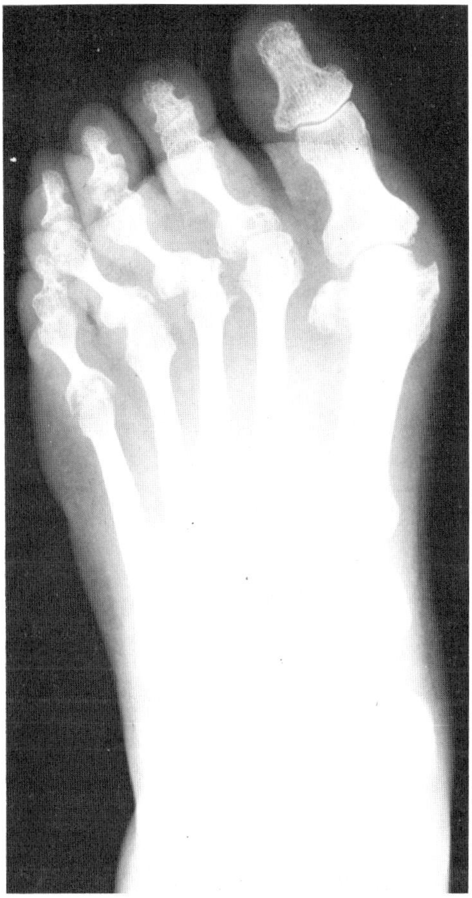

Fig. 17.17. X-ray, rheumatoid arthritis. Note lateral deflection of toes. Atrophic loss of substance chondro-osseous margins of bone.

latory or trophic disease creating an excellent focus for infection and subsequent sinus or trophic ulcer. The great toe may overlap or underlap the second toe. Callous tissue develops at such points of pressure as the second metatarsophalangeal joint, the dorsum of the proximal interphalangeal joint, and the distal end of the toe. Contractures of the extensor and flexor tendons, fascia and glenoid and collateral ligaments are noted. The skin on the plantar surface is contracted and very often fissured. The joints are enlarged and deformed. Ankylosis, usually of a fibrous nature, may result.

X-ray examination may disclose a calcified sinus or calcification of the bursa in long-standing lesions. Sequestration and a focal necrosis of bone may be in evidence. Lipping, osteophytes and loss of substance at the chondro-osseous margins are common.

Treatment. The treatment of hammertoe may be conservative or surgical. Conservative treatment may include wearing of different footgear to eliminate pressure on the affected part or use of complicated toe shields to relieve compression on the deformed toe. Conservative treatment is desirable in those cases that present poor surgical risks as only surgical intervention can correct an established hammertoe. In the early stages and especially in children, the use of adhesive materials to straighten deformed toes is often sufficient. Polokoff (1959) described his original double ring hammertoe device constructed from 1/16-in. Polokoff felt. Budin splints are helpful to keep the toe in alignment.

Plaster impressions and latex, plastic or silicone shields constructed over the cast have been used by podiatrists for many years. Moldable plastic materials and silicone products are currently being used along with tubegauze to create accommodative appliances for hammertoes. Inlay depth shoes allow freedom in the forefoot and relief of pressure. These shoes have a removable insole about 1/4 in. thick that

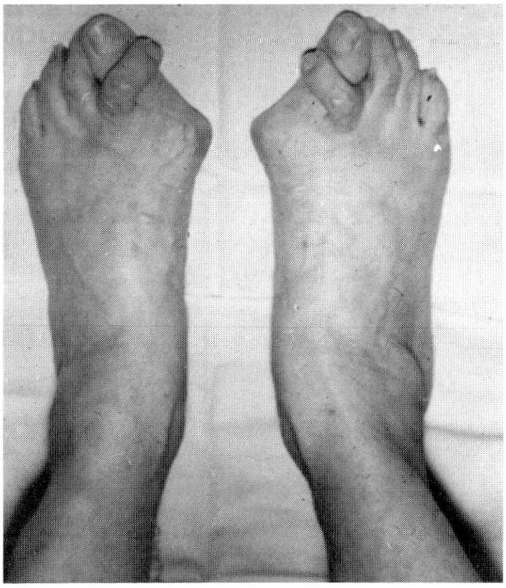

Fig. 17.18. Hallux valgus—overlapping second toes.

can be ground down to accommodate dorsiflexed toes.

Surgical treatment of hammertoe is described in the treatment of chronic corns. The initial incision may be longitudinal, elliptical, or curvilinear depending on the pathology. A transverse incision is made through the dorsal capsule and incision of the lateral collateral ligaments is then made close to the bone. Upon making the dorsal and lateral incisions of the articular capsule and ligaments, the head of the proximal phalanx is delivered into the surgical wound. The joint is resected through the neck of the proximal phalanx using a bone forceps or Stryker reciprocal saw or ultra-high-speed airdrills. Very small bites are made into the bone through the neck in order to preserve the integrity of the shaft of the bone and to reduce the possibility of splintering. The head and its articular cartilage is delivered into the wound and removed. The cut surface through the neck of the proximal phalanx is then rasped smooth and closure of the capsule is affected by the use of skin sutures that also include the capsule.

Another technique I use is making a transverse semi-elliptical incision around the painful excrescence overlying the joint and excising the excrescence and its underlying bursa. The joint is exposed and the same procedure described above is followed.

In some cases it is necessary to perform a tenectomy or tenotomy on the extensor tendon to the affected toe. In the severe cases where there is a subluxation or dislocation at the metatarsophalangeal articulation, it is helpful to do a capsulotomy at the metatarsophalangeal joint. Another technique where there is a dislocation at the metatarsophalangeal joint is to make an incision at the medial or lateral aspect of the toe exposing the entire proximal phalanx and dissecting out the proximal phalanx or removing the base of the proximal phalanx in order to realign the toe. I find that it is best to remove the entire proximal phalanx in order to correct both the metatarsophalangeal deformity and the deformity at the proximal interphalangeal joint.

When the deformity exists without enlargement of the joint margin, removal of the middle phalanx may be in order. The middle phalangectomy has been most successful when the middle phalanx is short resulting in good closure and little evidence of postoperative flaccidity. The treatment of choice with involvement at the distal interphalangeal joint is middle phalangectomy. In this procedure, a longitudinal incision is made over the middle phalanx and the entire phalanx is dissected from its attachments. Closure is made in the usual manner.

It is essential in some instances to create a bony ankylosis in order to straighten the affected toe. To do this, the head of the proximal phalanx is dissected out and the base of the middle phalanx is resected. The parts are apposed either by s.c. suturing to affect good apposition of the part or by pinning the bones with a Kirschner wire or Steinman pin. My experience indicates that pinning is unnecessary for interphalangeal joints and creates unnecessary trauma. A bony ankylosis will result if the part is splinted and maintained in close apposition following removal of the base of middle phalanx and the head of the proximal phalanx.

Where only soft tissue is involved in hammer-

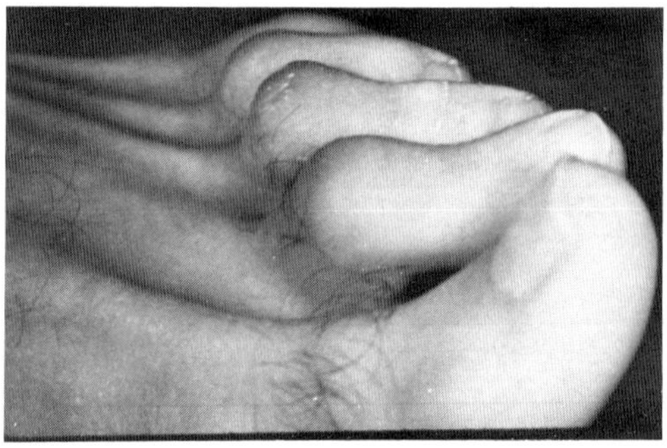

Fig. 17.19. Multiple hammertoes with contraction of extensor tendons.

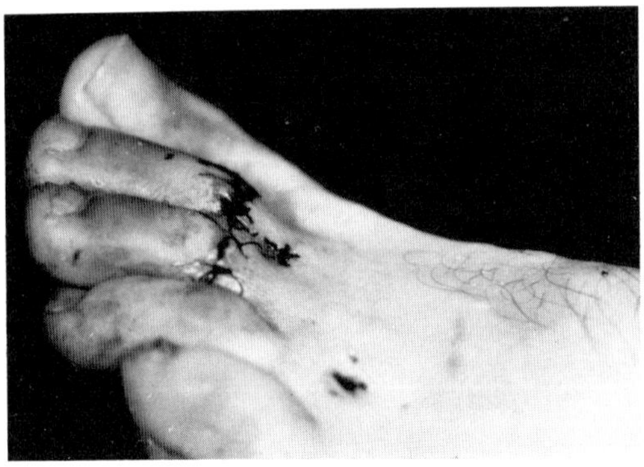

Fig. 17.20. Transverse semi-elliptical incisions removing ellipse, exposing extensor tendons, joint resection of the head of the proximal phalanx of second and third toes. Note site of tenectomy of extensor tendons to the fourth toe. Same patient as in Fig. 17.19.

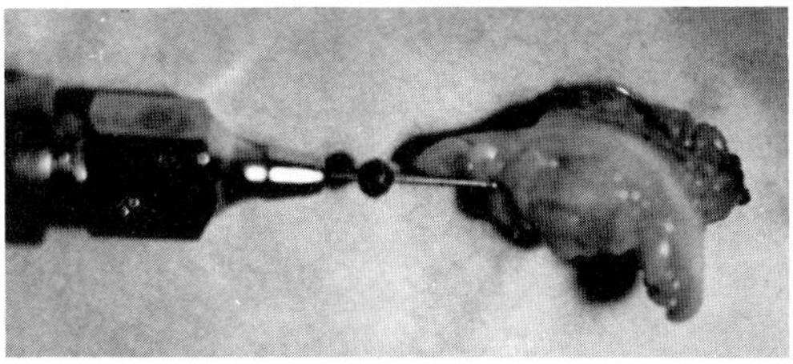

Fig. 17.21. Distended subhelomal bursa beneath elliptical section removed during surgical correction of hammertoe.

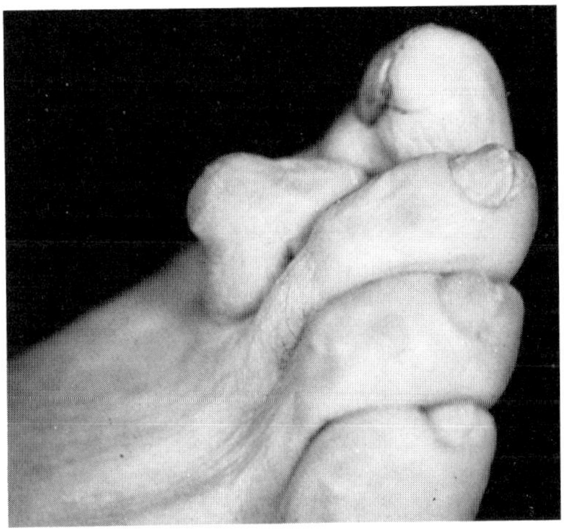

Fig. 17.22. Hammertoe.

toe deformity, cutting the plantar capsules and flexor tendons may correct the condition. This has been called "phalangeal set" by Roven (1969).

Hallux Flexus hallux malleus. This deformity is a hammertoe of the great toe characterized by a dorsiflexed proximal phalanx on the first metatarsal head with plantar flexion of the distal phalanx. This often is spoken of as a trigger toe. Lewis (1940) feels that this condition is usually due to a stenosing tenosynovitis, a synovioma or sesamoiditis.

Hallux flexus has been observed in adolescents when the child develops rapidly before shoes are changed to compensate for increased foot size. In conditions of foot strain, the compensatory contracture of the extensor hallucis longus tendon makes an attempt to support the arch by dorsiflexing the great toe. The flexor hallucis longus tendon is the antagonist in this case resulting in the deformity of hallux flexus.

Drop foot deformities from poliomyelitis or spastic paralysis result in great pull on the extensor muscles resulting in hallux flexus deformity.

Pes cavus, Schaeffer's foot, or so-called non-deforming clubfoot produces con-

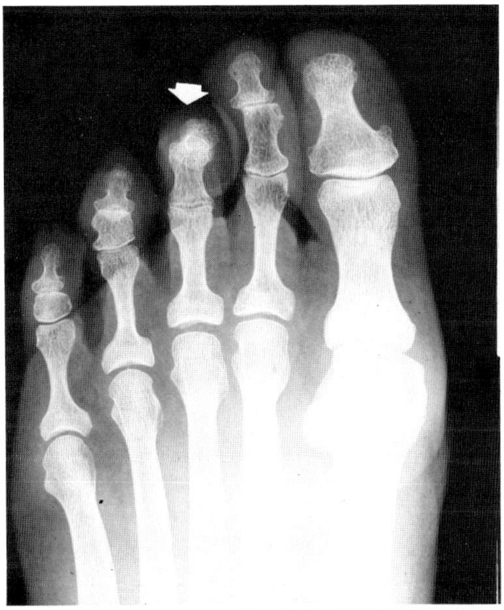

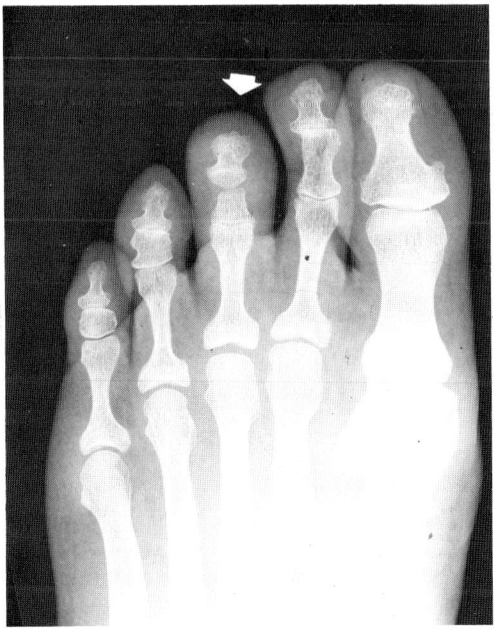

Fig. 17.23. Preoperative mallet toe. (top).
Fig. 17.24. Correction of mallet toe, distal interphalangeal joint (bottom).

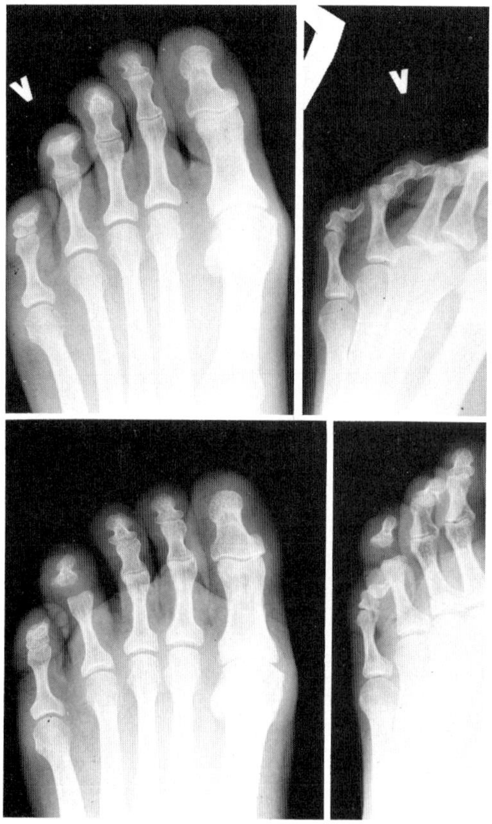

Fig. 17.25. Middle phalangectomy for correction of hammertoe.

tractures of the extensors with clawing of the lesser toes and hallux flexus.

A corn, callus or bursa may develop on the dorsum of the hallux with degenerative changes in the interphalangeal joint.

I have noted hallux flexus in children who present an improperly developed interphalangeal joint. The articulating surfaces are not transverse but angulated leaving an imbalanced joint and causing the toe to rotate in a slightly medial direction on its long axis.

Treatment of hallux flexus may be conservative and palliative or surgical and corrective. The congenital or hereditary deformities which result in a strong pull on the extensor hallucis longus tendon should be treated. The podiatrist must decide whether simply lengthening the extensor hallucis longus muscle would correct the deformity or if a complete surgical procedure involving the interphalangeal joint as well is necessary. If a lengthening of the tendon is indicated, a longitudinal incision is made to one side of the extensor tendon. The incision is deepened to expose the tendon and a Z-shaped lengthening of the tendon is performed. DuVries (1937) has developed a technique whereby he makes a small longitudinal incision at the medial plantar aspect of the interphalangeal joint, passes a small blade into the soft tissues adjacent to the bone and makes a transverse incision through the plantar capsular ligamentous tissues. The contracted tissues are released and the toe straightens out from its flexed position. However, where bony changes have taken place on the dorsal aspect of the interphalangeal joint it is necessary to remove the head of the proximal phalanx to affect a cure.

Treatment requires correction of stresses and strains which create pull on the extensor hallucis longus tendon. This is followed by lengthening of the extensor tendon, incision of the plantar capsule at the interphalangeal joint, and often a resection of the head of the proximal phalanx. Traction is of little help in treatment of this deformity.

Hallux flexus can be accommodated by an extra-depth shoe or the affected digit may be protected on its dorsal surface by a molded shield. Although this is a conservative approach it may also be beneficial after surgery in some cases.

Digiti Quinti Flexus. This is a flexion or hammertoe deformity of the fifth toe. The changes and symptoms are the same as those in digiti flexus. The digital branch of the extensor digitorum brevis tendon appears as a bow string on the

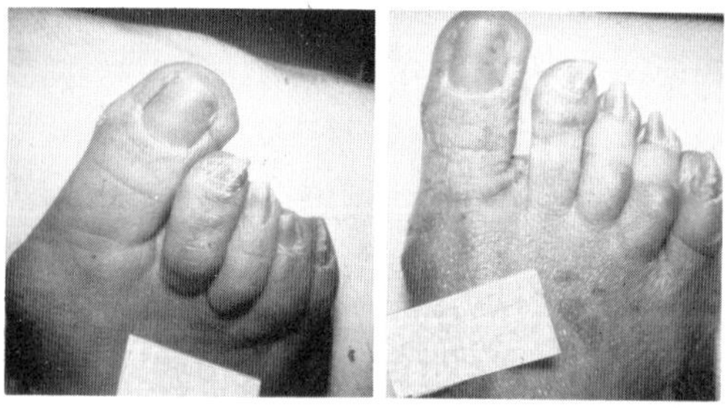

Fig. 17.26 and Fig. 17.27. Correction of hallux and lesser toes by osteotripsy and phalangeal set.

dorsum. I have observed several cases of tenosynovitis affecting the extensor tendons in severe cases of digiti quinti flexus. A painful heloma with underlying bursitis is common. A sinus infection may be present with periostitis of a phalanx visible on the radiograph. The sinus tract may be calcified if chronic. The margins of the articulating surfaces of the underlying joint present lipping and osteophytes with posterior displacement of the fat pad beneath the fifth metatarsal.

Treatment. The treatment of digiti quinti flexus is the same as that of hammertoe on other toes as described above.

Lengthening of the extensor tendon or incision of the dorsal capsule at the metatarsophalangeal joint and of the plantar flexors may be indicated.

Excision of a bursa or protection of the prominence of bone by temporary or permanent shields often relieves pain. Treatment of sinus tracts depends upon the extent of inflammation.

Goldhirsch (1957) describes the following technique for correction of digital deformities. The dorsal skin and subcutaneous tissue around the extensor tendon is anesthetized. No. 15 blade is used to puncture the skin. The blade is turned to contact the extensor tendon and the tendon is cut. On occasion, the dorsal capsule is incised.

Digiti quinti flexus as well as other flexion deformities of the phalanges are now easily corrected when soft tissue contractures are etiologic.

Roven (1969) developed a semi-closed surgical technique for reduction of malaligned digits. He coined the term "phalangeal set" to describe the realignment of phalanges. Under local anesthesia a stab incision is made at the level of interphalangeal joints to release contracted structures. Manipulation of the digits into a corrected position follows resulting in correction of the deformity. This technique is especially useful where bony deformity is

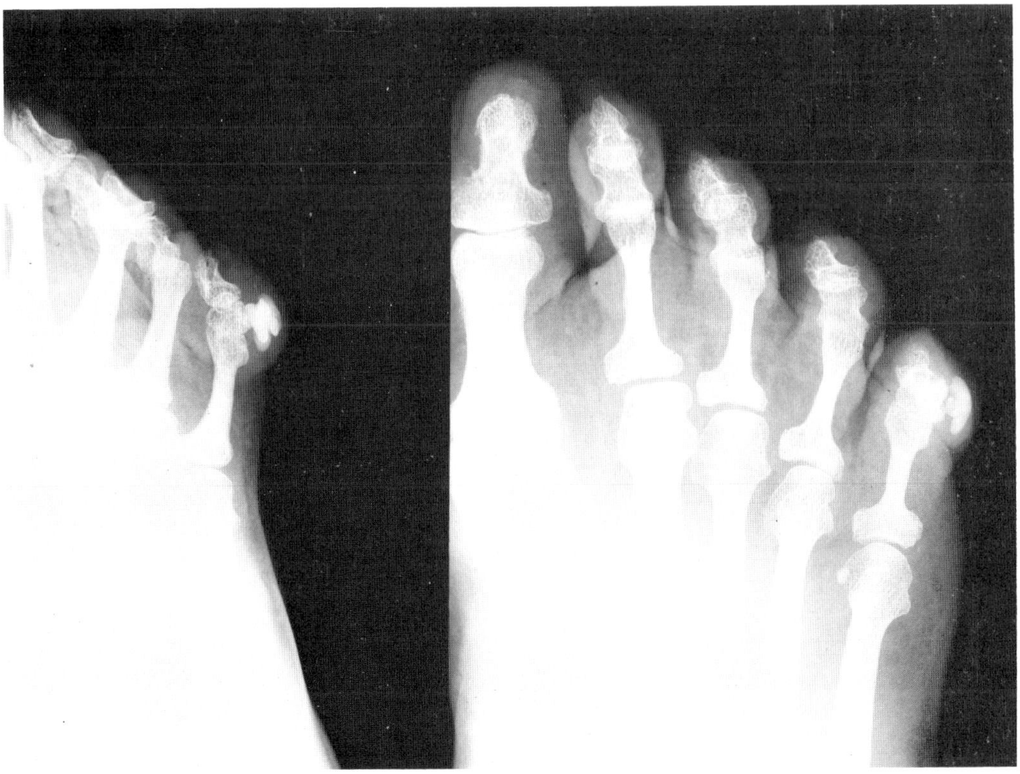

Fig. 17.28. Digiti quinti flexus complicated by subhelomal calcification.

minimal in a digiti quinti flexus or other flexion deformities of the lesser toes.

Hallux Valgus (hallux abducto valgus). This is a term given to the deformity in which the great toe is everted to an exaggerated degree and is kept in this position by accommodative changes in the cartilage, articular ligaments, joint capsule, sesamoids and tendons forming the first metatarsophalangeal joint. Its development is aided by short, narrow shoes with pointed toes. Ill-fitting socks or stockings may create abnormal stress while the deformity is increased by a shortening of the extensor and flexor hallucis longus muscle which, in their backward pull, evert the hallux commensurate with the obliquity of the first metatarsocuneiform joint.

Any inflammation of the joint may be a predisposing cause. Metatarsus primus varus may predispose to hallux valgus. The deformity is induced by changes following gout, rheumatism, infectious arthritis, traumatic arthritis and nervous lesions. The pronated gait of subtalar valgus may cause a hallux valgus.

As a rule, both feet are affected, although the deformity and symptoms are usually more marked on one side. About 30% of hallux valgus deformities are of congenital origin or of hereditary predisposition. I have seen several cases in which members of three generations in the same family exhibited hallux abducto valgus.

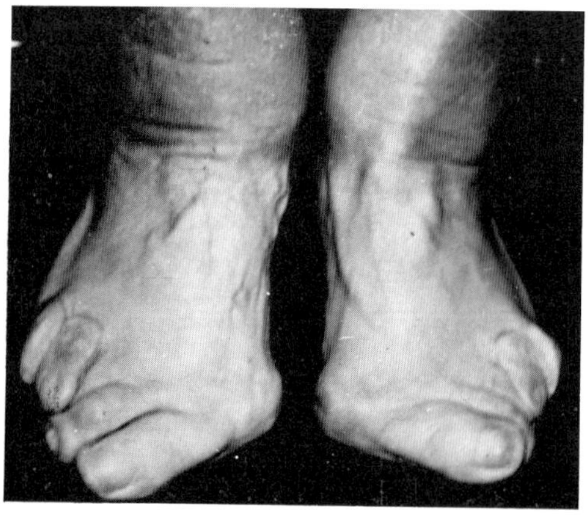

Fig. 17.29. Severe hallux valgus bilateral.

Pathology. The first metatarsal adducts and the great toe abducts; the second and third metatarsals usually adduct slightly while the fourth and fifth metatarsals abduct. The first metatarsal bone and the proximal phalanx may articulate on their lateral side by 50% or less. The cartilage on the exposed condyles of the metatarsal and phalanx usually becomes atrophied. Sesamoids are displaced laterally with the lateral bone lying between the first and second heads in the first intermetatarsal space. The tissues on the lateral side of the hallux joint undergo accommodative shortening and the tissues on the inner side are stretched and lengthened. Metatarsus primus varus with a compensatory pronation is noted.

The surface of the bone beneath the irritated periosteum becomes roughened and irregular; occasionally, exostoses due to irritation and pressure develop, thus aggravating the effects of lateral pressure by the shoe. The muscles around the great toe maintain and increase the deformity of hallux valgus. Once the deformity is begun—almost always as a result of improper footgear or genetic influences—the muscles complete the deformity. Muscles are continually contracting and when the resistance of bones is partially removed, as in the case of hallux valgus, the deformity progresses. The extensor and flexor hallucis longus muscles lie in the first intermetatarsal space rather than above and below the first metatarsal.

The flexor hallucis longus lying between the heads of the flexor hallucis brevis holds this muscle from under the first metatarsal head along with the sesamoid developed in each of its tendons. The adductor hallucis holds the proximal phalanx laterally being unresisted by the abductor hallucis which has slipped under the head of the first metatarsal bone or has been stretched by the shoe and pronation.

Symptoms. Hallux valgus is a condition present in many individuals to a

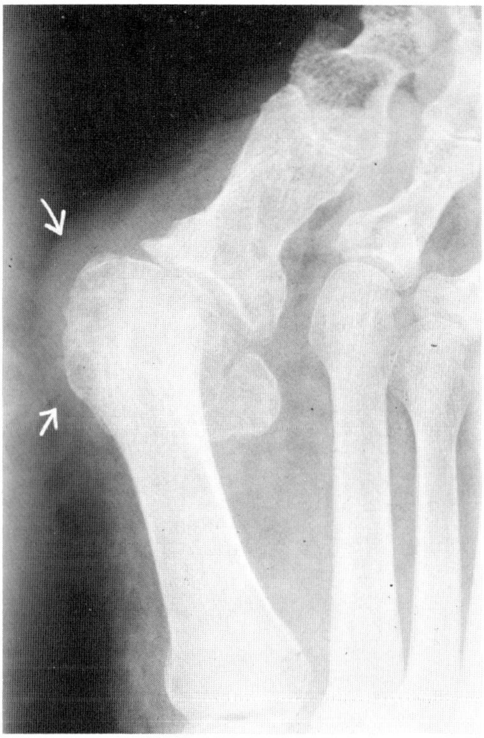

Fig. 17.30. Severe hallux abducto valgus.

point where it is not considered an acquired deformity. It is negligible if there are no symptoms of pain. The complications are more significant than the structural deformity itself. When the deformity is more pronounced the pressure of shoe causes pain, tenderness, and swelling. This eventually leads to the development of corns, calluses, bunions, septic bursitis, and, when it penetrates the joint, septic arthritis. Infected sinuses are common over the deformed joint.

The forefoot is hypermobile and spreads to allow for imbalance of the anterior metatarsal segments. Acute or chronic sesamoiditis may develop. Neuralgia caused by pressure on sesamoids and the periarticular structures may be present. Correction by the podiatric surgeon minimizes the complications of this deformity.

Roentgen Features. Marked lateral luxation of hallux on the first metatarsal head with either an imbalanced joint space or narrowing of the articulation is visible on x-rays. The lateral aspect of the articulating surface of the metatarsal head is being impinged upon by the lateral aspect of the base of the proximal phalanx which is rotated on its long axis.

A subarticular sclerosis is noted just distal to the base of the proximal phalanx. This consists of a dense, sclerotic, irregular line extending completely across the base underneath the articulating cartilage. The sclerotic trabeculae mingle with the rest of the bone. Effusion may be evident within the articular capsule while soft tissue swelling is present around the joint. A bursa is seen as a soft tissue mass or increase in soft tissue density overlying the deformed joint.

The head of the metatarsal may be altered in shape to a broad, flat, irregular, articulating surface instead of the smooth, rounded surface normally seen. The margins of th joint may present osteophytes, such as lippings and sometimes spurs. Hypertrophy of the trabeculae may be noted at sites of great stress. In the acute stages superficial demineralization from hyperemia or cellulitis often develops at the metatarsal head. Occasionally the overlying bursa may degenerate and become calcified presenting amorphous calcareous density overlying the joint on its medial aspect.

The sesamoids present degenerative changes such as degenerative periostitis, spurs and osteophytes. They are usually displaced into the first intermetatarsal space.

Care must be taken to rule out gout and rheumatoid or gonorrheal arthritis.

Treatment. Correction of hallux valgus deformities depends on the degree of deformity, the extent of pathology and the presence of complicating factors. It is essential to appreciate all the pathology that exists in hallux valgus while attempting correction. In the early stages, conservative treatment can be moderately effective with the use of hallux valgus active and passive exercises and splinting of the joint by use of night splints as prescribed. Special low-voltage stimulation, stretching and traction

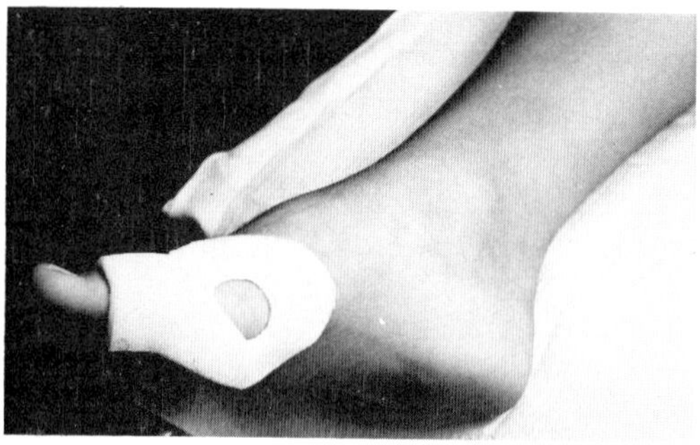

Fig. 17.31. Bunion shield—tube foam. May be impregnated with liquid latex or silicone gel for construction of a permanent shield.

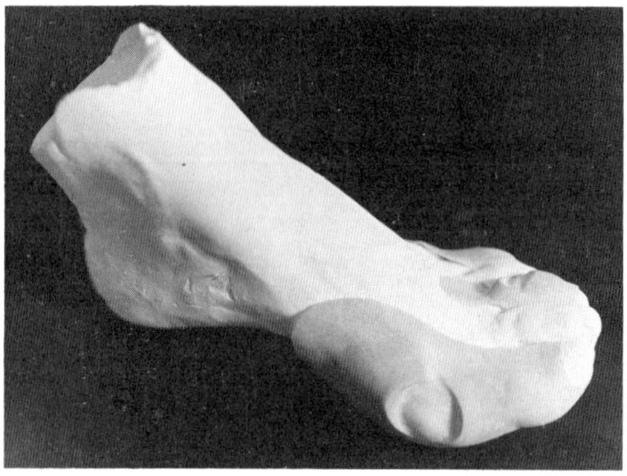

Fig. 17.32. Latex shield for protection of bunion over hallux valgus. Note shields on third and fifth toes. Courtesy of Liquid Rubber Appliance Laboratory.

devices, latex shields and splints, together with accommodative footgear may be helpful in the early stages.

Where marked deformity exists and bony proliferation and pathology involving the joint is noted, surgical intervention is indicated. The various surgical techniques for correction of hallux valgus have been described extensively in surgical texts. Modifications by podiatrists have resulted in a high percentage of good to excellent results.

Surgery must be sophisticated enough to attempt correction of most of the gross pathology. Simple corrective surgical procedures are often suitable for relief of pain and elimination of obvious minor deforming states.

Melillo (1972) has discussed the criteria for selection of a particular corrective hallux abducto valgus technique over others. He establishes his choice by considering the metatarsus primus angle, the presence or absence of motion at the first metatarsophalangeal joint, mild or severe axial rotation of the hallux and the degree of forefoot valgus.

The Silver-type technique is performed where the metatarsus primus angle is small, hallux valgus is minimal and the bones appear to be well aligned.

The McBride bunionectomy is performed when the metatarsus primus angle is less than 14 degrees and the hallux valgus angle less than 35 degrees.

Melillo notes that the Akin procedure is desireable when there is less than 14 degrees of metatarsus primus angle, a great degree of hallux valgus angle, a congruous first metatarsophalangeal joint and closure of the epiphysis of the proximal phalanx of the hallux.

The Keller-type bunionectomy is most successful where the hallux joint is painful, rigid, presents a degenerative joint disease, and extreme hallux valgus angle, a metatarsus primus angle of less than 15 degrees, and an elongated first metatarsal. Melillo has outlined preoperative, surgical and postoperative management for the above techniques, as well as the Stone and Mayo bunionectomies, Mitchell osteotomy and the closed and open wedge osteotomies of choice.

Digiti Quinti Varus (overlapping or overriding fifth toes; tailor's bunion). This is a deformity of the fifth toe,

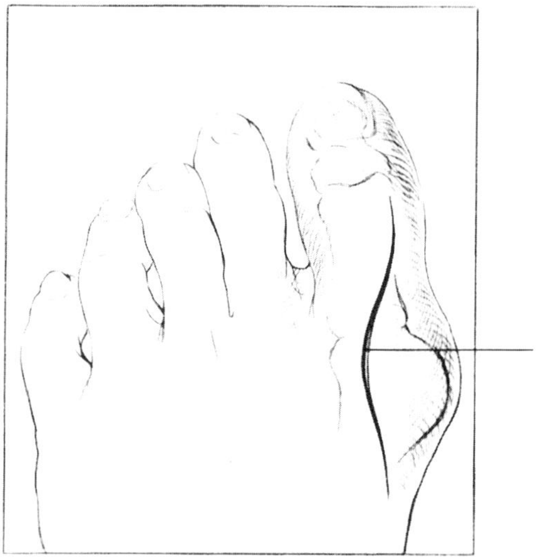

Fig. 17.33. Incision used for exposure of great toe joint. Courtesy of Hall International.

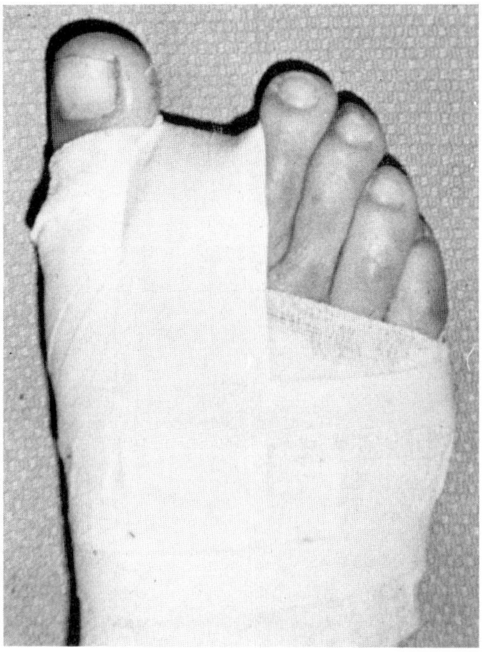

Fig. 17.34. Postoperative bandage—hallux abducto valgus.

similar to hallux valgus, in which the fifth metatarsal is abducted and the fifth toe is adducted and usually rotated outward on its long axis. The deformity may be caused by pointed, narrow, inflared shoes and is usually associated with hallux valgus as a result of increased lateral pressure. Trauma and occupational stress are principal causes of tailor's bunion. Genetic factors are to be considered when deformities show up early in life in the absence of trauma.

Pathology. Friction on the lateral side of the head of the fifth metatarsal gives rise to corns, calluses, bursitis and bony prominences on the fifth metatarsal head. Contraction of the soft structures on the inner side of the joint—the third plantar interosseous muscle, medial joint ligament, fourth lumbricalis muscle, fascia and skin—result in adduction and rotation of the fifth toe.

Symptoms. Pain is evident from irritation of the shoe on the fifth metatarsal head. The fifth toe may lie over or under the fourth toe. The lateral aspect of the fifth toe adjacent to the nail may be calloused and painful and a sinus tract infection or bursitis may be present beneath the painful callus.

Roentgen Features. A hypertrophied fifth metatarsal head and an overlying soft tissue mass are apparent. Superficial demineralization of bone with marked inflammation are noted. Effusion and soft tissue swelling may be present. Very often an infection may be evident to obscure the usual soft tissue response. A soft tissue calcification may be present in a chronic bursa or sinus tract over the enlarged joint.

Treatment. Digiti quinti varus does not necessarily present an overriding or overlapping fifth toe. However, the overlapping fifth toe may occur alone or with a digiti quinti varus. The treatment of choice in those cases that are poor surgical risks is accommodation of the lesion. This may require an alteration in footgear or the use of a shield to fit over the fifth toe and the prominence at the lateral aspect of the fifth metatarsophalangeal joint to protect it from injury. A shield can be constructed of felt, latex or plastic compounds. A plaster cast of the part is necessary and a latex or plastic shield is created over the cast by the dip method.

It is often a simpler procedure to construct the shield on the toe in dynamic fashion. A shield may be constructed with a toe ring around the fifth toe overlapping the fifth metatarsophalangeal joint laterally with a cut-out for the prominence. This can be coated with latex or silicone gel to give it firmness and

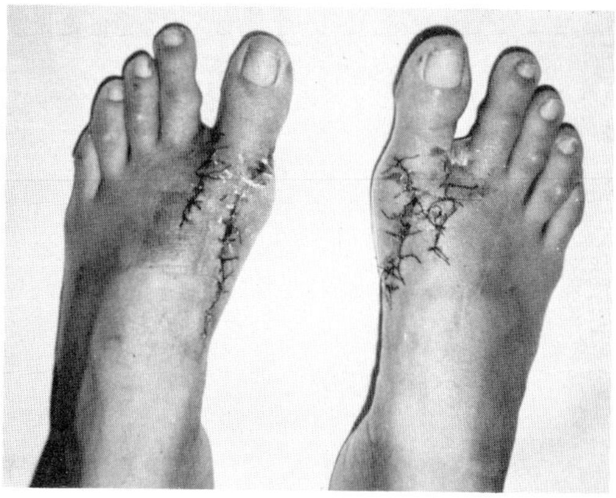

Fig. 17.35. Modified McBride bunionectomy 2 weeks postoperative. Courtesy of J. F. Yale.

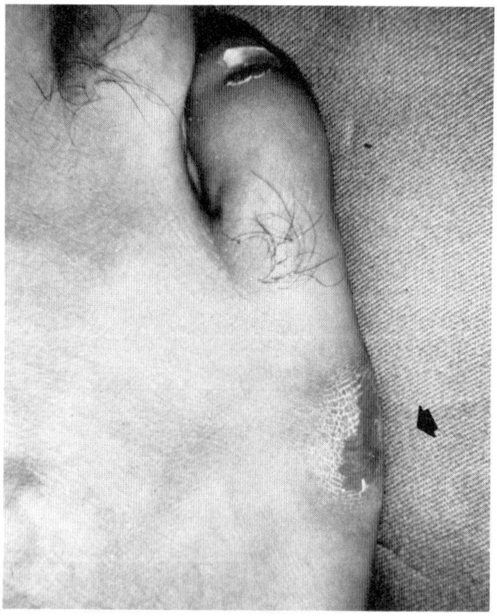

Fig. 17.36. Digiti quinti varus. Note overlying callus.

memory. The patient is provided with a covering—such as Saran wrap or other plastic substances—for the latex shield and is allowed to walk. The pad is dynamically shaped to the affected part.

Surgical correction of the digiti quinti varus should be conservative because of the importance of the digit in weightbearing. If surgical intervention is necessary, the following procedure is used. A semi-elliptical incision is made above the fifth metatarsophalangeal joint and is deepened to expose the articulation. A lateral transverse incision is made through the joint capsule exposing the prominent head of the fifth metatarsal. The joint capsule is reflected back and preserved. This prominence of the head of the fifth metatarsal is removed by a Stryker bone saw propelled by nitrogen gas, bone rongeur, bone forceps or chisel. Bone resection follows the surface of the neck of the metatarsal forward to the articular cartilage. The rough bone surface is rounded off with a fine bone rasp. The use of a Hall Surgairtome, an ultra-high-speed air drill, is especially suitable for rounding off the margins of bone.

Exostoses on the base of the proximal phalanx are rasped off without damaging the articular cartilage. Subcutaneous sutures are used to close the articular capsule; closure by layers is followed by skin closure. Where there is a contraction of the tendon of the extensor digitorum longus to the fifth toe, it is necessary to do a tenectomy on this tendon followed by a capsulotomy. A "Z" plasty to correct the contracted skin may also be in order if the toe is extremely contracted. Where calcification of a sinus tract leading into a chronic bursa is present, it is advisable to remove the sinus tract by a circumscribed excision around the tract down to the bursal area. Dissection of the bursa is essential and closure is accomplished in the usual manner.

Hallux Limitus is a painful affliction of the great toe characterized by a restriction of motion, particularly of dorsiflexion at the first metatarsophalangeal joint. It may occur in young adults or at any age and is caused by trauma such as stubbing the toe, a fall from a height, kicking a hard object or by a low-cut

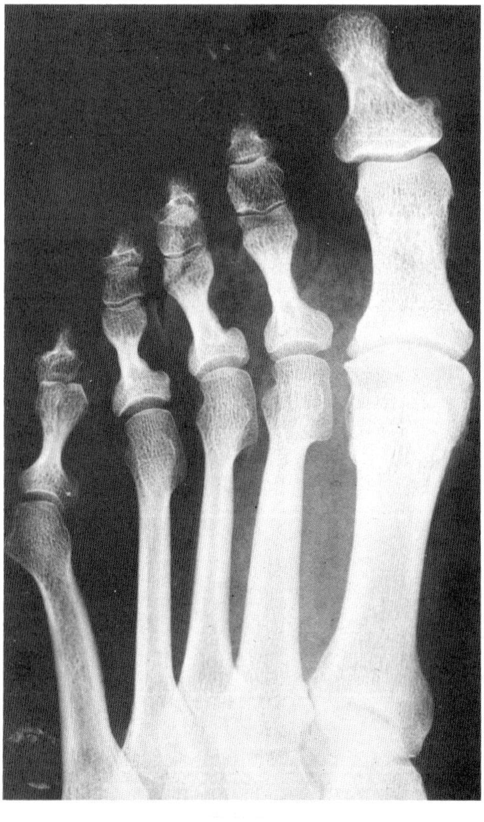

Fig. 17.37. Digiti quinti varus. Note prominent lateral aspect head of fifth metatarsal exostosis.

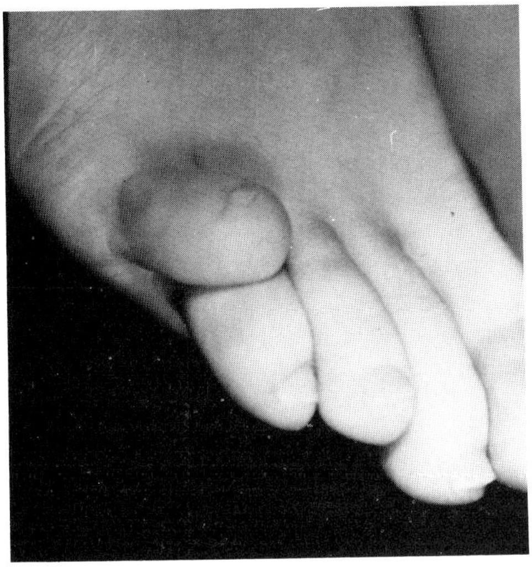

Fig. 17.38. Digiti quinti varus with overlapping fifth toe.

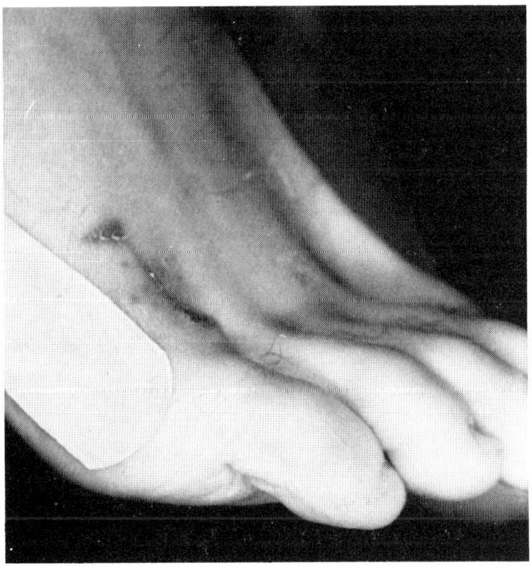

Fig. 17.39. Corrective surgery for overlapping fifth toe. The extensor tendon and dorsal capsule of the fifth metatarsophalangeal joint are incised. A "Z" plasty incision allows for stretching of the contracted skin. Repair of ends of "Z" by third intention. Same patient as in Fig. 17.38.

shoe producing impingement and limitation of function.

Infection, osteoarthritis, rheumatoid arthritis and post-traumatic arthritis may result in the limitation of function. Acute flare-up of monoarticular pain and swelling may be due to pseudo-gout such as hyperuricemia caused by thiozide diuresis.

Pathology. The affliction appears to be a form of periarticular fibrositis. The restriction of motion is caused by muscular spasm and accomodative changes of ligaments and tendons. In a recently treated case, I found that a marked soft tissue calcification was limiting function of the hallux joint. Protective spasms of soft tissues in recently traumatized joints may limit the motion of the hallux.

Symptoms. There is pain on motion and tenderness to touch, usually at the dorsolateral aspect of the joint. Swelling and redness is seen on the dorsum of the joint and there is limited motion and pain on flexion and extension of the joint.

The podiatrist may palpate an enlarged metatarsal head or bony growths about the articulate margins. Very often the distal phalanx is dorsiflexed from accommodative use as the fulcrum in walking.

Roentgen Features. There is a diminu-

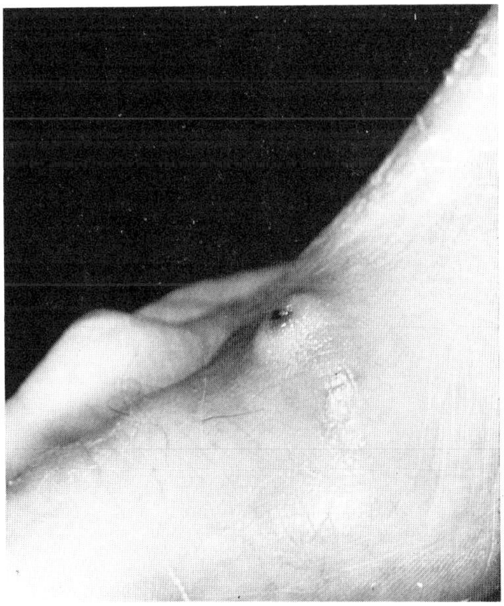

Fig. 17.40. Dorsal bunion—sinus tract, bursitis, dorsal exostosis. Hallux joint limited in dorsiflexion, often associated with tyloma, plantar surface of the hallux interphalangeal joint and plantar surface of the fifth metatarsal head as described by Locke (1952).

tion of articular cartilage; osteophytes and lippings may be present at the articular margins and a dorsal spur on the first metatarsal head extending upward and backward from the dorsal aspect of the head is common. The osteophytes are commonly seen at the external aspect of the articulating margins of the first metatarsophalangeal joint. I have seen complete ankylosis of this articulation with loss of function. Osteochondromas and osteochondritis have also been observed to produce this clinical picture of a rigid hallux joint. Calcareous deposits in the adjacent soft tissues, infection or tumor may cause hallux rigidus. An active tuberculosis of the joint may cause stiffness from spasms and contractures in the surrounding soft tissues. Acute gout may present effusion and limited function. Chronic gout produces destruction at the chondro-osseous margins of the joint limiting function. Loose bodies, chondromatosis or giant cell tumors may restrict normal function of the hallux joint. Gamble and Yale (1966) give definitive descriptions of the roentgen features.

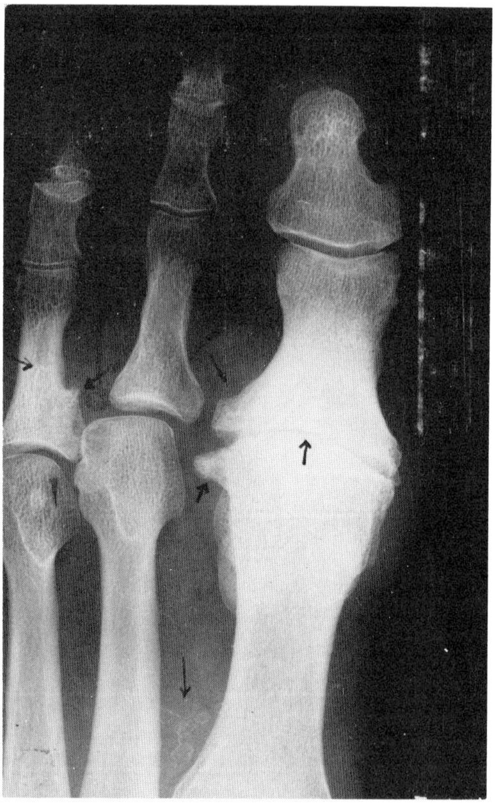

Fig. 17.41. Hallux limitus. Note narrowed joint space, lipping, osteophytes, exostosis and sclerosis.

Treatment. Limitation of function of the hallux may be due to fibrous ankylosis, complete bony ankylosis or contractures of the periarticular tissues. The purpose of therapy in most cases is to improve the functions of the foot as well as the affected part. In most cases in which there is slight motion in the joint, greater motion can be created with proper treatment. Improvement of function can be initiated by using a local anesthetic to relax the periarticular tissues. This is followed by traction on the first metatarsophalangeal joint accomplished with traction machines standard in most podiatry offices.

In addition to traction devices, foot appliances are used to relieve undue weightbearing on the affected part. This may require a steel plate placed between the inner sole and the outer sole to splint and relieve function of the joint to give it an opportunity to relax. In acute pain and swelling, Grovit and Block (1968) have shown that pain secondary to hyperuricemia due to thiozide diuresis can be relieved by injection of betamethasone acetate and betamethasone disodium phosphate into the affected monoarticular lesion.

Another technique is to use a balanced inlay appliance with a high longitudinal raise extending to just behind the sesamoids to transfer the weight from the affected joint to the lateral aspect of the foot. A rigid metal or acrylic orthotic properly posted can relieve pain. The use of various bars on the sole of the shoe such as a Jones bar and Denver heel is helpful. I have found that where a hallux limitus exists, relief can be obtained with a Thomas heel, rigid shank and extended counter, which shifts the weight laterally.

Joints that are completely ankylosed require entirely different care and treatment. Complete splinting of the joint by the use of a steel insole to keep the part from functioning is of great benefit in the relief of pain. However, if it is necessary to improve function where no function exists, surgical intervention may be necessary. This may involve the removal of any unusual exostoses, lipping or osteophytic changes around the margins of the joint. Resection of the base of the proximal phalanx is justified in extensive ankylosis.

If infections are present, they must be properly treated with antibiotics and drainage. The presence of tumors and exostotic overgrowths require surgical excision of these lesions to improve function. It may be necessary to remove the base of the proximal phalanx to establish a better functioning joint. The technique observed here is similar to that used for hallux valgus. I do not suggest total resection of the head of the first metatarsal to increase mobility of the hallux joint.

18

Orthotics, Appliances, Molds and Shields

Biomechanical foot disorders result in abnormal weight distribution with secondary alterations in supporting structures. The stress on an affected part is capable of disturbing structure beyond physiologic limits and creating pathologic changes in the skin, subcutaneous tissue and bony architecture. Many times the resultant pathology is not reversible and correctable. Yet, the patient requires relief from pain. This can often be accomplished by a thorough study of the problem followed by an evaluation of what is and what is not amenable to treatment.

It is not the purpose of this book to delve into the principles of orthopedics as they relate to the correction of foot deformities. The reader is referred to the fine texts on foot biomechanics. However, the day-to-day practice of podiatry includes the construction of appliances and orthotics to accommodate and correct abnormal structure and function. Prosthetic devices may be constructed in laboratories by technicians in accordance with the podiatrist's instructions. Some prosthetic devices are made by the podiatrist himself in the office laboratory and proper construction requires highly specialized skills. The podiatrist must construct, reconstruct and correct orthotic devices in his office if he is to practice his profesion to the fullest. In order to do this, he must be well-trained and well-supplied with quality materials and equipment. To this end, he is dedicated to seeking improved techniques and materials that lend themselves to quality foot care.

The type of orthotic devices constructed for the patient is only limited by the skill, ingenuity and creativity of the podiatrist who makes corrective orthotic devices as well as appliances, molds and shields. For the purpose of this chapter, the term *orthotics* refers to any device of sufficiently rigid construction to maintain the foot and its superstructure in a normal functional state in stance and in gait. *Appliance* refers to any device constructed of a flexible or semi-rigid material the purpose of which is to accommodate a foot deformity or lesion and limit pain. A *mold* is essentially an appliance that is molded over a foot or a part of the foot. It may also be constructed over a cast of the foot or a last. A *shield* is simply a protective device constructed of any flexible or moldable material over the foot, toe or a model of the foot or toe the purpose for which is to limit pressure, friction and extrinsic irritation.

Appliances Constructed in Shoes

Basic Insole Shells. Leather, foam, plastic and Celastic may be shaped to allow for heel cupping, for medial and lateral flanges and for complete heel-to-toe length basic shells. Leather insoles with or without 1/8 in. foam or impressable synthetic materials are placed in the shoe and the patient is asked to wear this for 1 week. At the end of this period the insoles are removed and the sites of pressure are evaluated.

Thermoplastic materials may be heated and placed in shoes. The unshod foot or the foot with smoothly fitting hose is placed in the shoe and laced firmly. The patient is asked to stand erect and alternately raise and lower his body weight from toe to heel. The material may be allowed to remain in the shoe for several days or can be removed, trimmed and cut to provide accommodations for plantar lesions.

Celastic insoles cut to size and shape with or without flanges and cupped heel are activated in acetone. They are tacked to a shelf and allowed to dry partially. Powder is placed in the shoe and the partially dry Celastic shell is inserted. The contact surface is powdered, and the unshod foot with indelible skin markings at sites of pressure is inserted into the shoe. After a few minutes of walking on the Celastic, the foot is carefully withdrawn. The formed shell is now removed and hung up to dry. Corrections and cutouts are made from the markings in the shell to remove pressure from the affected parts. Reinforcements of Celastic or corrections made of Celastic, rubber, cork, felt or other synthetic materials are applied to accommodate problems.

All the above shells may serve as the base for an accommodative appliance that is shoe-molded. They may be skived, ground down, cut out or built-up. The tops can be covered by leather or plastics.

Celastic Felt-Latex Molds. A 1/16-in. piece of felt is cut to fit into the Celastic shell on its contact surface, extending from the cupped heel forward to the toes. The felt is saturated with synthetic latex, squeezed out and molded with gloved fingers to the top of the shell. The entire unit is covered with strong but flexible plastic wrap and replaced in the shoe. The unshod foot is placed in the shoe and the patient walks about the office for about 15 min. The foot is carefully withdrawn and the formed mold is allowed to dry. To avoid shrinkage, the patient should wear the mold. This facilitates molding to the exact treading surface of the foot. After 48 hr. the entire appliance can be removed from the shoe. Cutouts and additional corrections may be applied to accommodate lesions and the top is covered with leather.

Thermoplastic Molds. Recently, several versatile thermoplastic materials have become available which have greatly simplified the task of the doctor and his assistants in fabricating foot molds. Rohadur, Prenyl and Neolite are a few of the newest of these materials. In field use, thermoplastics have enabled personnel with little experience to devise quickly and easily and to construct foot molds, foot prostheses, corrrective de vices, splints and braces, both statically and dynamically.

Thermoplastic material is available in large sheets or as a semi-finished foot orthotic. It is semi-rigid at normal room temperature, but becomes completely pliable when heated to approximately 140° F., average hot tap water temperature. Some materials require higher temperatures in a dry oven or over a hot plate.

Other Shoe Molds. Many mixtures of latex with cork, hardwood dust, fiber leather or plastic filings can be spatulated on shells or molded directly into a shoe. The material is mixed in a ratio of 3 of fiber, cork dust, etc. to 1 of latex. The use of synthetic latex is advisable to prevent shrinkage. A full foot mold with crest requires 12 level teaspoons of other material to 4 of latex. The unshod foot is placed on the mixture-filled insole and molded by weight bearing to the contour of the foot. A spray of equal parts of white vinegar and alcohol may be used on damp latex mixtures to accelerate curing. Rosoff (1953) pioneered mold therapy, including the contact mold, a contact pad for dresswear, a contact sandal and a shoe mold prepared by contact of the dynamic foot.

The mold can be removed from the shoe, covered with leather, trimmed, ground down or built-up according to the need.

Pre-formed insoles of impressable material, such as Molo and Contour-A-Mould may be placed in shoes for a week and corrected gradually to accommodate the pathology. These molds come covered with moisture-resistant material or may be recovered to suit individual needs.

A dorsoplantar radiograph of the feet, with a wire encircling the painful site, will assist the examiner in establishing the type of mold necessary for relief of symptoms.

Krantz (1954) described dynamic molding of a semi-rigid appliance; his technique is a modification of molds described by Rosoff (1953). The technique or modifications of the Krantz technique may afford a broad distribution of weight. The appliance is constructed of an acetone wet-down Celastic shell with cupping of the heel and medial and lateral sides which is placed in a shoe. The Celastic may be saturated with acetone and allowed to dry for a few minutes or it may only be sprinkled with acetone. The shell is placed in the shoe over wax paper and molded upon the sides and around the heel. The top is sprinkled with powder and the unshod-bare foot is inserted in the shoe. The patient walks on this shell for several minutes and the shell is removed and trimmed. The shell is painted on its top side with rubber cement. A mixture of rubber butter (equal parts of latex rubber and wood flour) is spatulated onto the top side of the shell. The material is covered with monks' cloth adhering the margins to the edge of the shell and overlapping it by ¼-in. The shell and its covered mass is placed back in the shoe and the top is powdered well. The unshod foot is slipped gently into the shoe and the patient walks about without stockings for about 1 hr. Stockings may be used following this impression period. A leather covering may be cemented to the weight-bearing surface of the appliance to complete the dynamic mold.

Schecter (1956) cites numerous researchers who have described the "fundamental physiologic and kinetic principle of a walking surface which takes on the exact contours of the foot and accommodates as well as supports

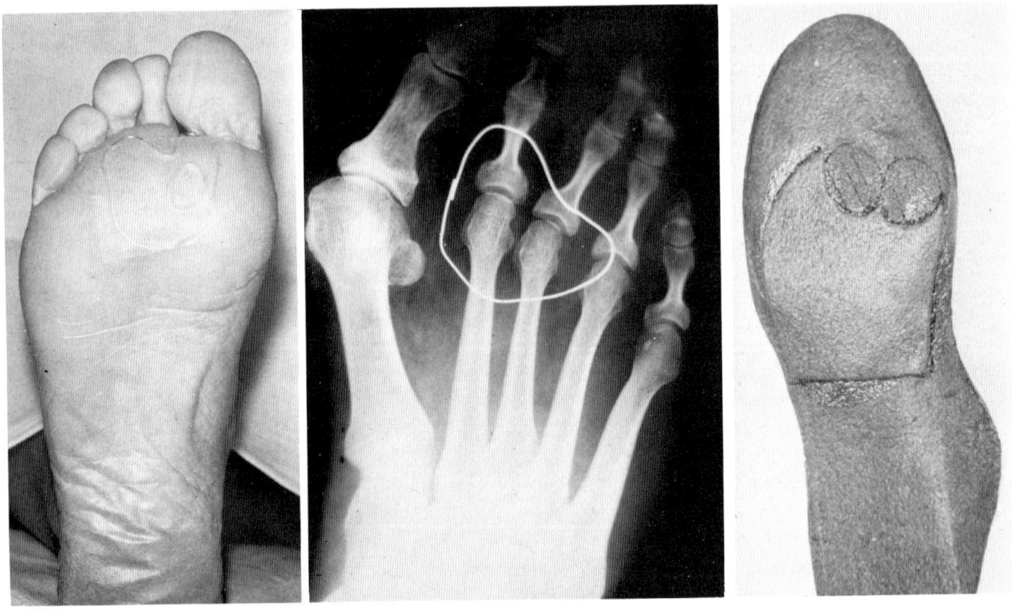

Fig. 18.1. *Left*, wire technique to isolate skin lesion prior to diagnostic radiography. Wire shaped to size of lesion and attached with plastic tape. Fig. 18.2. *Center*, radiograph depicting site of lesion. Fig. 18.3. *Right*, a Molo insole is constructed to remove pressure from the offending part. Courtesy of L. Hymes.

any imbalance." He states that ideally, the Levy mold technique should be accomplished by dynamic weightbearing on a new "impression" material rather than a cast. The adhesive resin does not dry, shrink, or set. The "impression" material is enclosed in a thin leather covering to form a shoe insert 1/8 in. and 3/8 in. thick. When placed in the shoe, repeated weightbearing results in a shaped mold. Corrections can be added to the under surface to provide additional support.

The finished appliance has a crest and cupped heel with adequate encompassing of the entire weightbearing foot surface. It is a self-conforming, self-molding, corrective and accommodative device. Many commercial impressable materials are now available for this purpose. Like all materials they are not panaceas, and their usefulness varies with the creativity and skill of the foot specialist.

Celastic Corrections in Shoes. I use Celastic shells cut out to size in a Whitman brace design for maintaining children's feet in a structurally acceptable position. The improvement of function generally relieves abnormal weight distribution through the rearfoot. It consists of a longitudinal medial flange with a lateral clip and cut-out heel. This approach to correction serves the foot specialist well as a means for early treatment of those feet requiring rigid orthotics. Celastic extensions under the 1st or 5th segments and a variety of elevations may be placed in the shoe to control the malfunctioning foot.

The Celastic shell is dipped in acetone and placed in the shoe. It is smoothed out with the gloved fingers using a heavy grade plastic glove to prevent finger irritation. The longitudinal area may be raised in subsequent visits by adding Celastic to the original shoe correction. The shoe is dried by a heat blower and powdered to relieve tackiness prior to wearing. This is not to be construed as a corrective device to replace foot orthotics made to casts.

Felt Pads Cemented in Shoes. There are many techniques for the construction of accommodative felt raises in shoes. These may include the placement of pre-cut and knife skived felt pads in the shoe to limit subtalar varus and compensatory forefoot problems in a manner conducive to relief of pain. Pads are adhered with rubber cement. The skived side is adhered to the inner sole and the pad may be covered with cover leather. The design of felt pads for shoes must consider the biomechanical advantages.

Plastazote for Accommodation of Foot Lesions. Plastazote, an expanded polyethylene, may be used without plaster cast models of the foot. The polyethylene appliance is constructed by making an outline of the foot on the sheet material (3/16, 5/16 or 3/8 in. in thickness). This is cut out allowing for a medial flange. The polyethylene is heated over a flame or hot plate and molded into a shoe. The foot is placed in the shoe and weightbearing for a few minutes provides an image of the dynamic foot. The shaped insole is trimmed and serves as a base for a permanent appliance. Corrections may be added to the Plastazote as needed. Cellulose acetate may be rubbed into the material to provide additional firmness. Rigidity is accomplished through the use of successive layers of gauze and cellulose acetate. When dry, leather or synthetic coverings may be adhered to top and bottom surfaces. Silicone gel may be used instead of cellulose acetate for a semi-rigid sturdy construction.

Dynamic Plantar Mold. The vinyl foam insole primarily is used to give more depth to the mold. It also smooths the inside sole of the shoe and can be used as the finishing undercover of the mold. Such themoplastics as Prenyl, Neolite and several rubber compounds are useful.

A vinyl foam insole is placed in the shoe and the heated thermoplastic material is placed on top of the vinyl. The patient then puts his foot into the shoe and walks around. If a metatarsal raise is to be incorporated in the mold, place a rubber pad of an individual design on the insole of the shoe before the vinyl foam insole is placed into the shoe. The pad will make a convexity into the plantar mold; the rubber metatarsal pad can then be removed.

If an excrescence on the foot is to be accommodated, place a ¼-in. piece of felt, cut to the size of the excrescence, on the excrescence. Put on the stocking and have the patient walk about on the heated insole. When the patient walks, the felt will make an indenture in the thermoplastic material. The felt piece is removed from the foot after about 10 to 15 min. when the thermoplastic becomes firm.

The procedure for duplicating an existing comfortable pad or shield on the foot is as follows. Outline the pad on the foot with an indelible pencil. Then moisten the inside of the shoe and have the patient walk barefooted in the shoe for a few minutes. The indelible outline will appear in the shoe. Remove the pad or shield from the foot and place it into the shoe within the outline. The pad can be held in place with a piece of adhesive tape. Place the vinyl foam and warm Prenyl insole into the shoe and have the patient walk about in the shoe. The pad will make a convexity in the mold. Remove the mold and pad from the shoe and adhere the pad to the underside of the mold in the concavity with cement. Adhere the vinyl foam to the Prenyl mold covering the pad on its undersurface.

Impression Techniques for Construction of Orthotics, Appliances and Shoes

Plaster of Paris, artist's wax and many moldable plastics may be used to take impressions for the purpose of diagnosis.

The most popular methods of taking impressions are done after indelible markings are placed on the skin over painful excrescences. Corns or calluses marked off will transfer their outlines from the skin to the negative cast on impression and then to the positive cast after the model is poured.

Slipper Cast. Plaster of Paris splints or bandages are dipped in water and molded about the affected foot off weightbearing. About three layers of the material are necessary for a strong slipper cast which extends over the toes from the plantar surface, about the heel, under the malleoli and about the dorso-medial and dorso-lateral aspects of the foot. For subtalar joint neutral control, the subtalar joint is stabilized while the forefoot is abducted and everted as the cast dries.

Toe Casts are made in a similar way by marking off the deformity or excrescence and either pouring plaster around the toe using impression trays or applying wet strips of plaster of Paris splints around the toe. Toe castings are used in diagnosis and for the construction of pads, shields and latex devices.

The entire foot or a single toe may be dipped in melted artist's wax after covering the part with a lubricant. The wax is cooled off by dipping the foot in cold water. This method is quite accurate for preparing study models in evaluating deformities of the foot. Pedi-Cast or dental impression compounds may be spatulated over the part to make a negative impression. A positive is poured and the impression material is removed when the cast is dry.

Foot Impression Technique (Grease Method). The grease compound impression technique first described by Adler and Babbitt has proved most successful in making plantar models of the feet. The materials used are: water pump grease, cup grease No. 3, two pans (each about 6 x 13 x 2½ in. deep), two pieces of cloth (larger than the pans, the cloth should be similar to that used in a man's T-shirt, a cotton bed sheet or a smooth face towel and a 3-in. metal spatula. Cover the bottom of the pans with 1 1-in. layer of water pump grease. On top of the water pump grease place a 1½-in. layer of cup grease No. 3. (This only has to be done the first time (except when replenished) because the same preparation is used over and over again after being smoothed out with the spatula.)

Wring out the cloths in water and apply smoothly over the compound. Allow the patient to stand, with moderate weight-bearing, in the compound and flex the toes back and forth slightly. Then have him sit down with the foot and knee at right angles and work the compound through the cloth under and around the foot making the amount of correction you feel is necessary. After the foot is removed from the compound, further corrections may be made, such as depressions for heel spurs, cysts or particularly sensitive bony prominences before pouring the plaster for the positive cast. No separating medium is required. The positive is easily removed and if the impression was properly taken, the cast will be perfectly balanced, and further correction on the positive is unnecessary. The procedure takes no more than 2 min. of the podiatrist's time, is accurate and the patient's foot remains clean.

Remove the cloths, smooth out the compound with the spatula and it is now ready for another impression. Hundreds of casts may be taken with the same batch of compound. Yale (1952 and 1960) described this technique and I am using it today for 99% of patients' casts. It is especially suitable for the Root techniques. Levine (1971) described a similar technique and gives credit to Skliar and Schuster.

With careful analysis of the plaster casts of feet of patients suffering from biomechanical disturbances, a proper orthotic device can be designed. Corroborative weight-bearing points, marked off excrescences, and weight-bearing radiographs are used to assure accuracy in construction. The use of the plaster

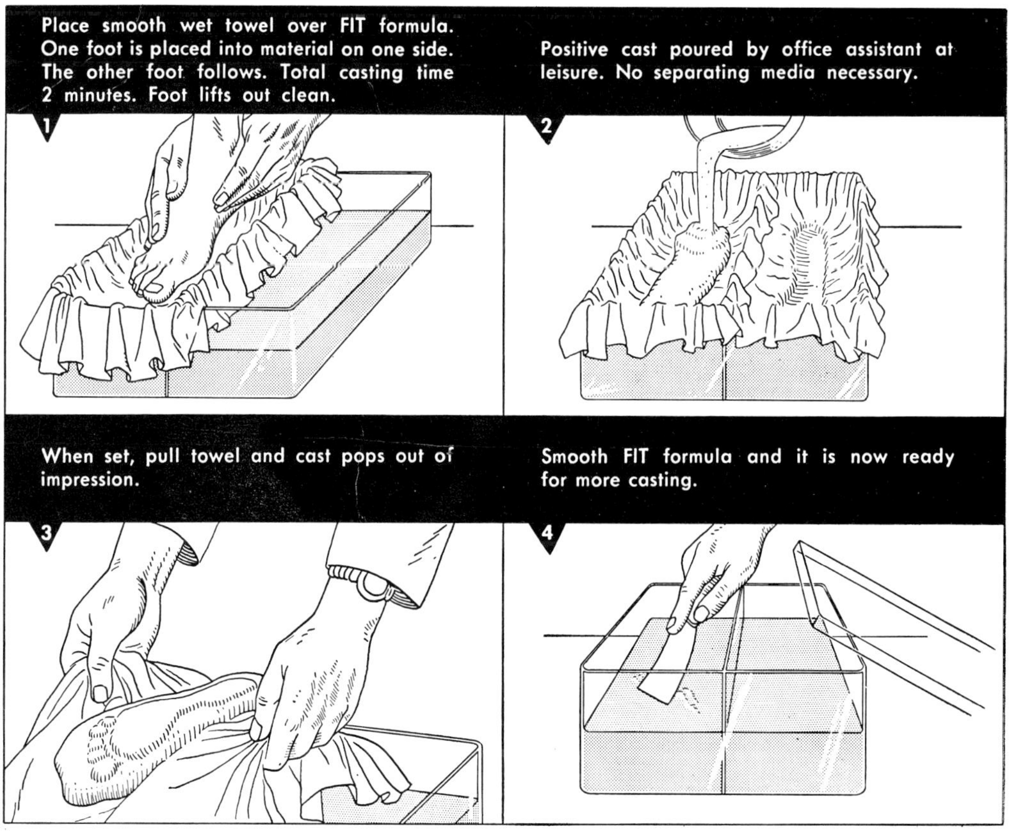

Fig. 18.4. Foot impression technique.

cast has been in disrepute until recent years. The evolution of biomechanical principles has revived many plaster cast techniques. Heretofore, the casting methods were based on the doctor's ability to correct and balance the cast before designing the orthotics. With this method of correction the orthotic frequently was subject to the errors produced by human inaccuracies and lack of standardization. Very little correction of the positive cast is necessary with modern techniques of casting for foot deformities.

Unique Casting Technique for Shoes. Rossi (1951) described a unique casting technique being used by the National Shoe Foundation for Disabled Feet, Boston, Mass. This included a cast-making machine which results in a 99.9% accurate cast for construction of a shoe last. The foot is placed in a pan of tiny ball bearings. The foot with full body weight makes a solid impression. A switch "freezes" the bearings electromagnetically. The impression is frozen in cold steel.

The method of balancing feet rather than producing abnormal corrective forces has proven its value in the treatment of biomechanical problems. Castings are used by the laboratory technician with an eye to balance of the foot in the shoe. The excrescences marked off by skin pencil are indelibly reprinted on the negative cast and then transferred to the positive. Corrections are made with an effort to accommodation of faulty foot structure and corrective forces are placed where they do the most good for the pathology.

Simplified Casting Technique for Orthotics and Molded Shoes. Miller (1971) uses the following technique for molded shoes. It can also be used for construction of orthotic devices.

Materials Required include two Polyfoam blocks measuring 1½ in. thick, 6 in. wide and 14 in. long; plaster of Paris bandage splints, extra fast setting, sizes 8 x 14, 6 pieces, 5 x 15, 10 pieces. Separator material is optional. Water glass mixed 50% with water or a tincture of green soap solution may be used as a separator. Absorbent paper towels and a basin of water are also necessary.

The Polyfoam is covered with a paper towel.

To cast the plantar area and heel, wet three pieces of the 8 x 14-in. splint and place on top of the towel. Immediately place the foot on top of the splints. Fold a piece of the 5 x 15 splint in half making it 5 x 7½, wet it and place it on the heel of the foot, bringing it well above the malleolus. To reinforce this edge, fold the splint back on itself at the malleoli. Bring the splint up around the heel and the inner and outer borders of the foot. Depress the foam rubber in front of the toes, and with your fingers push the splints up into the crest area. Now do the other foot. When you have completed the other foot, the first cast

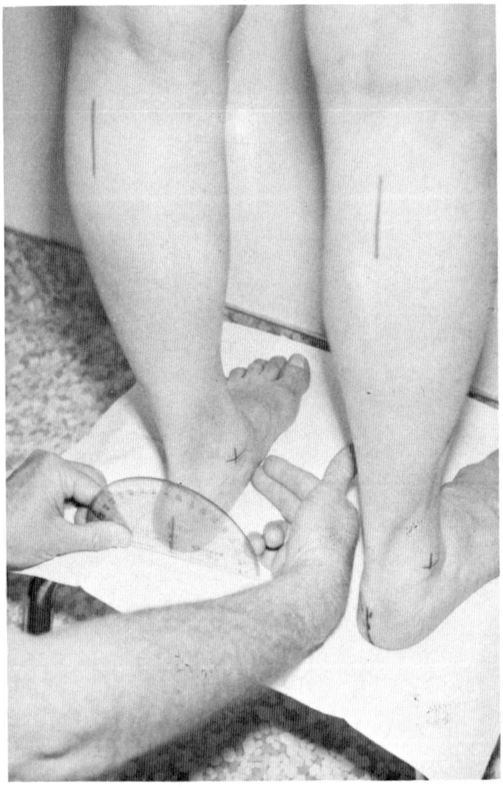

Fig. 18.5. Measuring heel rotation at rest and on weight bearing. Courtesy of Burns' Podiatric Laboratory, McCook, Neb.

will be dry enough to work the upper impression.

To cast the upper, paint the separating medium on the edges of the heel and plantar splints (optional). Using the 5 x 15 splints folded in half, build up the upper cast by laying one piece over the toes and overlapping the plantar impression. Then place a splint across the top of the foot from the malleolus forward, one on each side overlapping on the dorsum. The fourth piece should be placed on top of the foot from the top of the ankle to the toe. To reinforce the edges at the malleoli, fold the splint back on itself leaving an overlap of the heel splint of approximately ¼ in. Repeat this process on the other foot.

To remove the foot from the mold, loosen the edges that were reinforced at the malleoli and lift the front top piece upward. Pull gently away from the foot. Now lift the foot from the plantar and heel impression as gently as possible to prevent distortion. The upper and plantar negative casts are put together as a whole before sending them to the laboratory for processing.

Polyfoam Cast. Another method widely used is the non-plaster foot mold made in a solid tray of polyfoam. The foot is pressed carefully into the foam. When the foot is removed a beautiful, clean negative cast is ready in seconds. The disadvantage to this method is that the solid tray of foam can only be used once and is discarded.

Accommodative Orthotics and Shields Constructed to Plaster Models

Plaster casts may be used as models for the construction of foot appliances. The technique of casting feet varies. A negative slipper cast taken at rest with plaster of Paris splints, as previously described, is the most commonly used technique. When dry, a liquid soap or oily agent is used on the inside of the negative cast and a creamy plaster of Paris mix is poured into the negative cast to make the positive. The original negative is torn off the dry positive. The cast may have to be corrected. This can be done by scraping with a knife or by Screen-Pak.

Felt Latex Appliances. The positive cast is prepared by marking off excrescences with skin pencil. A light coating of paraffin is rubbed over the surface of the cast.

Longitudinal and metatarsal felt raises of suitable thickness are cut out and feather-edged by skiving. A strip of 1/8-in. felt is cut to a size which covers the entire treading surface and sides of the cast.

The felt is soaked in synthetic liquid latex and the excess is squeezed out. The 1/8-in. felt latex is molded over the positive cast allowing for cupping at the heel with medial and lateral flange.

The felt corrective raises after being dipped in latex are placed in position on the felt latex cast covering and molded into the material until it appears as one solid piece with corrections. The latex is self-vulcanizing and will be dry in a few days. The entire felt latex mold is removed from the cast, cut to shape and feather-edged by grinding. The mold is then covered with leather. Cut-outs are made to accommodate excrescences and bony prominences. Additional raises may be applied to the under surface of the felt-latex at a later date.

Synthetic Resins or Rubber Butter appliances. Synthetic resins or latex are combined with cork, plastic or hardwood dust to make a thick, creamy mass called "latex butter." The latex butter is spatulated on the cast to cover the bottom, sides and back of the heels. The arch and crest of the cast is filled with the rubber butter and the cast is placed sole-down on plate-glass or plastic to dry in a neutral position. After a few days the rubber is self-vulcanized and dry enough to be removed from the cast. The mold is covered with leather and the under surface is ground to fit the shoe. Additional wedges and elevations are applied to the undersurface of the appliance to control heel rotation and compensatory forefoot changes. The rubber butter appliance can be elevated at any time. Grinding out areas receiving pressure or stress can accommodate for excrescences and prominences. Balancing the applicance may correspond to measurements of structure and function of the foot at rest and on weight bearing.

Latex Shields. It is essential to use great care in taking the negative cast of a part. Impressions of deformed toes or other bony prominences on the foot are smoothed by fine sandpaper. The plaster cast is then dipped into natural latex several times and allowed to vulcanize and dry. A suitable foam, sponge or felt shield is adhered to the latex by rubber cement. The entire mass is then dipped into liquid latex two more times to cover the adhered shields and pads. This is allowed to dry for 24 hr. The shield on the cast is powdered well, removed from the cast and trimmed to fit the casted toe. Podiatrist laboratories are available for construction of latex shields to casts.

Tubegauze Shields. The toe cast or affected toe is covered with rubber cement or silicone gel. Tubegauze is cut to provide a covering for the entire toe with an overlap in back and forward of the toe. This is slipped on the toe or cast.

The bony prominences and excrescences are shielded with sponge rubber, foam, felt or other suitable material adhered by cement or silicone gel over the tubegauge. The tubegauze is coated with natural liquid latex or silicone gel and its distal overlapping tubegauze is turned back on itself to cover the shield. The entire shield is coated with more natural latex or silicone gel to a desired thickness, and allow to dry on the cast for 24 hr.

The prosthesis made on the toe is allowed to vulcanize on the toe as a dynamic shield. It is protected by household plastic wrap and covered with stocking and shoe. At the next visit the shield is removed from the positive cast or toe, trimmed, covered by more latex or silicone and dispensed as a replaceable shield.

Contact Appliance for Use in Conventional Footgear

Rosoff (1961) describes the fabrication of contact appliances for use in conventional footgear. He allows the patient to select a casual type of sandal. This is converted into a molded platform for the needs of the patient and for rehabilitative and therapeutic purposes. Rosoff states that the ultimate objectives of the contact sandal are to "create an environment simulating barefoot walking, and to create a type of footgear, protective and rehabilitative in nature, whose function is to induce toe flexion in varying and controlled degree."

The proper sandal selected must have front straps that are adjustable and long enough to accommodate additional bulk under the foot. The wedge height should be comfortable to wear.

Construction of a molded platform may vary with the individual practitioner. Rosoff's technique embodies a felt latex mold, the same size as the insole of the shoe over which is spatulated about 3 oz. of rubber butter. This is covered with a stockinette by slitting one side and placing it about the felt latex mold and rubber butter to make an envelope. Plaster of Paris, serving as an accelerator, is dusted on the under and top surfaces, and the entire envelope is placed on the insole of the sandal and the foot is gently placed in position. The straps are tightened and the patient stands in moderate weightbearing. The toes are alternately flexed to allow for disperson of the rubber butter. The foot is removed and the molded sandal is allowed to dry for 24 hr. The top of the mold is covered with a soft matching leather and the contact appliance is completed.

Pre-Molded Shells

I have used pre-molded shells to construct foot orthotics and appliances.

These are generally constructed of moldable leather or plastic compounds.

The proper size and style is selected for the individual type of foot problem.

The leather shell is softened in water and applied to the corrected cast and bound down firmly with an elasticized bandage. When the shell is dry, proper longitudinal and forefoot buildups are adhered to the under surface. The correction is ground to balance and distribute weight properly. The bottom is covered with leather. If the shell is a rubberized compound softened by heat, it is applied to the cast and bound down until firm and shaped. The bottom is balanced or cut out where indicated and covered with leather. Edges are ground down to a feather edge.

Premolded thermoplastics may be softened and bound down to the plaster cast. They may also be placed in the shoe and molded by the weightbearing foot. Celastic shells may be dipped in acetone and molded over a cast. Corrections may be added as necessary using rubber, leather, felt, cork or combinations of these materials and the entire orthotic device is covered with leather.

Orthodigital Correction by Molds and Shields

Fisher (1963) described a technique of taking impressions of deformities of the toes using dental impression techniques. This is followed by pouring a positive cast and the construction of a rubber and plastic orthodigital device under heat and pressure. The completed device can be ground down or increased in bulk to exert corrective forces on underlapping, varus and valgus of the toes, hammertoes, overriding toes, hallux valgus and a variety of forefoot deformities. The device is semi-rigid, durable and easily adjusted.

Polyurethane in a block about 3 x 3 x 1 in. can be used for a customized orthodigital correction for overlapping or underlapping toes. Small holes are punched in the material to correspond to and for insertion of the second, third and fourth toes. A hole may be lower or higher for an individual toe depending on the need to lower or raise the toe. The polyurethane is placed in a plastic bag with some liquid latex and squeezed repeatedly to allow for absorption of the liquid rubber. When the polyurethane is saturated the toes are placed through the previously cut holes. The entire mass is covered by a plastic bag and stocking. The foot is carefully placed in the shoe; the patient walks and shapes a flexible but firm forefoot mold over the deformed toes. This technique provides a polyurethane pad that will protect deformed toes and correct minor deformities where surgical correction is contraindicated. A plantar crest and dorsal pressure pad are formed to retain the parts in apposition.

Whitney (1963, 1965) described and illustrated urethane mold therapy.

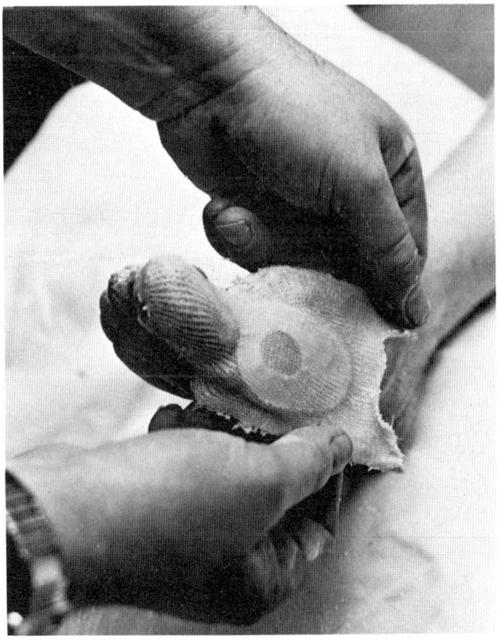

Fig. 18.6. Tubegauze applied to hallux and overlapping first metatarsophalangeal joint. Shield is adhered to protect bunion. Tubegauze folded back and adhered with silicone gel. Entire shield covered with silicone-gel to construct permanent shield. Cover with plastic wrap. Courtesy of S. Rosoff.

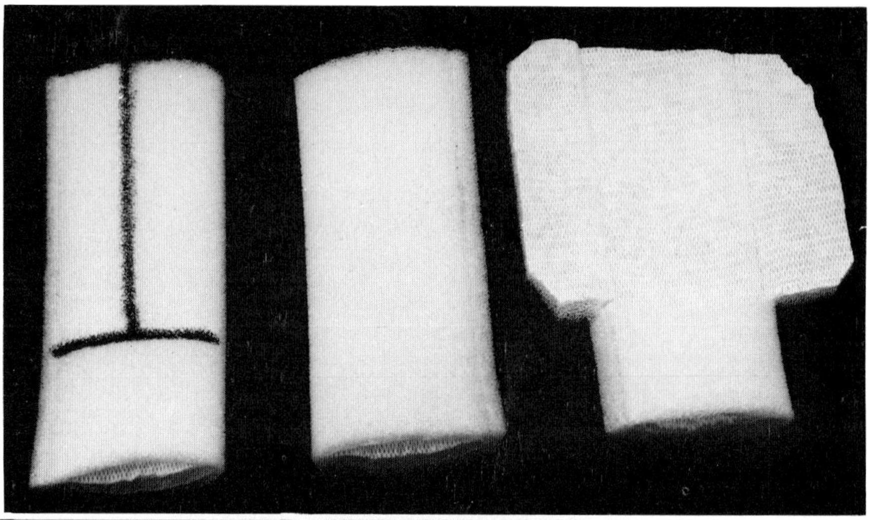

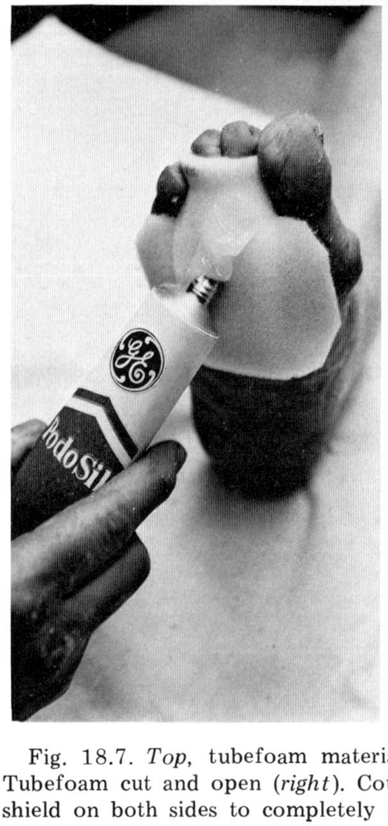

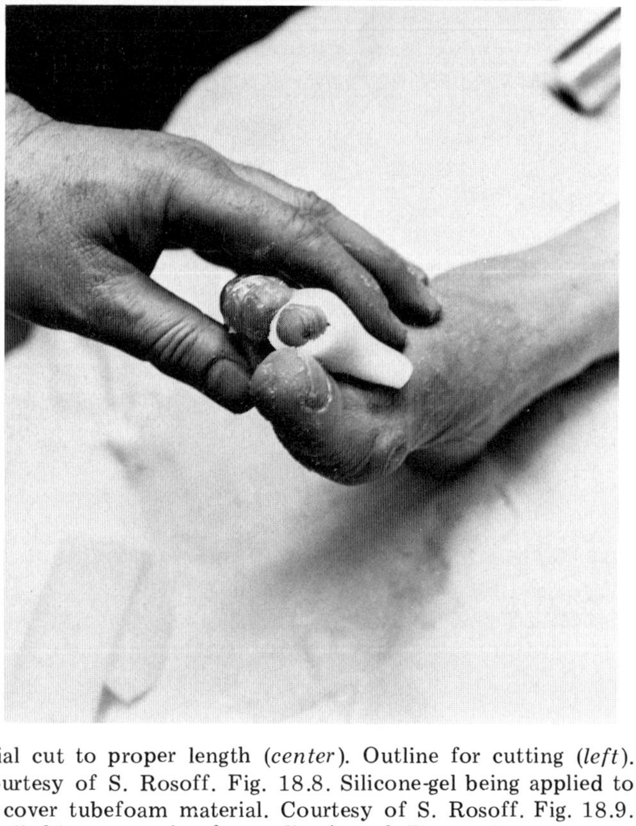

Fig. 18.7. *Top,* tubefoam material cut to proper length (*center*). Outline for cutting (*left*). Tubefoam cut and open (*right*). Courtesy of S. Rosoff. Fig. 18.8. Silicone-gel being applied to shield on both sides to completely cover tubefoam material. Courtesy of S. Rosoff. Fig. 18.9. *Bottom,* lesser toe sized tubefoam applied in preparation for application of silicone. Courtesy of S. Rosoff.

McGlamry (1968) later used these molds for postoperative retainers and rehabilitation. The methods used are essentially the same and the finished product is limited only by the creative skill of the operator. Metal punches for the toe holes, urethane foam 1 and 2 in. thick, Vultex rubber (General Latex and Chemical Co.), urethane mold coating (Vinyl) for finishing and a small sanding drum for carborundum disks is all that is needed.

Silicone Gel. Rosoff (1970) described a variation of the techniques of Pollack and Silverman in constructing shields by using a new silicone gel, PodoSil as a "butter" over stockinette, felt or most my material. A hallux shield is described, which is constructed in the following manner.

Tubular gauze is cut and fit over the hallux and its joint. The skin is coated with a thin layer of the silicone gel. A relief pad is skived and adhered to the gauze over the affected part. The pad is covered with the gel and a gauze cover is applied. The entire shield is then covered with the gel to construct a strong, flexible device. The entire shield is then covered by a sheet of plastic wrap and allowed to shape and dry on the shod foot.

It is removed and trimmed in 24 hr. and more of the gel is applied to complete the pad.

The same silicone gel can be applied to felt, foam, polyurethane or a variety of materials.

Coates (1971) described the use of silicone interdigital wedges and the construction of a variety of shields. His techniques were not unlike those that podiatrists have used for many years with natural and synthetic latex. The silicone product proposed has had wide acceptance in England and it is conceivable that many new silicone products will become available for such use.

Moldable Podiatric Compound. Schuster (1972) described a new Moldable Podiatric Compound (G.E. Medical Systems) for orthodigital corrections, protection and stress dispersion which seems to be acceptable and provides effective therapy. The material consists of a custom-compounded, silicone polymer and liquid curing agent contained in a pre-measured pliable mix package. The contents are mixed within the package, removed and kneaded for 10 to 20 sec.

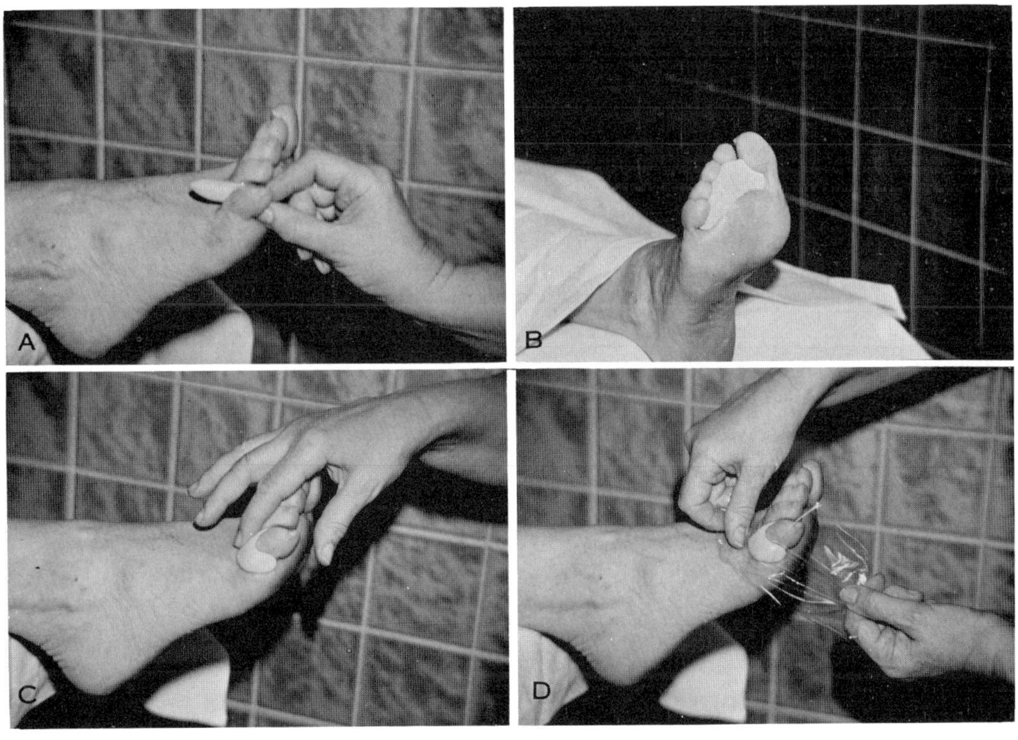

Fig. 18.10. Construction of moldable podiatric compound shield. Courtesy of R. O. Schuster.

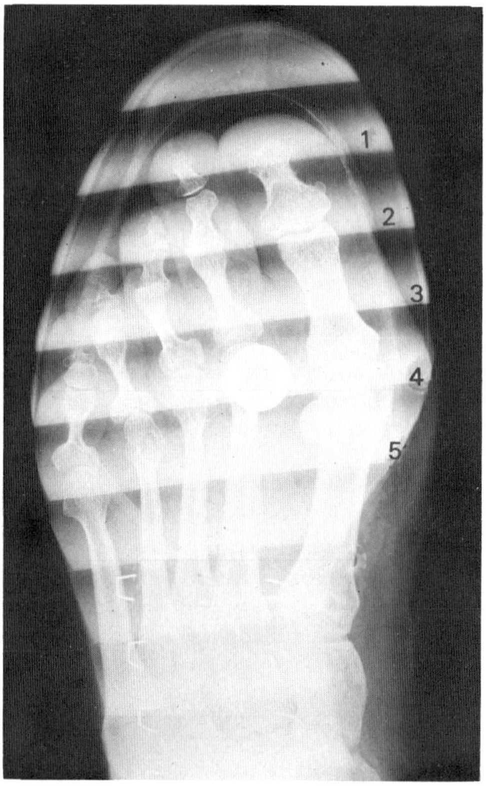

Fig. 18.11. Locating lesions on foot for accommodation in Ripple sole shoes.

into a soft putty-like consistency. Within 5 min. the material begins to cure into a rubbery state. It can now be molded between the toes, over painful sites for protection, for bunions and for crests. The mass is covered with a pliable film, the foot is placed in the shoe for compression, and it self-cures into an orthotic device within 15 to 20 min.

Shoe Sole Technique for Accommodation of Foot Pathology

The podiatrist provides relief from pain through accommodation of objective lesions in the foot. A plantar skin lesion, degenerative joint disease, a bony prominence, a malfunctioning forefoot, gravitational stress and many foot deformities have been relieved through adequate shielding, padding and wedging of the part. It has been proven time and again that duplicating our foot therapy through construction of an accommodative or corrective orthotic is yet another treatment. Permanent shields of plastic, leather, latex, and felt have served as excellent therapeutic agents for many chronic foot ailments. I describe here another technique capable of accomodating foot pathology.

A sturdy leather, rigid-shanked, firm or extended counter, straight last shoe is most desirable. This shoe must have a Ripple sole through which all accommodations are made.

The shoe must fit well, allowing for freedom of the forefoot with a snug fit in the arch and heel.

Diagnostic Techniques. A dorsoplantar and lateral radiograph is taken of the foot using a radiopaque material such as zinc oxide paste, metallic tape or other metallic substance on a deformity or pressure point. Metal washers as described by Sansone are very effective when adhered over a corn, callus or painful site prior to taking a foot radiograph. A radiograph is taken of the foot in the Ripple sole shoe.

The radiopaque material will show on the radiograph underlying one or more flexible ribs in the sole. Thus the site of the painful lesion is localized and easily accommodated.

This technique promises excellent results in the treatment of deep-seated helomas, tylomas and verrucae. Bursae, degenerative joint disease, sesamoiditis and deformities of the toes may be accommodated. Calcaneal spurs, plantar heel bursae, hallux limitus and a variety of structural and functional disturbances can be treated with ease. Obviously it is necessary to appreciate the foot structure as a vehicle of both stance and locomotion.

Technique of Treatment. When the site of discomfort has been identified, a small section of a ripple or ripples in the sole is removed to accommodate the condition. Thus, if a deep callus is noted directly below the seventh ripple under the first metatarsal head, a section of the seventh ripple is removed. This necessitates removal of only the section beneath the lesion at the medial side of the sole.

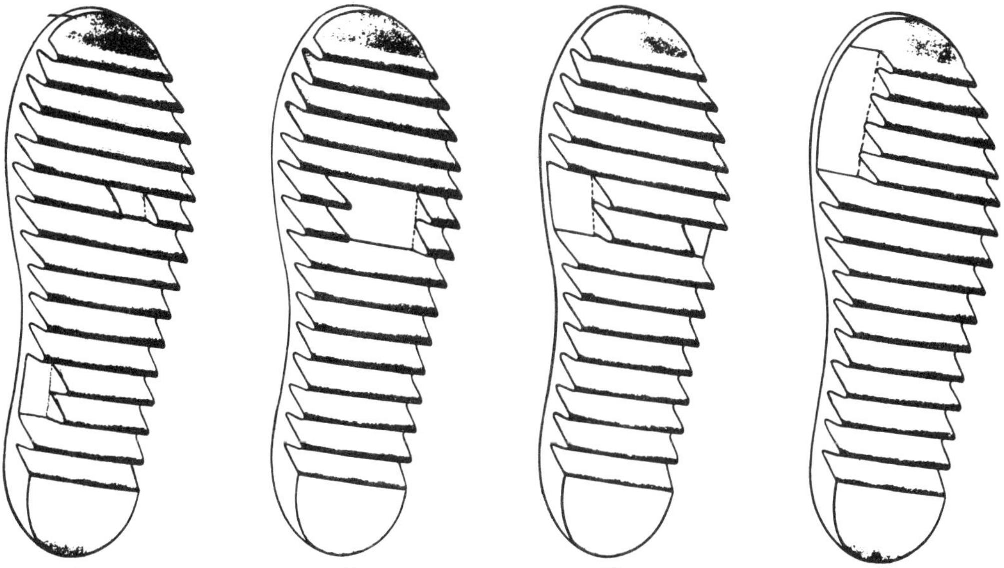

Fig. 18.12. *A*, removal of Ripple under third metatarsal head and at spur site, medial tubercle, plantar surface calcaneus. *B*, removal of Ripple to accommodate second, third and fourth metatarsophalangeal joints. *C*, cutout Ripples for sesamoiditis and deep-seated tylomas, plantar surface, head of first and fifth metatarsal heads. *D*, removal of Ripples to relieve stress from hallux joint in hallux rigidus.

This same technique applies to lesions under any of the metatarsal heads and it is possible to suspend all the metatarsal heads between ripples if necessary. Corns on the distal ends of toes seen in digiti flexus may be helped by removing a ripple. Similar cutouts can be used in alleviating pressure on the painful heel or under sesamoids.

References

Acker, I.: Subcutaneous implantation of a soft tissue substitute for the relief of heloma. J. Am Podiatry Ass., *54:* 623—625, 1964.

Adam, J. E.: Exfoliative dermatitis. Canad. Med. Ass. J., *99:* 661—666, 1968.

Adams, E.: Surgery with special reference to podiatry. Int. J. Surg., *45:* 339, 1932.

Addante, J.: Metatarsal osteotomy as a surgical approach for the elimination of plantar keratosis. J. Foot Surg., *8:* 36—38, 1969.

Aho, C. O.: Case report: Plantar cystic tumor of first toe. J. Am. Coll. Foot Surgeons, *4:* 13—14 1968.

Allen, A. C., and Spitz S.: Malignant melanoma: A clinic-pathological analysis of criteria for diagnosis and prognosis. Cancer., *6:* 1—45, 1953.

Allen, E. van Nuys, Barker, N. W., and Hines, E. A.: *Peripheral Vascular Disease.* Philadelphia, W. B. Saunders Co., 1947.

Amberry, T.: Sesamoid surgery of the great toe. J. Am. Podiatry Ass., *45:* 9, 1955.

American Rheumatism Association: Primer on the rheumatic diseases. J. Am. Med. Ass., *139:* 1068—1076, 1949.

Anderson, W. A. D.: *Synopsis of Pathology.* 2nd ed. St. Louis, C. V. Mosby Co., 1946.

Antahades, L. M.: Refrigeration anesthesia in the surgical excision of a plantar verruca. J. Am. Podiatry Ass., *53:* 662—663, 1963

Apt, A. C.: Diagnostic mycology, an introduction. J. Am. Podiatry Ass., *57:* 271, 1967.

Apt, A. C.: Mycology—some immunological considerations. J. Am. Podiatry Ass., *57:* 515—517, 1967.

Arancia, B. S., and Montgomery, R.: The management of cutaneous moniliasis with nystatin. J. Am. Podiatry Ass., *49:* 1—5, 1959.

Arner, O., Lindholm, A., and Grell, S. R.: Histologic changes in subcutaneous rupture of the Achilles tendon. Acta Chir. Scand., *116:* 484—490, 1958-1959.

Arner, O., Lindholm, A., and Lundvall, N.: Roentgen changes in subcutaneous rupture of the Achilles tendon. Acta Chir. Scand., *116:* 496—500, 1958-1959.

Asboe-Hansen, G.: Hypertrophic scars and keloids: Etiology, pathogenesis and dermatologic therapy. Dermatologica, *120:* 178—184, 1960.

Ashby, B. S.: Primary carcinoma of the nail bed. Brit. J. Surg., *44:* 216, 1956.

Ashur, M., and Farrar, R.: Griseofulvin in the treatment of tinea pedis and onychomycosis. J. Am. Podiatry Ass., *51:* 103—108, 1961.

Austin, D. W.: New concepts of etiology and treatment of helomata. J. Nat. Ass. Chir., *40:* 1927, 1950.

Babbitt, M. P.: Summary of grease compound impression technique. Personal communication., 1949.

Bailey, H.: Infections of the foot. J. Int. Coll. Surgeons., *27:* 475—482, 1957.

Bailey, O. T.: The cutaneous glomus and its tumors-glomangioma. Am. J. Path., *11:* 915, 1935.

Balkin, S. W.: Liquid silicone for plantar keratoses, case reports. J. Am. Coll. Foot Surgeons J., *5:* 114—115, 1966.

Balkin, S. W.: Silicone injection for plantar keratoses. J. Am. Podiatry Ass., *56:* 1—11, 1966.

Balkin, S. W.: Villonodular tenosynovitis—a case report. J. Am. Podiatry Ass., *53:* 282—283, 1963.

Balkin, S. W.: Plantar keratosis: treatment by injectable liquid silicone (report of an 8 year experience). Clin. Orthop., 235—247, 1972.

Balu, S.: Surgical planing for skin lesions of the foot. J. Nat. Ass. Chir., *47:* 277—278, 1957.

Banninga, H. S.: Musculoskeletal disorders: treatment of pain and spasm. Med. Times., *88:* 1440—1443, 1960.

Barré, J. A., and Masson, P.: Anatoma-Clinical study of certain painful subungual tumors (Tumors of the neuro-myoarterial glomus of the extremities). Bull. Soc. franc. de dermat. et. syph., *31:* 148—159, 1924.

Bart, R. S., Andrade, R., and Kopf, A. W.: Cutaneous horns. A clinical and histopathologic study. Acta Derm. Vener., *48:* 507—515, 1968.

Bartlett, R. W.: A conservative operation for care of so-called ingrown toenail. J. Am. Med. Ass., *108:* 1257, 1937.

Beerman, H.: Some aspects of cutaneous malignancy. Am. J. Med. Sci., *233:* 456—472, 1957.

Bereston, E. S.: Diseases of the nails. Clin. Med., *57:* 238, 1950.

Berger, R. A., Auerbach, R., and Orentreich, N.: Basal cell epithelioma of the sole. Arch. Derm., *94:* 317—319, 1966.

Bergeron, J. R., and Stone, O. J.: Koilonychia: a report of familial spoon nails. Arch. Derm., *95:* 351—353, 1967.

Berman, A., and Gartlan, J.: Metatarsal osteotomy for the correction of adduction of the forepart of the foot in children. J. Bone Joint Surg., *53-A:* 498—506, 1971.

Best, C. H., and Taylor, N. B.: *The Physiological Basis of Medical Practice.* 3rd ed. Baltimore, The Williams & Wilkins Co., 1943.

Betts, L. O.: Mortons metatarsalgia: neuritis of the fourth digital nerve. Med. J. Australia., *1:* 514, 1940.

Billig, H. E., and Brennan, R. L.: Foot pains. J. Nat. Ass. Chir., *33:* 34—35, 1943.

Blank, I. H., Smith, J. G., Roth, F. J., and Zaias, N.: Griseofulvin for the systemic treatment of dermatomycoses. J. Am Med. Ass., *171:* 2168, 1959.

Blank, I. H.: Protection against the invasion of bacteria and fungi. Symposium A.A.A.S., December, 1970.

Blau, S.: Conservative therapy in treatment of gangrenous ulcerations. J. Am. Podiatry Ass., *50:* 195—199, 1960.

Blau, S. H.: Surgical skin planing. J. Am. Podiatry Ass., *49:* 202—203, 1959.

Block, I.: Treatment of verruca plantaris with ultrasound. J. Am. Podiatry Ass., *57:* 330—331, 1967.

Bloomquist, G.: Xanthoma of the tendo achilles. Acta Radiol., *57:* 45—48, 1962.

Blooms, N.: Peripheral vascular disease. J. Nat. Ass. Chir., *46:* 371—375, 1956.

Blumer, G.: *History Taking.* New Haven, Conn., Associates of the Yale Medical Library, 1949.

Bodian, E. L.: Oral treatment of dermatomycosis and onychomycosis with griseofulvin. Int. Rec. Med., *173:* 85—87, 1960.

Bodine, G.: Subungual coagulum. J. Am. Podiatry Ass., *57:* 377—378, 1967.

Boesenberg, C., and Haas, M.: Vitamin A as an antikeratinic factor. J. Am. Podiatry Ass., *49:* 255—256, 1959.

Bonavilla, E. J.: Histopathology of the heloma durum: some significant features and their implications. J. Am. Podiatry Ass., *58:* 423—427, 1968.

Booher, R. J.: Lipoblastic tumors of the hands and feet. J. Bone Joint Surg., *47-A:* 727—740, 1965.

Bornstein, B.: Effects of oral chymotrypsin on surgical sequelae. J. Am. Podiatry Ass., *53:* 349—351, 1963.

Bourns, H. K., and Sanerkim, N. G.: Mucoid lesions (mucoid cysts) of the fingers and toes: clinical features and pathogenesis. Brit. J. Surg., *50:* 860—866, 1963.

Bowler, C. W.: Nail techniques. Brit. J. Chir., *32:* 85—87 1967.

Brachman, P.: *Mechanical Foot Therapy.* Ann Arbor, Mich., Edwards Bros., 1940.

Brady, B. J., and Brezak, S.: A report on the alleviation of nocturnal cramps by the combined use of Quinine sulfate and aminophylline. J. Am Podiatry Ass., *50:* 203—206, 1960.

Breneman, J. C.: Postoperative thromboembolic disease computer analysis leading to statistical prediction. J. Am. Podiatry Ass., *197:* 576—580, 1965.

Broder, H. M., and Caughran, J. H.: Traumatic arteriovenous aneurysm of the foot. J. Bone Joint Surg., *39-A:* 427—430, 1957.

Brohner, M. D.: Morton's toe or Morton's neuralgia. J. Nat. Ass. Chir., *39:* 18—26, 1949.

Bronston, G.: A soft tissue approach for plantar lesions. J. Am. Podiatry Ass., *57:* 331—332, 1967.

Brown, J.: Erythrasma and identification with Wood's light. J. Am. Podiatry Ass., *60:* 322—323, 1970.

Bruno, J.: Gross muscle evaluation by the podiatrist. J. Am. Podiatry Ass., *57:* 309—315, 1967.

Budin, H.: Pain the great toe joint. J. Exp. Podiatry, *1:* 1940.

Buneson, T. E.: Neuroma of the first metatarsal interspace—a case history. J. Am. Coll. Foot Surg., *5:* 35, 1966.

Burnstein, I. A.: The role of the podiatrist in the prevention of varicose vein disabilities. Podiatry J., *2:* 18, 1941.

Burnstein, I. A.: Prevention of discomfort and disability in the treatment of varicose veins. Am J. Surg., *54:* 362—370, 1941.

Burwell, E. N.: An unusual tumor of the foot. Brit. J. Surg., *52:* 708—711, 1965.

Buske, E. G.: Local parenteral and oral bismuth therapy for verrucae. J. Am. Podiatry Ass., *53:* 269—271, 1963.

Cameron Co.: Visualizer technique. pp. 20—24, Brochure.

Cameron, D. J.: A new rapid and prolonged acting steroid for intra-articular inflammatory disorders. J. Am. Podiatry Ass., *56:* 317—319, 1966.

Campanelli, M.: Juvenile melanoma (a case report). J. Am. Podiatry Ass., *56:* 461—463, 1966.

Carleton, F. J.: An effective applicance for calcaneal spur. J. Nat. Ass. Chir., *44:* 35—36, 1954.

Carleton, F. J.: *Shoes and Feet.* West Chester, Pa., Charles H. Andress, 1940.

Carlino, J.: Removal of a penetrating foreign body, a case report. Current Pod., 13—14, 1971.

Carpenter, W. E.: an evaluation of injectable vitamin A concentrate in the treatment of corns and calluses. J. Am. Podiatry Ass., *52:* 120—121, 1962.

Carpenter, W. E.: Preliminary results of a study to develop a treatment regimen for onychomycosis. J. Am. Podiatry Ass., *52:* 343—347, 1962.

Carpenter, W. E.: Results of a four year study of injection therapy in the treatment of plantar warts. J. Am. Podiatry Ass., *51:* 407—409, 1961.

Carpenter, W. E.: Tolnaftate, its effectiveness in pedal mycosis, a preliminary report. J. Am. Podiatry Ass., *56:* 541—546, 1966.

Carter, R. T.: Verruca, some impressions from a study of 118 cases. J. Am. Podiatry Ass., *59:* 336—339, 1969.

Castaldi, E.: Experience with local vitamin A

injection in the treatment of helomata and verrucae. J. Am. Podiatry Ass., *49:* 203—206, 1959.

Cecil, R. LaF., and Kennedy, F.: *A Textbook of Medicine.* 3rd ed. Philadelphia, W. B. Saunders Co., 1933.

Cecil, R. LaF., and Kennedy, F.: *A Textbook of Medicine.* 5th ed. Philadelphia, W. B. Saunders Co., 1940.

Cedrone, D.: A short review of classification and etiology of tumors. J. Am. Podiatry Ass., *50:* 19—23, 1960.

Chagas, C. P.: Carcinoma of the nail matrix. Brazil Medico, 233, 1921.

Charache, H.: Squamous cell carcinoma of extremities. Surg. Gynec. Obst., *68:* 1002—1006, 1939.

Chazan, D. V.: A comparison of the effects of reflex heat to local heat in patients with mild to moderate peripheral vascular disease. J. Am. Podiatry Ass., *61:* 125—131, 1971.

Churney, A. M.: Moles, warts and birthmarks. Pediatric Clinic North Am., *8:* 249—252, 1961.

Cinzio, J. R.: Myofascial syndromes in the lower extremity and their diagnosis. J. Am. Podiatry Ass., *53:* 195—198, 1963.

Citron, J.: Case report: benign mummifying epithelioma. J. Am. Coll. Foot Surg., *4:* 42, 1965.

Clarke, B. F., and Dillanger, K. A.: Surgical treatment of ingrown toenail. Surgery, *21:* 919—924, 1947.

Coates, J. S.: Personal communications., 1972.

Cohen, W., and Sheely, W. B.: Ankle ulcer or Werner's syndrome. Arch. Derm., *87:* 86—89, 1962.

Collens, W. S., Vulahos, E., Dobkin, G. B., Neuman, E., Rakow, R. R., Altman, M., Siegman, F.: Conservative management of gangrene in the diabetic patient. J. Am. Med. Ass., *181:* 692—698, 1962.

Collins, H. L.: Surgical nail flap operation. Clin. J. Chir. Podiatry Pedic Surg., *9:* 220, 1937.

Colson, G. M., and Wilcox, A.: Phalangeal metastases in bronchogenic carcinoma. J. Am. Med. Ass., *137:* 995, 1948.

Commack, K. V.: Moles—benign or potentially malignant? J. Mich. State Med. Soc., *55:* 1353—1354, 1956.

Conant, N. F., Smith, D. T., Baker, R. D., Callaway, J. L.: *Manual of Clinical Mycology.* Philadelphia, W. B. Saunders Co., 1971.

Conrad, N. L.: Response of various fungi to specialized media and some chemic irritants. J. Am. Podiatry Ass., *55:* 109—112, 1965.

Conrad, N. L.: Some experiments involving modifications of fungus culture media. J. Am. Podiatry Ass., *51:* 121—125, 1961.

Conway, D.: Postoperative development of an epidermal cyst. J. Am. Coll. Foot Surg., *4:* 7—8, 1965.

Cornell, J. A.: Malignant growths of the feet. Chiropody Record, *20:* 234—235, 1937.

Corsaro, J. A.: Ulcers and injection therapy. Footprints, Florida Chir. Ass., *4:* 2, 1958.

Cortese, C. J.: Clinical signs in differential diagnosis of bacterial infections. J. Am. Podiatry Ass., *62:* 287—297, 1972.

Cortese, T. A.: Treatment of friction blisters. Arch. Derm., *97:* 717—721, 1968.

Costello, J. A., and Costello, J. O.: Chronic ulcerations of the lower extremities differential diagnosis and treatment. J. Am. Osteo. Ass., *55:* 732—735, 1956.

Cozen, L.: Neuroma of the plantar digital nerve; a new method of treatment. Clin. Orthopaed., *11:* 224—226, 1958.

Cramer, L. L.: Parenzyme injection for plantar warts. J. Am. Podiatry Ass., *48:* 526—528, 1958.

Cranley, J. J.: Clinical grading of the severity of obliterative arterial disease of the lower extremities. Geriatrics, *11:* 91—96, 1956.

Dallek, A.: *Podiatric Time Savers* (brochure). Bronx, N. Y.

Das Gupta, T.: Subungual melonoma, 25 year review of cases. Ann. Surg., *161:* 545—552, 1965.

Davies, R. R., Everall, J. D., and Hamilton, E.: Mycological and clinical evaluation of griseofulvin for chronic onychomycosis. Brit. J. Med., *3:* 464—468, 1967.

Davis, A. N.: A new dermatologic agent for hyperidrosis and brominrosis—a preliminary report. J. Am. Podiatry Ass., *50:* 901—906, 1960.

DeBakey, M. E., Crawford E. S., and Cooley, D. A.: Chronic arterial insufficiency of the lower extremities. D. M., pp. 1—45, 1957.

DeCarlo, R.: Sinuses. Chiropody Record, *18:* 3, 1935.

Deffinger, T. L.: Neuroma accompanying heloma durum. J. Am. Podiatry Ass., *52:* 27—32, 1962.

Delaney, H. N., and Travis, L. O.: A clinical evaluation of one hundred cases of infection of the lower leg and foot in military personnel. Milit. Med., *130:* 184—190, 1965.

Delaney, J. M.: A simple plastazote insole. Brit. J. Chir., *35:* 77, 1970.

Delaney, J. M.: Chairside appliances of plastazote. Brit. J. Chir., *34:* 101, 1969.

Dell, J. M.: Demonstrations of sinus tracts, fistulas and cavities by lipoidal. Am. J. Roen. Rad. Ther., *61:* 223—231, 1949.

DeLorimer, A. A.: *The Arthropathies, a Handbook of Roentgen Diagnosis.* Chicago, Year Book Publishers, 1946.

Dencer, F. E.: Lecture notes on diseases of nails. Illinois College of Chiropody and Foot Surgery, 1937.

Denny-Brown, D.: *Handbook of Neurological Examination and Cast Recording.* Cambridge, Mass., Harvard University Press, 1946.

Des Champs, E. R.: Tricophytosis. Chiropody Record, *17:* 47, 1934.

DeWeese, J. A.: Pedal pulses disappearing with

exercise. A test for intermittent claudication. New Eng. J. Med., *262:* 1214—1217, 1960.

Dickenson, P. H.: The managment of lower limb ischemia. Current Med. Drugs, *7:* 10—18, 1967.

Dickson, F. D., and Diveley, R. L.: Functional disorders of the foot. Philadelphia, J. B. Lippincott, 1939.

Dieter, R. A., and Graziano, J. L.: Proteolytic enzyme—antibiotic preparations in the treatment of stasis ulcers. Clin. Med., *77:* 20, 1970.

DiPiero, H.: A device for measuring foot deviations. J. Am. Podiatry Ass., *51:* 203—205, 1961.

Dix, R., and Soan, B.: An evaluation of a local and oral medication in the treatment of onychomycosis, J. Am. Podiatry Ass., *56:* 450—454, 1966.

Dixon, F. C., and Mastin, M. N.: The use of pantothenylol in lower extremity lesions. J. Nat. Ass. Chir., *47:* 61—62, 1957.

Dixon, M.: Keratosis palmaris and plantaris (a case report). J. Am. Podiatry Ass., *56:* 376—377, 1966.

Downie, E., and O'Connor, M.: Infection and gangrene in the foot of diabetic patients; value of conservatism. Aust. New Zealand J. Surg., *26:* 194—197, 1957.

Drummer, B.: Keramin injection in the treatment of helomata. J. Am. Podiatry Ass., *48:* 99—101, 1958.

Dubois, E. J.: Gangrene as a manifestation of systemic lupus erthematosus. J. Am. Podiatry Ass., *181:* 366—374, 1962.

Dueriling, W. M.: Cutaneous neuroma. Arch. Derm. Syph., *19:* 226, 1929.

DuVries, H.: Hypertrophy of the unguilabia. Chiropody Record, *17:* 33—35, 1934.

DuVries, H.: Lectures in Surgery., Illinois Coll. Chiropody Foot Surg., 1936.

DuVries, H.: *Surgery of the Foot.* St. Louis, C. V. Mosby Co., 1959.

DuVries, H. L.: Hypertrophy of unguilabia. Chiropody Record *16:* 11, 1933.

DuVries, H. L.: Ingrown toenail. Chiropody Record, *27:* 155—159, 1944.

DuVries, H. L.: New approach to the treatment of intractable verruca plantaris. J. Am. Podiatry Ass., *44:* 26, 1954.

DuVries, H. L., and Cascino, J. P.: Massive neurofibroma (neurinoma). J. Int. Coll. Surg., *18:* 5, 1952.

Dyer, A. M., and Cohen, M. F.: A report on the use of negative galvanic current for the correction of incurvated nails. J. Nat. Ass. Chir., *45:* 21—22, 1955.

Eads, W. J.: Non-specific tendonitis of flexor longus hallucis tendon. J. Am. Podiatry Ass., *44:* 32—44, 1954.

Eastman Kodak Co, Rochester, New York: *The Fundamentals of Radiography.* 6th ed. Rochester, N. Y., Eastman Kodak Co., 1946. pp. 61—67.

Edmonson, A. S., and Calandruccio, R. A.: Drug therapy for Causalgia. Mississippi Doctor., *34:* 239—241, 1957.

Eibel, P.: Unguis Incarnatus Complicated by Glomus Tumor.

Eichenholtz, S. N., and DeAngelo, C.: Squamous-cell carcinoma of the nail bed. J. Am. Med. Ass., *191:* 1080—1083, 1965.

Eisenberg, H. S.: *Orthodigita.* Brooklyn, N. Y., 1939.

Eisenberg, L. A.: Physiologic rest through a rigid immobilization in the treatment of foot problems. J. Am. Podiatry Ass., *51:* 485—487, 1961.

Ekbom, K. A.: Restless legs. Acta Med. Scand. Suppl., *158:* 123, 1945.

Elliot, J. A.: Recurrent primary varicose veins. Canad. Med. Ass. J., *74:* 388—389, 1956.

Emmert, C.: Operations for ingrown nail. Arch. F. Klin. Chir., *11:* 268—277, 1869.

Engman, M. F., Jr., and Mook, W. H.: Melanotic whitlow. Arch. Derm. Syph., 1174, 1931.

Epstein, E.: Shoe contact dermatitis. J. Am. Med. Ass., *209:* 1487, 1969.

Estersohn, H.: An effective oral antifungal for chronic infections in the aged. J. Am. Podiatry Ass., *56:* 117—119, 1966.

Everall, J. D., and Truter, E. V.: New approach to the problem of epidermal contact hypersensitivity. Arch. Derm., *75:* 428—436, 1957.

Everett, M. A., and Alston, H. D.: Griseofulvin therapy of superficial cutaneous mycoses. J. Oklahoma Med. Ass., *52:* 793—795, 1959.

Evison, G., and Price, C. H. G.: Subungual exostosis. Brit. J., Radio., *39:* 451—455, 1966.

Falknor, G.: Needleing—a new technique in varrucae therapy. J. Am. Podiatry Ass., *59:* 51—52, 1969.

Farley, R. D.: Medial arthroplasty for correction of heloma. J. Am. Podiatry Ass., *61:* 473—476, 1971.

Feder, H., and Feder, J.: Penetration of topical steroids. J. Am. Podiatry Ass., *58:* 388—390, 1968.

Feldman, A. C.: Lipoma, a case report. J. Am. Coll. Foot Surg., *5:* 36, 1966.

Feldman, B.: Dry skin its cause and treatment. J. Am. Podiatry Ass., *48:* 191—194, 1958.

Feldman, B.: Griseofulvin in podiatry. J. Am. Podiatry Ass., *50:* 292—296, 1960.

Ferguson, L. K.: *Surgery of the Ambulatory Patient.* Philadelphia, J. B. Lippincott., 1955. pp. 199—201.

Fields, A.: Leg cramps. California Med., *92:* 204—206, 1960.

Fisher, A. A.: Some practical aspects of the diagnosis and management of shoe dermatitis. Arch. Derm., *79:* 267—274, 1959.

Fisher, C.: A new technique in orthodigital correction and balance. J. Am. Podiatry Ass., *53:* 187—191, 1963.

Fisher, E. R.: Malignant blue nevus. Arch.

Derm., *74:* 227, 1956.
Fleck, C. J.: Verruca plantaris. Chiropody Record, *17:* 95—99, 1934.
Fletcher, T. J.: Nail fungus-the problem and its management. J. Am. Podiatry Ass., *49:* 311—314, 1959.
Foley, W. T.: Treatment of gangrene of the feet and legs by walking. N. Y. J. Podiatry., *8:* 10—18, 1958.
Fox, D. B.: A new approach to the treatment of leg ulcers. Brit. Med. J., *2:* 1370—1373, 1962.
Frank, I. H., and Silver, A. G.: Diabetic foot lesions-preliminary report on a method of healing. J. Am. Podiatry Ass., *52:* 596—598, 1962.
Frank, S. C.: Case report-plantar fibromatosis. J. Am. Coll. Foot Surg., *4:* 9, 1965.
Frankel, E., Henenfeld, M.: Dysbasia podo-dynia. *Modern Foot Therapy*, pp. 636—655. New York, Foot Therapy Publishing Co., 1948.
Franks, A. G.: Dermatologic use of baths. Am. Practitioner, *9:* 1998—2000, 1958.
Fred, H. L., Giesler, R. G., Berry, W., and Eiband, J. M.: Keratosis palmaris et plantaris. Arch. Internal Med., *113:* 866—871, 1964.
Freed, J. B.: Glomangioma: the physiologic effect of traumatized arteriovenous shunts. J. Am. Podiatry Ass., *55:* 198—200, 1965.
Freed, J. B.: Histologic post mortem evaluation of bone hyperplasia accompanying digital clavus. J. Am. Podiatry Ass., *59:* 467—472, 1969.
Freed, J. B.: Sesamoidectomy clamp. J. Am. Podiatry Ass., *56:* 371—372, 1966.
Freeman, D. W.: Case history-early squamous cell carcinoma. J. Am. Coll. Foot Surg., *51:* 142—143, 1966.
Freeman, D. W.: Prolonged local anesthesia in chiropody. J. Am. Podiatry Ass., *44:* 28—34, 1954.
Freigenberg, S.: Fibromatosis of the plantar fascia. J. Am. Coll. Foot Surg., *5:* 30, 1966.
Frohlich, H., Frons, W., and Cedar, T.: A reliable topical antifungal for podiatry. J. Am. Podiatry Ass., *57:* 177—178, 1967.
Frost, L.: A treatment for paronychia with concomitant onychocryptosis. J. Am. Podiatry Ass., *49:* 197—201, 1959.
Frost, L.: Digital calcinosis-a case report. J. Nat. Ass. Chir., *47:* 71—73, 1957.
Frost, L.: Mortons metatarsalgia unilateral multiple neurofibromata. J. Am. Podiatry Ass., *49:* 62—66, 1959.
Frost, L.: Onychomycosis-treatment by avulsion and onychophytex. J. Am. Podiatry Ass., *50:* 283—287, 1960.
Frost, L.: Root resection for incurvated Nail. J. Nat. Ass. Chir., *40:* 19, 1950.
Frost, L. A.: Surgical correction for the incurvated nail. Current Med. Digest, *29:* 119—121, 1962.
Gafafer, W. M. (Editor): Occupational diseases—a guide to their recognition. Public Health Service Pub. #1097:28, Washington, D.C., U.S. Government Printing Office, 1964.
Galinski, A.: Cutaneous herniations. J. Am. Podiatry Ass., *60:* 128—129, 1970.
Gamble, F. O.: Attitudes of subjects' feet in foot roentgenology. Chiropody Record, *22:* 149—150, 1939.
Gamble, F. O., and Yale I.: *Clinical Foot Roentgenology.* Baltimore, Williams & Wilkins Co., 1966.
Ganley, J. V.: An effective topical fungicidal agent for use in podiatry. J. Am. Podiatry Ass., *56:* 121—124, 1966.
Gardner, P.: Negative galvanic current in the surgical correction of onychocryptotic nails. J. Am. Podiatry Ass., *48:* 555—560, 1958.
Gasser, F. J.: Report of two unusual neoplastic cases. J. Am. Coll. Foot Surg., *4:* 26—27, 1965.
Gelfarb, M., and Michaelides, P.: Plantar fibromatosis. Arch Derm., *85:* 278—281, 1962.
Geller, S. D.: Foreign body removal with the aid of a metal locator. J. Am. Podiatry Ass., *51:* 502—503, 1961.
Gemmett, R. A.: Plexiform neuroma (a case report). J. Am. Podiatry Ass., *56:* 330—331, 1966.
Genovese, V. H.: An unusual neuroma site. J. Am. Coll. Foot Surg., *4:* 33, 1965.
Gerbert, J.: The location of the terminal branching of the posterior nerve and its effect on administering a posterior tibial nerve block. J. Am. Podiatry Ass., *61:* 8—11, 1971.
Gerbert, J., and Melillo, T.: A modified skin procedure for the correction of hallux valgus. J. Am. Podiatry Ass., *61:* 132—136, 1971.
Gertner, J. J.: Treatment of superficial thromobophlebitis. J. Am. Geriat. Soc., *4:* 834, 1956.
Gesell, A., and Ilg, F. L.: *The Child from Five to Ten.* New York, Harper & Brothers, 1946.
Giannattasio, R. C.: Dactylophallotomy spontanea. N. Y. J. Med., *70:* 568—569, 1970.
Gibbs, R.: Differential diagnosis of plantar verrucae. J. Am. Podiatry Ass., *59:* 90—92, 1969.
Gibbs, R. C.: Pitfalls in differential diagnosis and treatment of tinea pedis. J. Am. Podiatry Ass., *60:* 125—128, 1970.
Gibbs, R. C., and Frank, S. B.: Keratoma hereditaria mutilans. Arch. Derm., *94:* 619—625, 1966.
Gibson, S. H., Montgomery, H., Woolner, L. B., and Brunsting, L. A.: Melanotic whitlow (subungual melanoma). J. Invest. Derm., *29:* 119—129, 1957.
Gicker, J. W.: Differential diagnosis of diseases of the foot. Chiropody Record, *22:* 151—154, 1939.
Gilbert, R. S., and Williams, M. J.: Local injection of vitamin A (keramin) for plantar verrucae. U. S. Armed Forces Med. J., *10:* 843—847, 1959.
Gilman, M.: Excision of ganglionic cyst and

exostosis. J. Am. Coll. Foot Surg., *5:* 41—42, 1966.

Godfrey, C. E.: Case report-vascular leiomyoma. J. Am. Coll. Foot Surg., *4:* 19, 1965.

Goff, C.: Gait and posture: a symposium. Clin. Ortho., *25:* 7—109, 1962.

Goldberg, H. C.: Clinical observations on the use of griseofulvin by mouth in fungus diseases. J. Am. Podiatry Ass., *50:* 290—291, 1960.

Goldberg, H. C.: Laboratory re-evaluation of fungus growths in shoes, socks and skin. J. Am. Podiatry Ass., *49:* 433—437, 1959.

Goldfarb, N. J., Rosenthal, S. A., Bock, A., Borota, A., Dick, L., Qurnari, D., Fraser, C.: Dermatomycosis treated with griseofulvin. Antibiotic Ann., *7:* 693—700, 1959—1960.

Goldhirsch, S.: Tenotomy as an aid in orthodigita. J. Nat. Ass. Chir., *47:* 463, 1957.

Golding, D. N.: Polyarteritis presenting with leg pains. Brit. Med. J., *1:* 277, 278, 1970.

Goldman, L., and Palmero, J.: A podophyllin lotion for warts. Arch. Derm., *84:* 505—506, 1961.

Goldman, L., and Stillman, L.: Combined cryotherapy and electrodesiccation in the management of verrucae. Pod. Q., *2:* 16—19, 1963.

Goldman, L., and Unger, L.: A comprehensive treatment for monilial infections of skin and nails. J. Am. Podiatry Ass., *49:* 371—373, 1959.

Goldstein, S.: Office management of intermetatarsal neuralgias. J. Am. Podiatry Ass., *48:* 529, 530, 1958.

Goodman, J. M.: Liquid nitrogen therapy of warts and other skin lesions. Canad. Med. Ass. J., *82:* 628—630, 1960.

Goldy, H.: Oscillographic interpretations. J. Nat. Ass. Chir., *46:* 826—830, 1956.

Goldy, H., and Steinberg, M.: Etiological factors in multiple infected onychocryptosis. J. Nat. Ass. Chir., *46:* 769—771, 1956.

Gottlieb, A.: The foot during pregnancy and postpartum. J. Nat. Ass. Chir., *30:* 5—8, 1940.

Gottlieb, M. M., and Gottlieb, J. J.: The permanent removal of nails by avulsion and chemical cauterization. Chronical Pod., *3:* 17—18, 1953.

Grady, E. D.: A simple method of removing plantar warts. General Practioner, *25:* 89, 1962.

Graham, H. F.: Ingrown toenail. Am. J. Surg., *6:* 411, 1929.

Gray, H.: *Anatomy of the Human Body.* 22nd Ed. Philadelphia, Lea & Febiger Co., 1930.

Grayson, M.: Corneal manifestations of keratosis of plantaris and palmaris. Am. J. Ophth., *59:* 483—486, 1965.

Green, A. L.: Case report of a typical Kaposi's hemorrhagic sarcoma. J. Am. Coll. Foot Surg. *4:* 21—22, 1965.

Greenberg, W.: Hereditary callosities. J. Nat. Ass. Chir., *46:* 327—328, 1956.

Greene, A. A.: A modification of the phenol-alcohol technique for toenail correction. Chronical Pod., *13:* 20—25, 1964.

Grolich, H., Irons, W., and Ceder, E.: A reliable topical antifungal for podiatry. J. Am. Podiatry Ass., *57:* 177, 1967.

Gross, R. H.: *Modern Foot Therapy.* New York, Foot Therapy Publishing Co., 1948.

Gross, R. H., and Burnett, E. K.: *The Practice of Podiatry.* New York, Harriman Printing Co., Inc., 1933.

Grovit, M., and Block, P.: Pedal manifestations of hyperuricemia due to thiazide diuresis. J. Am. Podiatry Ass., *58:* 176—177, 1968.

Haas, M., and Boesenberg, C.: Treatment of onychomycosis and dermatophytosis with griseofulvin. J. Am. Podiatry Ass., *50:* 814—817, 1960.

Haber, H., and Wells, G. C.: Subcorneal pustular dermatosis of the soles. Brit. J. Derm., *71:* 243—245, 1959.

Hall, V.: An improved method for the injection of Keramin in the treatment of heloma neurofibrosum. J. Am. Podiatry Ass., *48:* 97—98, 1958.

Hara, B.: Cavernous hemangioma. J. Am. Coll. Foot Surg., *5:* 30—31, 1966.

Harris, L.: Combined electro desiccation and chemo-surgery for plantar verrucae. J. Am. Podiatry Ass., *56:* 160—161, 1966.

Hauser, E. D. W.: *Disease of the Foot.* Philadelphia, W. B. Saunders Co., 1939.

Hauser, E. D. W.: Neurofibroma of the foot. J. Am. Podiatry Ass., *121:* 1217, 1953.

Haverhill fever (erythema arthriticum epidemicum), Editorial. J. Am. Med. Ass., *113:* 941—942, 1939.

Hazan, M.: Proteolytic enzymes in podiatry. J. Am. Podiatry Ass., *50:* 207—208, 1960.

Heiss, H. B., and Gross, P. R.: Keratosis palmaris et plantaris treatment with topically applied vitamin A acid. Arch Derm., *101:* 100—103, 1970.

Helfand, A. E.: The pathologic physiology of edema. J. Am. Podiatry Ass., *49:* 374—375, 1959.

Helfand, A. E., Hirt, P. R., Madresh, A. C., and De Vincentis, A.: Triamcinolone acetonide in the treatment of bursitis and other foot disorders. J. Am. Podiatry Ass., *61:* 174—179 1971.

Heller, A. G.: A prophylactic surgical procedure. J. Am. Podiatry Ass., *48:* 258—259, 1958.

Hendler, S. S.: Management of onychomycosis. J. Am. Podiatry Ass., *44:* 57—60, 1954.

Henenfeld, M.: Balance and imbalance. J. Nat. Ass. Chir., *46:* 817—825, 1956.

Henenfeld, M., and Walkes, M. H.: A modification of the DuVries plantar condylectomy. J. Am. Podiatry Ass., *50:* 24—27, 1960.

Henenfeld, M., and Walkes, M. H.: Subluxations of the metatarsophalangeal joints. N. Y. State J. Pod., *20:* 1959.

Higashi, N.: Melanocytes of toenail matrix and

nail pigmentation. Arch. Derm., *97:* 570—574, 1968.
Hirschberg, S.: A "missing link" in the treatment and control of epidermophytosis. J. Am. Podiatry Ass., *49:* 14—17, 1959.
Hiss, J. M.: *Functional Foot Disorders.* Los Angeles, University Publishing Co., 1937.
Hlavac, H., and Schoenhaus, H.: The plantar fat pad and some related problems. J. Am. Podiatry Ass., *60:* 151—155, 1970.
Hoffmeister, F. H.: Dynamic balance therapy. J. Am. Podiatry Ass., *48:* 19—20, 1958.
Hoffner, M. L.: Case report: excision of plantar fibroma with secondary painful internal scar formation. Am. Coll. Foot Surg., *5:* 38—39, 1966.
Holmes, J. G.: Diagnosis of ringworm. Lancet, *2:* 62—63, 1956.
Homans, J.: *Circulatory Disease of the Extremities.* New York, Macmillan Co., 1939.
Howard, W. R.: Ingrown toenail, its surgical treatment. N. Y. Med. Surg. J., *57:* 579—581, 1893.
Hubay, C. A.: Sesamoid bones of the hands and feet. Am. J. Roent. Radiol. Ther., *61:* 500—505, 1949.
Hunter, G. A., and Hellier, F. F.: Tumors of the palm and sole resembling basal cell epithelioma. Brit. J. Derm., *72:* 285—287, 1960.
Hyman, A. B., and Michaelides, P.: Basal-cell epithelioma of the sole. Arch. Derm., *87:* 481—485, 1963.
Hymes, L.: Personal communication. 1971.
Ignatoff, W.: Dermatology in geriatrics. J. Am. Podiatry Ass., *48:* 183—188, 1958.
Ignatoff, W. B.: Reactions to adhesive tape. J. Nat. Ass. Chir., *46:* 749—755, 1956.
Ignatoff, W. B., and Bleiberg, J.: A new therapy for onychomycosis. J. Am. Podiatry Ass., *48:* 359—363, 1958.
Ilowite, N. H.: Experimental production of tinea pedis. J. Am. Podiatry Ass., *57:* 120—122, 1967.
Ingersoll, T. E.: Sesamoidalgia. J. Am. Podiatry Ass., *45:* 15—24, 1955.
Jablon, V. A.: Epithelioma. Chiropody Record, *20:* 232—234, 1937.
Jacobs, J.: Mobilizing adhesions with negative pressure. J. Am. Podiatry Ass., *50:* 116—117, 1960.
Jahsman, W. E.: An approach to the etiology, diagnosis and management of peripheral arteriosclerosis. Henry Ford Hosp. Med. Bull. (Detroit), *4:* 56—61, 1956.
Janik, A.: Tumors of tendon sheathes. Ann. Surg., *85:* 897—911, 1927.
Jarrett, A., and Spearman R. I. C.: The histochemistry of the human nail. Arch. Derm., *94:* 652—657, 1966.
Jaskoski, B. J.: Treatment of onychomycosis in a foot clinic. J. Am. Podiatry Ass., *59:* 230—233, 1969.
Jaskoski, B. J., Jacobs, J. F., and Carr, D. L.: Some mycotic problems in a podiatry clinic. J. Am. Podiatry Ass., *52:* 825—828, 1962.
Jenkinson, Edwin O.: Sound-seen source of safe surgery. Interview Podiatry News., *8:* 1—2, 1970.
Jennett, J. H.: Persistent hereditary edema of the legs-Milroys disease. Clin. Orthop., *8:* 122—123, 1956.
Jesser, J.: Disease of the hand. Classroom lectures, Illinois College of Chiropody and Foot Surgery, Chicago, 1937.
Jillson, O. F.: Allergic dermatitis produced by pathogenic and saprophytic fungi. Ann. Allergy, *15:* 14—24, 1957.
Job, C. K., Riedel, R. G., et al: Squamous cell carcinoma arising in leprosy. Int. J. Leprosy *32:* 37—44, 1964.
Johnson, A. V.: Onychoclavus a fifth toe problem. J. Am. Podiatry Ass., *52:* 436—438, 1962.
Johnson, E. W., Ghormley, R. K., Dockerty, M. B.: Hemangioma of extremities. Surg. Gynec. Obstet., *102:* 531—538, 1956.
Johnson, S. A. M., and Tuura, J. L.: Glyceryl triacetate (triacetin) as a fungicide. Arch. Derm., *74:* 73—75, 1956.
Jones, C. L.: The cutaneous virulence of candida albicans of the foot. J. Foot Surg., *7:* 22—24, 1968.
Jones, C. L. Skin graft following avulsion of nail, a preliminary report. J. Am. Podiatry Ass., *55.* 191—193, 1965.
Jones, R. F., Watson, D. O., and Tracy, G. D.: "Cold injury" in a temperature climate. Med. J. Aust., *1:* 323—327, 1970.
Kaplan, E., and Weinstock, R.: Corticosteroid instillation by jet spray and check of penetration. J. Am. Podiatry Ass., *57:* 409—411, 1967.
Kaplan, E., and Weinstock, R.: Local anesthesia of the foot using jet injection. J. Am. Podiatry Ass., *57:* 370—373, 1967.
Kaplan, E. G.: A new approach to the surgical correction of overlapping toe. J. Am. Coll. Foot. Surg., *3:* 24—25, 1964.
Kaplan, E. G.: Elimination of onychauxis by surgery. J. Am. Podiatry Ass., *50:* 111—113, 1960.
Kaplan, E. G., and Kashuk, K. Disclaiming the myth of use of epinephrine local anesthesia in feet. J. Am. Podiatry Ass., *61:* 335—340, 1971.
Karsner, H. T.: *Human Pathology.* Philadelphia, J. B. Lippincott Co., 1955.
Kasden, P. R.: The environmental effects on the morphology of three strains of trichophyton mentagrophytes, and a study of two of their enzymes. J. Am. Podiatry Ass., *60:* 109—115, 1970.
Kaump, D. H.: Laboratory tests in general practice. J. Am. Med. Ass., *132:* 253—258, 1946.
Keck, C.: The tarsal tunnel syndrome. J. Bone Joint Surg., *44-A:* 180, 1962.
Keefer, C. S.: Some clinical features of deficiency disorders. N. Y. State J. Med., *32:* 1405—1413, 1932.

Keyes, E. L.: Surgical treatment of ingrown toenail. J. Am. Med. Ass., *102:* 1458, 1934.
Kheng Khoo, T., and Ban Tze, Khong: A sweat gland tumor of the mixed salivary type of the right middle toe. Med. J. Malaya., *2:* 128—133, 1964.
Kierland, R. R.: The problem and treatment of pruritis. Rocky Mountain Med. J., *55:* 44—49, 1959.
Kilberg, A. J.: Surgical treatment of onychocryptosis. Clin. J. Chir. Pod. Pedic. Surg., *7:* 222—224, 1935.
King, E. S. J.: Malignant tumors of tendon sheathes. Aust. and New Zealand J. Surg., *10:* 338—353, 1941.
Kingland, H. D.: Cryotherapy in treatment of verrucae. J. Am. Podiatry Ass., *52:* 435, 1962.
Kipping, H.: A case of eccrine poroma. J. Bull. Millard Fillmore Hosp., Buffalo, N. Y., *9:* 95—97, 1962.
Kirton V., and Price, W.: Black heel. Trans. St. John Hosp. Derm. Soc., *51:* 80—84, 1965.
Kleger, S. J., and Feldman, B.: Larva migrans. J. Am. Podiatry Ass., *56:* 324—325, 1966.
Kleiman, M. A.: Some observations concerning the phenol-alcohol nail technique. Footprints, Fla. Pod. Ass., *19:* 6, 1964.
Kleiman, M. A.: Treatment for heloma milliare. Footprints, Fla. Pod. Ass., *4:* 1, 1958.
Kleinberg, S.: Angioma of the foot. J. Bone Joint Surg., *24:* 367—371, 1942.
Knox, J. M., and Spiller, W. F.: Eccrine poroma. Arch. Derm., *77:* 726, 1958.
Knudsen, E. A., and Amdrup, E.: Verrucae vulgares et plantares treated with ultrasoft x-rays. Acta Dermato-vener. Scand., *35:* 379—389, 1955.
Kopell, H. P., and Thompson, W. A. L.: Peripheral entrapment neuropathies of the lower extremity. New Engl. J. Med., *262:* 56—60, 1960.
Kovacs, R.: *Electrotherapy and Light Therapy.* 3rd ed. Philadelphia, Lea & Febiger, 1938.
Kozie, L. J., Ballard, R., Buividas, A.: A clinical evaluation of diphemanil methylsulfate in the treatment of hyperhidrosis. J. Nat. Ass. Chir., *47:* 398—400, 1957.
Krausz, C. E.: A nail survey of 4,600 patients. J Nat. Ass. Chir., *40:* 5—11, 1950.
Krausz, C. E.: Nail survey (1942—1970). British J. Chir. *35:* 117, 1970.
Krammer, D. W.: *Manual of Peripheral Vascular Disorders.* Philadelphia, Blakiston Co., 1940.
Krantz, M. K.: Converting a commercial sandal into a molded sandal. J. Nat. Ass. Chir., *47:* 555, 1957.
Krantz, M. K.: Dynamic moulding of a semirigid appliance. J. Nat. Ass. Chir., *44:* 55—59, 1954.
Kravette, M. A.: Peripheral nerve entrapment syndromes in the foot. J. Am. Podiatry Ass., *61:* 457—472, 1971.
Kravity, H., and Boehm, J. J.: Rhythmic habit patterns in infancy: their sequence, age of onset, and frequency. Child Development, *42:* 399—414, 1971.
Kulchar, G. V.: Benign and malignant tumors of the foot. Am. Med. Ass. *124:* 761—766.
Kurzweil, M.: A new instrument for digital surgery. J. Am Podiatry Ass., *51:* 274—175, 1961.
Kwittken, J., and Negri, L.: Malignant blue nevus. Arch. Derm., *94:* 64—69, 1966.
Landau, A.: Microsedimentation (Linzenmeier-Raunert method) Am. J. Dis. Child., *45:* 691—734, 1933.
Lanham, R. A.: Plantar fibromatosis of the foot. J. Am. Coll. Foot Surg., *4:* 37—38, 1968.
Lapidus, P. W.: Dorsal bunion. J. Nat. Ass. Chir., *29:* 9—13, 1939.
Lassen, N. A., Larson, O. A., Sorenson, A. W., Hallbrook, T., Dohn, I., Nilsen, R., Westling, H.: Conservative treatment of gangrene using mineralocorticoid induced moderate hypertension. Lancet, *1:* 606—609, 1968.
Laurence, K. R.: Treatment of verrucae with small pox vaccine. J. Am. Podiatry Ass., *61:* 12—19, 1971.
Law, P.: Neurologic tests. Lectures in neurology. Chicago, College of Chiropody and Foot Surgery, 1938.
Layman, C. W.: Use of liquid oxygen in dermatology. Minnesota Med., *29:* 151—152, 1956.
Lerner, L.: Management of plantar verrucae via excision and curretage. J. Am. Podiatry Ass., *49:* 11—14, 1959.
Lerner, M. R., and Lerner, A. B.: *Dermatologic Medications.* 2nd ed. Chicago, Year Book Publishers, 1960.
Levene, M., et al.: Distribution of skin tumors of the sole of the foot. The Chiropodist, *14:* 11, 1959.
Levey, M.: Formaldehyde and vitamin A in treatment of verrucae. Curr. Podiatry., *7:* 14, 1958.
Levin, B.: Heloma surgery. J. Am. Podiatry Ass., *48:* 244—245, 1958.
Levine, D. P.: An improved casting technique. Footprints, Fla. Pod. Ass., *125:* 5—6, 1971.
Levinson, S. A., and McFate, R. P.: *Clinical Laboratory Diagnosis.* Philadelphia, Lea & Febiger Co., 1939.
Levitus, I. M., and Scheimer, O. M.: Gout as a complication. J. Nat. Ass. Chir., *28:* 36—38, 1938.
Levy, S. E.: A controlled evaluation of subdermal corticosteroid injections. J. Am Podiatry Ass., *48:* 403—407, 1958.
Lewin, P.: *The Foot and Ankle.* Philadelphia, Lea & Febiger Co., 1940.
Lewis, H. M., Stensaas, C. O., Okun, M. R.: Basal cell epithelioma of the sole. Arch. Derm., *91:* 623—624, 1965.
Lewis, L. L.: Podal propulsive hinge as a key to normal foot function. J. Am. Podiatry Ass.,

56: 103—109, 1966.
Lewis, M., and Lutterbeck, E.: Verrucae: a clinical review. J. Am. Podiatry Ass., *57:* 263—268, 1967.
Lewis, Sir T.: *Vascular Disorders of the Limbs.* New York, The Macmillan Co., 1936.
Lieberman, H.: An empirical treatment for mosaic verrucae. J. Am. Podiatry Ass., *50:* 737, 1960.
Lindenberg, L. M.: Treatment of tinea pedis and tinea unguium with griseofulvin: preliminary report. Curr. Podiatry., *8:* 11, 1959.
Lloyd-Davis, R. W., and Brill, G. C.: The etiology and management of ingrown toenails. Brit. J. Surg., *50:* 592—597, 1963.
Locke, R. K.: Arthridities and allied disorders as factors in everyday chiropody practice and their treatment. J. Nat. Ass. Chir., *46:* 756—777, 1956.
Locke, R. K.: Bone clamp for forefoot surgery. J. Am. Podiatry Ass., *56:* 368—370, 1966.
Locke, R. K.: Corticosteroid injections therapy in the foot. J. Am. Podiatry Ass., *48:* 505—511, 1958.
Locke, R. K.: Local injection of combined dexamethasone 21-phosphate-lidocaine in non-articular foot disorders. J. Am. Podiatry Ass., *53:* 510—514, 1963.
Locke, R. K.: Local steroid injection therapy. Podiatry Quart. Summer 1961.
Locke, R. K.: Onychomycosis. J. Am. Podiatry Ass., *45:* 15—28, 1955.
Locke, R. K.: Personal communication, 1971.
Locke, R. K.: Shoe sponging—a new adjunct in treatment of plantar excrescenses. Chiropody Record, *25:* 105, 1942.
Locke, R. K.: Steroids in podiatric management of arthritis. J. Am. Podiatry Ass., *57:* 164—167, 1967.
Locke, R. K., and Strauss, H.: The reduction of post operative pain and edema in foot surgery through local instillation of corticosteroids. J. Am. Podiatry Ass., *54:* 703—708, 1964.
Locke, R. K., and Zang, K.: Controlled intralesional deposition of a sclerotic in verruca therapy. J. Am. Podiatry Ass., *59:* 377—384, 1969.
Lovett, R. W.: *The Treatment of Infantile Paralysis.* Philadelphia, P. Blakiston and Son & Co., 1917.
Lowenberg, R. I.: Use of the cuff pain test in the early diagnosis of phlebothrombosis. J. Am. Podiatry Ass., *48:* 141—143, 1958.
Luft, S.: Reactions to parenteral enzyme therapy. J. Am. Podiatry Ass., *50:* 209—210, 1960.
Luikart, R., Ayres, S., III, Wilson, J. W.: Surgical planing of the skin, dichlorotetrafluoro-ethane as a freezing agent. Calif. Med., *84:* 151—154, 1956.
Lyell, A., and Miles, J. A.: The Myrmecia, a study of inclusion bodies in warts. Brit. Med. J., *1:* 912, 1951.
Mackee, G. M., and Cipallaro, A. C.: *X-Ray and Radium in the Treatment of Diseases of the Skin.* 4th ed. Philadelphia, Lea & Febiger Co., 1946.
Madden, J. J.: Inflammatory disorders of skin of the feet. J. Am. Med. Ass., *124:* 743—747, 1944.
Maibach, E. I., and Kligman, A. M.: Short-term treatment of onychomycosis with griseofulvin. Arch. Derm., *81:* 733—734, 1960.
Marples, R. R., and Kligman, A. M.: Growth of bacteria under adhesive tapes. Arch Derm., *99:* 107, 1969.
Maskin, I. L., Taschdjian, C. C., and Franks, A. C.: Etiology of dermatophytosis. Arch. Derm., *75:* 66—69, 1957.
Mason, S.: Case report of calcified bursa. J. Am. Coll. Foot Surg., *4:* 12, 1965.
McCarthy, D. J., Habowsky, J. E. J.: A cytological survey by strata of skin in heloma durum using electron microscopy. J. Am. Podiatry Ass., *62:* 239—249, 1972.
McCarthy, D. J., Habowsky, J. E. J.: Alterations in skin morphology in heloma dura utilizing maceration technique for examination of epidermal-dermal interface. J. Am. Podiatry Ass., *62:* 303—307, 1972.
McElvenny, R. T.: The etiology and surgical treatment of intractable pain about the fourth metatarsophalangeal joint. J. Bone Joint Surg., *25:* 675, 1943.
McGlamry, E. D., and Kitting, R.: Postoperative urethane molds. J. Am. Podiatry Ass., *58:* 169—175, 1968.
McGlone, J. J.: The tarsal tunnel syndrome. J. Am. Podiatry Ass., *58:* 435, 1968.
McGregor, R. R.: New stretch nylon shoe lace as a therapeutic aid. J. Am. Podiatry Ass., *51:* 497—500, 1961.
Meadow, E. N.: Myxoma on the plantar surface (a case report). J. Am. Podiatry Ass., *56.* 463—464, 1966.
Melillo, T. V.: Gastrocnemius equinus—its diagnosis and treatment. Proc. Res. Alumni Ass., Calif. Pod. Med. Center, *1:* 37—54, 1972.
Meyerding H. W., and Stuck, W. G.: Painful heels among children (apophysitis). J. Am. Med. Ass., *102:* 1658—1660, 1934.
Meyers, H. L.: New elastic support for stasis and stasis ulcers of the legs. Vascular Dis., *5:* 188—193, 1968.
Michael, B. H.: Juvenile melanoma. J. Am. Coll. Foot Surg. *5:* 135—136, 1966.
Michael, B.: Management of calcaneal spur Inflammation with triamcinolone acetonide. J. Am. Podiatry Ass., *51:* 801—803, 1961.
Michael, C. A.: Pruritis, what it is and some suggestions for management. J. Am. Podiatry Ass., *52:* 432—435, 1962.
Michota, S.: Standard weight bearing platform. Personal communication. 1972.
Moatz, J. D.: Reflexes of the feet and their significance. J. Nat. Ass., Chir., *29:* 5—8, 16—18, 1939.
Mogull, P.: Acrylic nail plate and onychomy-

cosis. J. Nat. Ass. Chir., *47:* 401—402, 1957

Mogull, P.: Uses of methyl methacrylate in the treatment of inverted nails. J. Nat. Ass. Chir., *44:* 35, 1954.

Montgomery, R. M., and Brezak, S.: Topical use of vioformhydrocortisone in podiatry. J. Am. Podiatry Ass., *48:* 364—366, 1958.

Montgomery, R. M., and Hyman, D.: Cutis., *3:* 1212—1215, 1967.

Montgomery, R. M., and Montgomery, A. H.: Common hyperkeratotic lesions of the foot. J. Am. Med. Ass., *124:* 756—761, 1944.

Morton, D. J.: *The Human Foot.* New York, Columbia University Press, 1935.

Morton, J. J., and Scott, W. J.: Methods for estimating the degree of sympathetic vasoconstriction in peripheral vascular disease. New Engl. J. Med., *204:* 955—962, 1931.

Mowbray, D. T.: Angiofibroma involving the short saphenous vein and sural nerve. Chiropody Record, *17:* 61, 1934.

Mulary, D. H., and Ubach, F.: Proteolytic debridement of hyperkeratoses of palms and soles. Arch. Derm., *78:* 758, 1958.

Mullens, B.: An effective treatment for heloma neurofibrosum. J. Nat. Ass. Chir., *46:* 772—774, 1956.

Mullens, B. C.: Claustrophobia. J. Nat. Ass. Chir., *39:* 21—22, 1949.

Nelson, G. W.: *Your Feet.* Minneapolis, 1947.

Newman, A. W.: Case report: juxta articular rheumatoid nodule. J. A. C. F. S., *4:* 10, 1965.

Newell, R. R.: Roentgenology: contrast media. In Glasser, O., ed., *Medical Physics.* Vol. 1. Chicago, Year Book Publishers, pp. 1269—1271, 1944.

Ney, G. C.: An operation for ingrowing toenails. J. Am. Med. Ass., *80:* 374, 1923.

Nickel, W. R.: Nevi: clinical and pathological evaluation. Plastic Reconstr. Surg., *22:* 123—138, 1958.

Nomland, R.: Cutaneous manifestations of the circulatory disorders of the foot. A symposium, foot disorders and their treatment. J. Am. Med. Ass., *124:* 747—750, 1944.

Norlander, N. B.: Restless legs syndrome. Brit. J. Physical Med., New Series, *17:* 160—162, 1954.

Nutt, J. J.: *Diseases and Deformities of the Foot.* 2nd ed. New York, E. B. Treat & Co., 1925.

Nyman, S. P.: The phenol-alcohol technique for toenail excision. J. Nat. Ass. Chir., *5:* 2, 1956.

O'Brien, F. L., et al.: Nutrition in chiropody. J. Nat. Ass. Chir. *47:* 601—608, 1957.

Ochsner, A., and Debakey, M.: Thrombophlebitis, the role of vasospasm in the production of clinical manifestations. J. Am. Med. Ass., *114:* 117—124, 1940.

Okun, M. R., and Ansell, H. B.: Eccrine poroma. Arch. Derm., *88:* 561—566, 1963.

Ornstein, D. E.: Orthopedics. Class lecture, Illinois College of Chiropody and Foot Surgery, Chicago, 1936.

Ormond, C. S.: Cantharone, a cantharidin tincture as a useful agent in treating intractable plantar lesions. J. Am. Podiatry Ass., *52:* 427—430, 1962.

Ottley, C. M.: Glomus tumor. Brit. J. Surg., *29:* 387—391, 1942.

Oughterson, W. W., and Tennant, R.: Angiomatous tumors of the hands and feet. Surger, *5:* 73—100, 1939.

Overcast, V. C.: Curetting verrucae with minimum hemorrhage. J. Nat. Ass. Chir., *47:* 187, 1957.

Owens, R. E.: Adenylic acid therapy for mechanical foot problems of varicose veins. J. Am. Podiatry Ass., *51:* 729—730, 1961.

Owens, R. E.: Surgical correction for onychauxis. J. Am. Podiatry Ass., *52:* 591—593, 1962.

Oyston, J. K.: Madura foot: a study of twenty cases. J. Bone Joint Surg., *43-B:* 259—267, 1961.

Pack, G. T.: Prepubital melanoma of skin. Surg. Gynec. Obstet., *86:* 374—375, 1948.

Pack, G. T.: The pigmentated mole and malignant melanoma. Virginia Med. Monthly, *84:* 111—119, 1957.

Pack, G. T.: *Tumors of the Hands and Feet.* 3rd ed. St. Louis, C. V. Mosby Co., 1939.

Pack, C. T., and Adair, F. E.: Subungual melanoma differential diagnosis of tumors of the nail bed. Surgery, *5:* 47—72, 1939.

Pack, G. T., and Oropenza, R.: Subungual melonoma. Surg. Gynec. Obstet., *124:* 571—582, 1967.

Packer, A.: Post traumatic neurofibroma a case report. J. Am. Podiatry Ass., *53:* 756—757, 1963.

Page, J. A.: Painful feet syndrome among war prisoners in the far east. Brit. Med. J., *2:* 709, 1946.

Palmer R., and Martz, C. D.: Recovery of power in leg muscles following poliomyelitis. Physical Ther. Rev., *36:* 466—473, 1956.

Pardo-Costello, V.: *Disease of the Nails.* Springfield, Ill., Charles C. Thomas Co., 1941.

Partels, C. C., and Rullo, F. R.: Unsuspected diabetes mellitus in peripheral vascular disease. New Engl. J. Med., *250:* 633—634, 1958.

Parven, H. A.: Excision of a fibroma of unusual size and location. J. Am. Coll. Foot Surg., *5:* 118—119, 1966.

Pascher, F., and Sims, C. F.: Basal cell epithelioma of the sole. Arch. Derm., *69:* 475—481, 1954.

Patel: Osteomés developés dans les tendons d'achille. Chiropody, *28:* 351, 1931.

Paul, G. R., Leach, R. E., Beetham, W. P.: Pulmonary carcinoma metastasis to the great toe. J. Am. Med. Ass., *208:* 2163, 1969.

Pearlman, L.: The importance of ankle edema in the diagnosis of cardiac and renal problems. J. Nat. Ass. Chir., *47:* 609—611, 1957.

Peck, S., and Klein, G.: *Therapy of Dermatological Disorder.* Philadelphia, Lea & Febiger, pp. 80—81, 1951.
Penneys, N. S., Fulton, J. E., Weinstein, G. D., and Frost, P.: Location of proliferating cells in human epidermis. Arch. Derm., *101:* 323—327, 1970.
Pepin, W. A., and Lauritzen, W. H.: Can peripheral vascular disease be helped by improving foot mechanics? An early report. J. Am. Podiatry Ass., *52:* 202—204, 1962.
Pepin, W.: Measurements of hip rotation and foot pronation and supination in school children. J. Am. Podiatry Ass., *53:* 181—186, 1963.
Perchuk, E., Weinreb, M., Aksu, A.: A new treatment for nocturnal leg cramps. Angiology, *12:* 102—184, 1961.
Perrone, M. A.: Nail matricectomy by onychotripsy with air motor. J. Am. Podiatry Ass., *60:* 92—93, 1970.
Perry, G. M.: Molluscum Contagiosum—a case report. J. Am. Podiatry Ass., *54:* 32—33, 1964.
Perry, G. M.: Villous synovitis, a case report. J. Am. Podiatry Ass., *53:* 757—758, 1963.
Phelps, W. M., and Kiphuth, R. J. H.: *The Diagnosis and Treatment of Postural Defects.* Springfield, Ill., Charles C. Thomas Co., 1932.
Pickett, N. J.: Gun shot wound in the heel. Chiropody Record, *22:* 27—29, 1939.
Pincus, A.: The syndrome of plantar metatarsal neuritis (mortons toe). J. Am. Podiatry Ass., *52:* 746—749, 1962.
Pinkus, H.: Examination of the epidermis by the strip method of removing horny layers. I. Observations on thickness of the horny layer, and on mitotic activity after stripping. J. Invest. Derm., *16:* 383—386, 1951.
Plotnick, D. L.: Glomus tumor. J. Am. Podiatry Ass., *50.* 126, 1960.
Pogonowska, M. J., Collins, L. C., Dobson, H. L.: Diabetic osteopathy. Radiology, *89:* 265—271, 1967.
Pohl, J. F.: *The Kenny Concept of Infantile Paralysis.* Minneapolis and St. Paul, Bruce Publishing Co., 1943.
Polokoff, M.: Ingrown toe nail and hypertrophied nail lip surgery by electrolysis. J. Am. Podiatry Ass., *51:* 805—808, 1961.
Polokoff, M.: Lesser toe latex shield made with tubular gauze. J. Am. Podiatry Ass., *48:* 432—433, 1958.
Polokoff, M.: Negative galvanic procedure for Morton's neuralgia. J. Am. Podiatry Ass., *51:* 31—36, 1961.
Polokoff, M.: Negative galvanism in nail surgery. Lecture Chiropodists Society of New Jersey, Feb. 1944.
Polokoff, M.: Raspostectomy—reduction of exostosis and hypertrophied condyles with files and rasps. J. Am. Podiatry Ass., *52:* 599—602, 1962.
Polokoff, M.: Removable shield for lesions about head of fifth metatarsal. J. Am. Podiatry Ass., *57:* 566—568, 1967.
Prentice, H.: Sublesional administration of corticosteroids, a new technique with broad applications in podiatry. J. Am. Podiatry Ass., *51:* 791—800, 1961.
Prentice, H., and Brezak, S.: An investigation of a water-miscible oil preparation for topical treatment of podiatric dermatoses. J. Am. Podiatry Ass., *48:* 197—200, 1958.
Pressman, D.: Ambulatory condylectomy for intractable plantar keratosis. Curr. Podiatry, 11—12, 1971.
Pullen, R. L.: *Medical Diagnosis.* Philadelphia, W. B. Saunders Co., 1944.
Purgett, D. L.: Surgical correction for dislocated joint. Chiropody Record, *21:* 52, 1938.
Pusey, W. A.: *The Principles and Practice of Dermatology.* 3rd ed. New York, D. Appleton & Co., 1911.
Quiring, D. P., Boyle, B. A., Borousch, E. L., and Lufkin, B.: *The Extremities.* Philadelphia, Lea & Febiger Co., 1945.
Rakow, R. B.: Leiomyoma of the foot (a case report). J. Am. Podiatry Ass., *56:* 24—25, 1966.
Rakow, R. B.: Obliterative arterial disease. J. Nat. Ass. Chir., *34:* 17—20, 1944.
Rakow, R. B.: The treatment of necrotic lesions in the diabetic patient. J. Am. Podiatry Ass., *57:* 412—421, 1967.
Reiss, F., and Kornblee, L.: Common mycotic infections of the lower extremities. N. Y. J. Med., *63:* 548—556, 1963.
Reyer, W. A.: Periorbital dermatitis following adhesive tape strapping of the lower extremity. Ann. Allergy, *15:* 144—149, 1957.
Riccitelli, M. L. (Illustrations, Yale, I.): Foot problems of the aged. J. Am. Geriatric Soc., *14:* 1058—1066, 1966.
Rice, J. R. D.: Psychosomatic manifestations seen in the foot. J. Nat. Ass. Chir., *46:* 27, 1956.
Ritchie, J.: Phenylbutazone for non-specific inflammation. J. Am. Podiatry Ass., *56:* 124—125, 1966.
Robin, Gerald M.: A typical callus—a case report. J. Am. Podiatry Ass., *60:* 212—213, 1970.
Robins, P.: Chemosurgery for skin cancer patients, a report, N. Y. U. Med. Center, 1970.
Robertson, W. E., and Robertson, H. F.: *Diagnostic Signs, Reflexes and Syndromes.* 3rd ed. Philadelphia, F. A. Davis Co., 1947.
Roetman, R. L.: Physical examination of the podiatric patient. J. Am. Podiatry Ass., *56:* 271—280, 1966.
Roetman, R. L.: Some factors in lower extremity edema. J. Am. Podiatry Ass., *58:* 385—387, 1968.
Rogachefsky, H., Rosenthal, S. A., Litt, J. Z., and Baer, R. L.: Trichophytin reaction after exposure to dermatophytes. Arch. Derm., *74:* 606—609, 1956.
Rosen, M. R.: An injectable steroid anesthetic

combination in disorders of the foot. J. Am. Podiatry Ass., *53:* 514—516, 1963.
Rosenberg, A.: Nodular fasciaitis-a case report. J. Am. Podiatry Ass., *59:* 400—402, 1969.
Rosoff, S.: Contact podiatry. J. Podiat., *10:* 1953.
Rosoff, S.: Fabrication of orthotic devices with the use of silicone gel. J. Am. Podiatry Ass., *60:* 313—321, 1970.
Rosoff, S.: Further uses of orthotic gel devices. Current Podiat., Feb., 1971.
Rosoff, S.: The fabrication of contact appliances for use in conventional footwear. J. Am. Podiatry Ass., *51:* 189—194, 1961.
Ross, E. B.: Ainhum, a case report. J. Am. Podiatry Ass., *48:* 255—256, 1958.
Ross, S. B.: Subungual granuloma pyogenicum. J. Nat. Ass. Chir., *45:* 17—18, 1955.
Roven, M.: Accommodating the overlapping second toes. J. Am. Podiatry Ass., *57:* 425—426, 1967.
Roven, M. D.: A latex forefoot device with threefold action. J. Am. Podiatry Ass., *48:* 417—418, 1958.
Roven, M. D.: A traction sling to affect an overlapping fifth toe. J. Am. Podiatry Ass., *49:* 376, 1959.
Rothman, S. K. G., and Windhorst, D.: Tinea pedis as a source of infection in the family. Arch. Derm., *75:* 270—271, 1957.
Rowe, L.: Granuloma pyogenicum differential diagnosis. Arch. Derm., *78:* 341—347, 1958.
Rubin, A.: Periarthritis, hydrocortisone and adaptation to stress in the foot. J. Am. Podiatry Ass., *45:* 17—30, 1955.
Rubin, A.: Somatic pain. Chiropody Record, *38:* 37—45, 1955.
Rubin, L. M., and Wess, S. G.: Complete nail eradication utilizing galvanic current. J. Am. Podiatry Ass., *54:* 401—403, 1964.
Runting, E. G. V.: *Practical Chiropody.* London, Faber & Gwyer, 1928. p. 61.
Russinoff, R. M.: Pathogenesis of depressed metatarsal heads. J. Nat. Ass. Chir., *20:* 5, 1940.
Rutledge, B. A., and Green, A. L.: Surgical treatment of plantar corns. U. S. Armed Forces Med. J., *8:* 219—234, 1957.
Sachs, W., MacKee, G. M., Schwartz, O. D., Pierson, H. S.: Junction nevus—nevocarcinoma. J. Am. Med. Ass., *135:* 216—218, 1947.
Sachs, W., Miller, C. S., and Gray, M. B.: Neurodermatic reaction. Arch. Derm. Syph., *54:* 397—407, 1946.
Sachs, W., Sachs, P. M., and Young, A. W.: Nummular eczema. Skin, *3:* 103—108, 1964.
Samuels, S.: Value of oscillometry. J. Am. Med. Ass., *88:* 1780, 1927.
Samuels, S. S.: Management of gangrene in the extremities. Angiology., *7:* 532—536, 1957.
Samuels, S. S.: Treatment of gangrene of the extremities. Clin. Med., *69:* 2635—2445, 1962.
Sandel, R. K.: Unilateral multiple glomus tumors. J. Am. Coll. Foot Surg., *4:* 130, 1966.
Sanders, S. C.: Acrylic nail groove protector by brush technique. J. Am. Podiatry Ass., *45:* 23—24, 1955.
Sano, S., Kuroda, M., Miyazawa, I.: Some biochemical aspects on pathological keratinization. Glycogen, pentose, hexosamine and beta-glucuronidase in normal and pathological horny layers. Kobe J. Med. Sci., *11:* 1—12, 1965.
Sansone, R. E.: Forefoot imbalance due to alteration of metatarsus parabola. J. Nat. Ass. Chir., *47:* 219—227, 1957.
Sansone, R. E.: Parallel strip padding for weight stress distribution and redirection. J. Am. Podiatry Ass., *60:* 193—198, 1970.
Sarkany, I., Taplin, D., and Blank, H.: Erythasma — common bacterial infection of the skin. J. Am. Med. Ass., *177:* 130—132, 1961.
Schaffer, B.: A clinical appraisal of pigmented nevi in the light of present day histopathologic concepts. Arch Derm. *72:* 120—132, 1955.
Schamberg, I. L., Askovita, S. I., and Greenberg, M.: Critical evaluation of the effects of steroid lotions on inflammatory dermatoses. Arch. Derm., *78:* 490—499, 1958.
Schecter, G. O.: A new self conforming self molding inlay compression insole. J. Nat. Ass. Chir., *45:* 325—326, 1956.
Scheimer, O. M.: Case report—invasive malignant melanoma. J. Am. Coll. Foot Surg., *4:* 18—19, 1965.
Scheimer, O. M.: Case report—massive Intermetatarsal inclusion cyst. J. Am. Coll. Foot Surg., *4:* 10, 1965.
Scheimer, O. M.: Chiropodical management of infantile metatarsus varus. J. Nat. Ass. Chir., *47:* 435—443, 1957.
Schwartz, L., and Peck, S. M.: The patch test in contact dermatitis. J. Nat. Ass. Chir., *36:* 7—16, 1946.
Scott, M. J., Costello, M. J., and Simuango, S. A.: Keratosis punctata palmaris et plantaris. Arch. Derm., *64:* 301, 1951.
Scotti, T. M.: The nature and pathogenesis of the lesion in Morton's metatarsalgia. J. Am. Podiatry Ass., *52:* 750—753, 1962.
Seifer, O., and Mueller, F.: *Manual of Physical and Clinical Diagnosis.* 2nd ed. Philadelphia, J. P. Lippincott, 1934.
Sgarlato, T. E.: A compendium of podiatric, biomechanics. California College of Podiatric Medicine, San Francisco, 1971.
Shaffer, B.: Pigmented nevi. Arch. Derm. *72:* 120, 1955.
Sharp, J. T.: Juvenile flat foot. J. Nat. Ass. Chir., *39:* 9—17, 1949.
Sharpe, A.: Pathology of traumatic callus and heloma. J. Nat. Ass. Chir., *33:* 6—10, 1943.
Shatin, H., and Reisch, M.: Dermatitis of the feet due to shoes. A. M. A. Arch Derm. Syph., *69:* 651—666, 1954.
Shaw, R. E.: Xanthoma tuberosum. J. Am.

Coll. Foot Surg., *4:* 14—15, 1965.
Sheribel: Class lectures in medicine. Illinois College of Chiropody and Foot Surgery, Chicago, 1936—1937.
Sherman, L. H.: Complicated onychocryptosis. J. Nat. Ass. Chir., *29:* 11—17, 1939.
Silver, S. H., Glickman, F. S., and Wanderer, G.: Granuloma annulare—a case report. J. Am. Podiatry Ass., *51:* 127, 1961.
Silverman, L. J.: Forefoot problems of the nondeforming clubfoot. J. Am. Podiatry Ass., *56:* 110—113, 1966.
Sivitz, S. C.: A new approach to dynamic molding techniques. J. Nat. Ass. Chir., *46:* 21—26, 1956.
Sivitz, S. C.: Acrylic resins: a preliminary report on the use of self curing plastic resins in nail groove therapy. J. Nat. Ass. Chir., *43:* 34—39, 1953.
Sivitz, S. C.: A new resilient plastic for orthodigital prosthetics. J. Nat. Ass. Chir., *47:* 172—175, 1957.
Smernoff, R.: A new treatment for verruca. Curr. Podiatry, *18:* 12, 1969.
Solomon, S.: Excision of a typical nodular hydradenoma. J. Am. Coll. Foot Surg., *5:* 80—81, 1966.
Solovay, J., and Solovay, H. W.: Paraplegic neuroarthropathy. Am. J. Roen. Radiol. Ther., *61:* 475—481, 1949.
Spence, W. R., and Sheilds, M.: Prevention of blisters, callosities and ulcers by absorption of shear forces. J. Am. Podiatry Ass., *58:* 428—434, 1968.
Spencer, A. M.: Report on a study of nylidrin HCl and vitamin E on the treatment of peripheral vascular disease. J. Am. Podiatry Ass., *51:* 341—344, 1961.
Spinelli, J. A.: Case report—Hemangiofibroma. J. Am. Coll. Foot Surg., *4.* 15 16, 1965.
Spoor, H. J.: Onychomycosis and corneal dystrophy. Arch. Derm., *95:* 427—428, 1967.
Stalbach, J. J.: The nail plate—a key to diagnosis. Chiropody Record., *22:* 184—187, 1939.
Stanley, W. J.: Koilonychia and polycythemia vera. Med. Illus., *10:* 399—400, 1956.
Steinberg, H. H.: Myalgia of the foot. J. Wis. Soc. Chir., *5:* 7—10, 1957.
Steinberg, M. D.: A simplified technique for surgery of ingrown toenails. Surgery., *36:* 1132—1137, 1954.
Steinberg, M. D.: Benign, multiple acanthoma of the toes a new concept entity. J. Nat. Ass. Chir., *40:* 50—54, 1950.
Steinberg, M. D.: Observations on the possible etiologic relationship between fungus infection of the human foot and rheumatoid arthritis. J. Nat. Ass. Chir., *46:* 589—592, 1956.
Steinberg, M. D.: The use of vitamin B12 in Morton neuralgia. J. Am. Podiatry Ass., *45:* 41—42, 1955.
Steinberg, M. D., and Block, Philip: The use and abuse of epinephrine in local anesthetics. J. Am. Podiatry Ass., *61:* 341—343, 1971.
Steinberg, M. D., and Taub, J.: Lecture. Los Angeles, American Society Clinical Pathologists, 1969.
Steindler, A.: *Mechanics of Normal and Pathological Locomotion in Man.* Springfield, Ill., Charles C Thomas Co., 1935.
Stem, J.: Ganglionic cyst produces symptoms of Morton's neuralgia—a case report. J. Am. Podiatry Ass., *54:* 720—721, 1964.
Stern, J.: Quinocaine injection therapy for verrucae. J. Am. Podiatry Ass., *51:* 413—415, 1961.
Stern, J.: Treatment standardization for iontophoresis. J. Nat. Chir., *45:* 39—40, 1955.
Stern, J., and Fletcher T.: Anti tineal effectiveness of a new topical agent. J. Am. Podiatry Ass., *56:* 162, 1966.
Stieglitz, J. O.: *Chemistry in Medicine.* New York, The Chemical Foundation, Inc., 1929.
Stiles, P. G.: *Human Physiology.* 6th rev. ed. Philadelphia, W. B. Saunders Co., 1932.
Stillman, E. G.: A new dynamic foot mold. J. Am. Podiatry Ass., *48:* 144—147, 1958.
Stoler, W. A.: Fibrolipoma with calcified organized thrombi. J. Am. Coll. Foot Surg., *5:* 35—36, 1966.
Stout, A. P.: Liposarcoma—malignant tumor of lipoblasts. Ann. Surg., *119:* 86—107, 1944.
Stout, A. P.: Tumors of soft tissues. Washington, D. C., Armed Forces Institute of Pathology, 1953.
Strahs, R.: Treatment of onychomycosis with a lacquer formulation of chloranil. J. Am. Podiatry Ass., *52:* 508—509, 1962.
Strang, J. M.: Obesity and diabetes. Am. J. Med. Sci., *236:* 405—418, 1958.
Streiker, F. B.: New uses of chymotrypsin in podiatry. J. Am. Podiatry Ass., *51:* 713—717, 1961.
Sturm, M.: A theoretical explanation of the etiology of cardiovascular states. Med. Record, *142:* 445—446, 1935.
Sturtz, H.: The management of excessive dry skin. Indiana State Podiatry J., *24:* 1959.
Subotnick, S. I.: The practical value and research potential of synovianalysis of joints within the human foot. Proc. Res. Alumni Ass., Calif. Pod. Med. Center, *1:* 1—16, 1972.
Suppan, R. J., and Besterman, G.: Currettage and chemo-cautery for verrucae. J. Am. Podiatry Ass., *53:* 265—258, 1963.
Suppan, R. J., and Ritchlin, J. D.: A non-debilitating surgical procedure for "ingrown toenail." J. Am. Podiatry Ass., *52:* 900—902, 1962.
Sutton, E. H.: Clinical J. Chir. Pedic Items. Nov., 1942.
Sutton, R. L., and Sutton, R. J.: *Disease of the Skin.* 10th ed. St. Louis, C. V. Mosby Co., 1939.
Sutton, R. L., and Sutton, R. L.: *Synopsis of Diseases of the Skin.* St. Louis, C. V. Mosby Co., 1942.
Sutton, R. L., and Sutton, R. L. Jr.: Calcifying

epithelioma. Arch. Derm., *31:* 48, 1935.
Swanbeck, G.: A new treatment of ichthyosis and other hyperkeratotic conditions. Acta Derm. Vener., *48:* 123—127, 1968.
Tai, P. L.: An investigation of clinical applications of mesomorphic cholesteric liquid crystals in podiatric medicine: a preliminary study. J. Am. Podiatry Ass., *63:* 119—128, 1973.
Tanenbaum, M. H.: Eccrine poroma. Am. Surg., *31:* 603—604, 1965.
Taub, J., and Steinberg, M. D.: Porokeratosis dermatopathological entity. Int. J. Derm., *9:* 83—90, 1970.
Tax, H. R.: Podopediatrics, Lecture notes, the care of children's feet. New York, 1948.
Taylor, P. C.: Case report—malignant melanoma of the great toe. J. Am. Coll. Foot. Surg., *4:* 45—46, 1965.
Temple, D. E., and Boardman, C. R.: Incidence of erythrasma of the toewebs. Arch. Derm., *86:* 518—519, 1962.
Thompson, S. G.: Epithelioma cuniculatum: an unusual tumor of the foot. Brit. J. Plastic Surg. *18:* 214—217, 1965.
Thompson, T. C.: A test for rupture of the tendo achilles. Acta Orthop. Scand., *32:* 461—465, 1962.
Tintocalis, C. A.: A measuring device for orthopedic evaluation. J. Am. Podiatry Students Ass., *12:* 8—15, 1968.
Toth S.: Perineural fibrosis—a case report. J. Am. Podiatry Ass., *53:* 755, 1963.
Toth, S. P.: Xanthoma—a case report. J. Am. Podiatry Ass., *53:* 600—601, 1963.
Tracy, G. D.: Management of peripheral gangrene in the aged. Postgrad. Med., *37:* 464—469, 1965.
Trapp, B.: Ultra-sound in verruca plantaris. J. Am. Podiatry Ass., *57:* 326—329, 1967.
Trice, E. W.: A new hypothesis on the etiology of heloma miliare. J. Nat. Ass. Chir., *45:* 28—29, 1955.
Trout, E. F.: A new sign of the climateric. J. Clin. Endocr., *6:* 515, 1946.
Vandenbos, K. Q., and Bowers, W. F.: Ingrown toenail: a result of weight bearing on soft tissues. U. S. Armed Forces Med. J., *10:* 1168—1173, 1959.
Van Scott, E. J., Reinertson, R. P., and McCall, C. B.: Prevalence histological types & significance of palmer & plantar nevi. Cancer, *10:* 363, 1957.
Varzos, P. N.: Hesperdin and ascorbic acid in conjunction with mechanotherapy for static foot problems. J. Am. Podiatry Ass., *51:* 861—865, 1961.
Vernon, S.: Ingrown toenail, operation by electrosurgery. Am. J. Surg., *42:* 396—397, 1938.
Verovitz, C. H.: Swellings of legs and ankles. J. Nat. Ass. Chir., *27:* 10—15, 1937.
Waddell, W. A.: The common corn clinically considered. Canad. Chir. J., Summer Issue, 1948. pp. 29—37.
Walker, M.: A study of griseofulvin as related to tinea pedis. J. Am. Podiatry Ass., *51:* 112—122, 1961.
Walker, M.: Report on griseofulvin. J. Am. Podiatry Ass., *50:* 297—303, 1960.
Walker, M. H.: A chronical of tinea pedis and chloroxylenal for control of tinea pedis. J. Am. Podiatry Ass., *52:* 737—745, 1962.
Walker, M. H.: An evaluation of some clinical data in the treatment of tinea pedis with copper sulphate iontophoresis and some fungicidal preparations. J. Am. Podiatry Ass., *49:* 303—311, 1959.
Walker, M. H. Etiology of carcinomas of the lower extremities. J. Nat. Ass. Chir., *45:* 22—24, 1955.
Walkes, M.: Parenzyme in podiatry. J. Podiatry, *2:* 9—13, 1957.
Walters, J. D.: The science of mycology. J. Nat. Ass. Chir., 1939.
Wartenberg, R.: *The Examination of Reflexes.* Chicago, Year Book Publishers, 1945.
Watkins, W. L., Cobb, S., Finesinger, J., Brazier, M., Shands, S. H., and Pincus, G.: Psychiatric and physiologic studies on fatigue. Arch. Phys. Med., *28:* 199—206, 1947.
Webb, J. L.: Diagnostic analysis, lectures in dermatology. Illinois College of Chiropody and Foot Surgery, 1936.
Webb, J. L.: Lectures in dermatology. Illinois College of Chiropody and Foot Surgery, Chicago, 1936.
Weed, John H.: Nocardiosis of the foot—a case report. J. Am. Podiatry Ass., *53:* 561—563, 1954.
Weiner, E.: Dermatitis of the feet due to wearing of impermeable shoes. J. Am. Podiatry Ass., *50:* 545—547, 1960.
Weiner, H.: Some comments on metatarsalgia. J. Nat. Ass. Chir., *47:* 460—462, 1957.
Weinstock, B.: An evaluation of the curettage treatment of plantar verrucae. J. Nat. Ass. Chir., *47:* 67—68, 1957.
Weinstock, R. C.: The wooden sole shoe in podiatry practice. J. Am. Podiatry Ass., *56:* 365—370, 1966.
Weisfeld, M.: Understanding porokeratosis plantaris discreta. J. Am. Podiatry Ass., *63:* 138—144, 1973.
Wheeless, J. V.: Porokeratosis of mibelli. Arch. Derm., *100:* 381—382, 1969.
White, C. J.: Disease of the nail. Chiropody Record, *32:* 115—119, 1949.
White, C. J., and Laipply, T. C.: Diseases of the nails. Chiropody Record, *41:* 6—7, 1958.
White, C. J., and Laipply, T. C.: Diseases of the nails: 792 cases, clinical microscopic findings, with resume of newer therapeutic methods. Indust. Med. Surg., *27:* 325—327, 1958.
White, C.: Diseases of the nails. Postgrad. Med., *8:* 43, 1950.
White, D. D.: Betamethasone in certain inflammatory states of the foot. J. Am. Podiatry Ass., *56:* 234—236, 1966.
White, H.: Some aspects of the neural integra-

tion involved in gait and posture. J. Am. Podiatry Ass., *57:* 157—163, 1967.
Whitney, A. K.: An illustrated labiomatricectomy procedure. J. Am. Podiatry Ass., *57:* 169—172, 1967.
Whitney, A. K.: Podokinetics. J. Nat. Ass. Chir., *47:* 383—387, 1957.
Whitney, A. K.: Total matricectomy procedure. J. Am. Podiatry Ass., *58:* 157—159, 1968.
Whitney, A. K.: Urethane moulds in podiatry. Podiatry Q., Spring, 1965.
Whitney, A. K.: Urethane mould therapy. New Engl. J. Podiatry, *42:* 17, 1963.
Wichman, B.: Subungual exostoses and nail border problems. J. Am. Podiatry Ass., *57:* 521—522, 1967.
Willis, R. A.: *Pathology of Tumors.* St. Louis, C. V. Mosby Co., 1948.
Winograd, A. M.: Modification in technique of operation for ingrown toenail. J. Am. Med. Ass., *92:* 229, 1929.
Winsor, T.: An evaluation of the plethysmograph for study of the peripheral circulation. J. Am. Podiatry Ass., *53:* 813—818, 1963.
Wittenberg, M.: Reactions to injected drugs and their emergency care. J. Am. Podiatry Ass., *48:* 516—522, 1958.
Wolf, D. S.: Cavernous hemangioma. J. Am. Podiatry Ass., *59:* 446—447, 1969.
Woolf, W. H.: Capillary tube acid applicator for verrucae. J. Am. Podiatry Ass., *49:* 18—20, 1959.
Woolf, W. H.: Verruca: its possible relationship to other neoplasms. J. Am. Podiatry Ass., *52:* 893—898, 1962.
Wright, E. W.: Compensating and corrective appliances. J. Nat. Ass. Chir., *46:* 312—315, 1956.
Yale, I.: A new injection technique for the treatment of verrucae as proposed for practice in the armed forces. J. Podiatry., *3:* 7—9, 1941 and *4:* 12—13, 1942.
Yale, I.: A new therapeutic approach for accommodation of foot pathology. J. Am. Podiatry Ass., *48:* 477—480, 1958.
Yale, I.: A statistical report on a review of 1290 foot radiographs. J. Nat. Ass. Chiropodists., 1957.
Yale, I.: A time for greatness (inaugeral address—President of American Podiatry Association). J. Am. Podiatry Ass., *57:* 436—440, 1967.
Yale, I.: Challenge and opportunity in podiatry. Commencement address., June 5, 1953.
Yale, I.: Clinical and roentgenological interpretations in the lower extremities. Am. Podiatrist, 517, 1950.
Yale, I.: Clinical and roentgenological interpretations in the lower extremities. Chiropody Lit., Ansonia, Conn., 1952.
Yale, I.: Clinical and roentgenological interpretations in the lower extremities. Chiropody Record, *32:* 186—187, 1949.
Yale, I.: Clinical and roentgenological interpretations in the lower extremities. Chiropody Record *33:* 319—223, 1950.
Yale, I.: Conn. Chiropodist. *11:* 45, 1951.
Yale, I.: Foot impression technique. Current Podiatry, 11—13, 1958.
Yale, I.: Foot protection device for use in athletic shoes. J. Am. Podiatry Ass., *48:* 53—56, 1958.
Yale, I.: Foreign bodies in the foot. Conn. Chiropodist, *10:* 3—4, 1954.
Yale, I.: Idiopathic osteochondrosis of the tarsal navicular. J. Nat. Ass. Chiropody, *41:* 41—44, 1951.
Yale, I.: Imagination and creativity. J. Am. Podiatry Ass., *55:* 288—290, 1965.
Yale, I.: Imbalanced forefoot. Conn. Chiropodist, *2:* 3—5, 1955.
Yale, I.: Non-deforming club foot. Chiropody Record, 1939.
Yale, I.: Podiatry faces the future. J. Am. Podiatry Ass., *56:* 72—73, 1966.
Yale, I.: Presidents message. J. Am. Podiatry Ass., *58:* 270—271, 1968.
Yale, I.: Radiographic study of calcification of the medial calcaneal branch of posterior tibial artery, age group 20—40. J. Nat. Ass. Chiropodists, *44:* 44—52, 1954.
Yale, I.: Vaso-motor imbalance. Chiropody Record, *21:* 133—134, 1938.
Yale, I. and Yale, J.: Kaposi cell sarcoma-report on two cases. J. Am. Podiatry Ass., *56:* 165—168, 1966.
Yale, J. F.: Cutaneous mucous cysts of the toes. J. Am. Podiatry Ass., *57:* 457—463, 1967.
Yasuda, T., Kawoda, A., and Yashuda: Eccrine poroma. Arch. Dem., *90:* 428—431, 1964.
Yater, W. M.: *Symptoms Diagnosis.* 4th ed. New York, D. Appleton-Century Co., 1942.
Yontef, R.: Treatment of dermatomycoses with griseofulvin. J. Med. Soc. N. J., 738—740, 1959.
Young, J. R., and DeWolfe, V. G.: Recurrent lymphangitis of the leg associated with dermatophytosis: report of 25 consecutive cases. Cleveland Clin. Quant. *27:* 19—24. 1960.
Young, J. R., Humphries, A. W., and DeWolfe, V. G.: Restless leg syndrome. Geriatrics, *24:* 167—171, 1969.
Zadik, F. R.: Obliteration of the nail bed of the great toe without shortening the terminal phalanx. J. Bone Joint Surg., *32-B:* 66, 1950. 1950.
Zaias, N.: Psoriasis of the nail. Arch. Derm., *99:* 567—579, 1969.
Zislin, S.: Intermetatarsal Bursa producing a neuroma syndrome. J. Am. Coll. Foot Surg., *5:* 62—63, 1966.
Zitzlsperger, S.: The mechanics of the foot based on the concept of the skeleton as a statically indeterminate space framework. Clin. Orthop., *16:* 47, 1960.
Zugerman, I.: Basal cell epithelioma of the sole. Arch Derm., *76:* 247—249, 1957.

Index

Page references in *italic* refer to illustrations.